The social history of medicine over the last fiftee   ...c
boundaries of medical history. Specialized papers aɪɪɑ monographs have
contributed to our knowledge of how medicine has affected society and
how society has shaped medicine. This book synthesizes, through a series
of essays, some of the most significant findings of this 'new social history'
of medicine.

The period covered ranges from ancient Greece to the present time.
While coverage is not exhaustive, the reader is able to trace how medicine
in the West developed from an unlicensed open market place, with many
different types of practitioners in the classical period, to the nineteenth-
and twentieth-century professionalized medicine of state influence, of
hospitals, public health medicine, and scientific medicine. The book also
covers innovatory topics such as patient–doctor relationships, the history
of the asylum, and the demographic background to the history of
medicine.

Medicine in society

MEDICINE IN SOCIETY
Historical essays

Edited by ANDREW WEAR

Lecturer in the History of Medicine, University College London and
Wellcome Institute for the History of Medicine

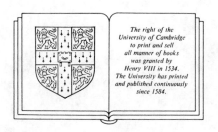

The right of the
University of Cambridge
to print and sell
all manner of books
was granted by
Henry VIII in 1534.
The University has printed
and published continuously
since 1584.

CAMBRIDGE UNIVERSITY PRESS
Cambridge
New York   Port Chester
Melbourne   Sydney

Published by the Press Syndicate of the University of Cambridge
The Pitt Building, Trumpington Street, Cambridge CB2 1RP
40 West 20th Street, New York, NY 10011–4211, USA
10 Stamford Road, Oakleigh, Victoria 3166, Australia

First published 1992

Printed in Great Britain at the University Press, Cambridge

A catalogue record for this book is available from the British Library

Library of Congress cataloguing in publication data

Medicine in society / edited by Andrew Wear.
　　p.　cm.
ISBN 0–521–33351–2 (hardback).　ISBN 0–521–33639–2 (paperback)
1. Medicine – History. 2. Social medicine – History. I. Wear, A. (Andrew), 1946–　.
[DNLM: 1. History of Medicine. 2. Social Conditions – history. WZ 40 H674]
R131.H564　1992
362.1′09 – dc20
DLC　　91–10962
CIP

ISBN 0 521 33351 2 hardback
ISBN 0 521 33639 2 paperback

Contents

Contributors

Elizabeth Fee, *School of Hygiene and Public Health, Johns Hopkins University, Baltimore*

Lindsay Granshaw, *Wellcome Institute for the History of Medicine, London*

Arthur E. Imhof, *Fachbereich Geschichtswissenschaften, Freie Universität, Berlin*

Jane Lewis, *Department of Social Science and Administration, London School of Economics and Political Science*

Irvine Loudon, *Green College, Oxford*

Vivian Nutton, *Wellcome Institute for the History of Medicine, London*

Katharine Park, *Department of History, Wellesley College*

Dorothy Porter, *Department of History, Birkbeck College, London*

Roy Porter, *Wellcome Institute for the History of Medicine, London*

Guenter B. Risse, *Department of the History of the Health Sciences, University of California, San Francisco*

Andrew Wear, *Wellcome Institute for the History of Medicine, London*

Paul Weindling, *Wellcome Unit for the History of Medicine, Oxford*

Introduction

ANDREW WEAR

The social history of medicine has come of age. It is now possible to see in some detail the way in which medicine has developed within society. Whereas before the history of great doctors, great discoveries and great ideas was the staple diet of the history of medicine, now this new but flourishing branch of history gives us a sense of how medicine has affected society and how society has shaped medicine. In the process the definition of 'medicine' has been extended and deepened.

The contributors to this book show these changes, but they are only incidentally concerned with historiography, with how to write history. Their main aim has been with writing history itself, with giving to the reader some of the results of the new social history of medicine. Their chapters are synthetic and draw upon recent work in their fields, but they are also based on the primary research that each contributor has carried out.

Overall, this book shows that health care has been of perennial concern to Western society, but the forms it took have been different over time with modern State-influenced health-care systems, hospitals and professionalized practitioners contrasting strongly with the smaller, more open systems that existed before the nineteenth century. Running through the contributions are various themes. The balance of power in the patient–doctor interaction has changed over time. When medical practitioners depended on patients' fees and trade and the patient had a greater choice in practitioners, the patient tended to dominate: later, in the environment of the hospital and asylum, the doctor took charge and the patient increasingly lost control of events. The role of the state in medicine is another recurrent topic. This increased with time from its small beginnings in the Roman period, when civic doctors were given tax immunities, and assumed large proportions in the nineteenth and twentieth centuries. Then the state came to legislate on the structure of the medical profession and to provide or oversee health-care schemes that delivered health care to all the population. Another thread that runs through the book is a concern with the demographic facts of life and death. In the pre-modern world the expectancy of life was low, infant and maternal mortality was high and for many it was in Katharine Park's phrase 'a universe of disease'. The ways in which this picture of mortality was improved is discussed in various of the contributions. Life and death are the ultimate concerns of medicine, and always have to be kept in mind in a social history of medicine.

In some ways the period from classical times up to and including the eighteenth century can be taken as a whole and seen as forming the first part of the book. In this period change was often slow and continuities abound. Highly original work has been done recently in this area. One of the innovations has been for historians to look at the multiplicity of medical providers that existed, without attaching to any one group a greater degree of significance than to any other. This mirrors the historical situation where an open, unregulated market place was the norm. In other words, the nineteenth- and twentieth-century values of the medical profession which in past history of medicine had been applied to earlier periods to condemn empirics, quacks, magical and religious practitioners have been discarded. In the process a much richer medical world has been uncovered.

Vivian Nutton in his chapter on the social history of Graeco-Roman medicine shows how at this time an open medical market place existed that was made up of a variety of religious, magical, empirical and medical practitioners. Anyone could be a healer, there was no licensing and patients drew on the services of what appear today to be practitioners holding radically different and contradictory belief. Self-help, especially in the countryside, was widespread. Illness was dealt with in the family: there were no hospitals in classical Greece. When in the Roman period hospitals were built they were designed to care only for two economically important groups, soldiers and slaves.

Katharine Park in her chapter on 'Medicine and society in medieval Europe, 500–1500' and Roy Porter on 'The patient in England: c. 1600–c. 1800' (the 'long' eighteenth century), indicate that very similar open medical market places existed in their periods. Before the industrialization of the nineteenth century change was often slow. However, there were some significant happenings.

The medicine of Hippocrates and Galen, the learned medicine taught by a lengthy process of education, tried to differentiate itself from other forms of healing during the classical period. It associated itself with philosophy which had high social status; it developed anatomical research, both as a spectacle and as a form of disinterested knowledge; and it gained patronage in royal courts such as Alexandria, and in fashionable Roman society. In the later medieval period the claims of learned medicine to form the elite part of the medical market place were strengthened by the rise of the universities with their medical faculties and set curricula, and by the establishment of city medical colleges or guilds which often claimed the right to control and license practitioners in their areas. Park points out that this marks the rudimentary beginning of 'professional medicine'; it did not have its nineteenth-century monopoly or power, and the rest of the medical market place remained largely unaffected. This situation continued to the eighteenth century.

Another event that influenced medicine was the arrival of Christianity. Charitable care of the sick was a peculiarly Christian idea and motivated the monastic care of the sick, and the building of hospices and hospitals. Moreover, as Christ had healed the sick so priests undertook the cure of the body as well as the soul.

The association of religion with medicine continued well into the eighteenth century if on a declining scale. The Catholic church had tried, from the time of the Middle Ages, to stop priests engaging in medicine for gain. The Reformation had stopped Protestants from healing by means of the sacraments which was regarded as Popish superstition (the age of miracles being thought to be long past). But until the processes of secularization in the eighteenth century began to reduce the significance of religion, Christianity remained a powerful force to be appealed to when ill, and rich and poor alike had recourse to religion even when they were using naturalistic medicine.

Porter's chapter describes the multiplicity of choice available in the medical market place in England during the 'long' eighteenth century, in which religion still played a role and when the vociferous claims of elite learned medicine to competence were met by the equally vociferous claims of the other members of the market place. Some changes in the continuity with the past did occur; the practitioners of regular, learned medicine increased from the end of the seventeenth century and made inroads into the numbers of certain types of lay healers such as wise women and cunning men (a process accelerated by the growing secularization of at least the middle and upper sections of society and the decline of magic amongst them). The increasing commercialization of society also affected how people got their medicines, which were no longer collected from the fields but bought from shops. However, self-help and lay healing continued unabated. Roy and Dorothy Porter, have pioneered a new approach. They have written the history of medicine from the patient's point of view, which before was largely ignored.[1] In his chapter Porter, not only discusses the medical market place, but shows how patients had great control over their treatment: they frequently treated themselves, they exchanged information about cures and saw themselves as the equals of their doctors. Journals like the *Gentleman's Magazine* printed letters on medical topics from lay people and medical practitioners without distinction. The English medical culture of the eighteenth century gave patients near equality with their doctors. To end his contribution Porter looks at the voice of the mad, mad peoples' writings about themselves. Their numbers are very small, but the different ways in which the mad described their experiences shows us the diverse forces acting to give meaning to sufferers' lives. Madness as a psychomachy between the Devil and God, 'madness' as the unreal and unjust persecution by jailors or doctors, these are some of the meanings given to their condition by the mad. Meanings that refer less to medicine and more to society at large.

Andrew Wear's chapter also focuses on some of the meanings of health and illness. After briefly discussing how the meanings of medical theories of childbirth and of death changed from the sixteenth to the mid eighteenth century the contribution centres on perceptions of health and the environment in early modern England. That an unhealthy environment helped to create disease was well known in the sixteenth and seventeenth centuries. Little however was done about it. Food markets might be regulated, cesspits cleaned, the rubbish collected by parish scavengers, building restrictions imposed to reduce overcrowding, but the problem of the environment was thought to be getting worse, especially as the cities grew larger. Towns and cities, in particular London, were perceived as being less healthy than the countryside. This chapter explores how the environment and health were related by the use of the broad divisions of countryside and city. Transcending the

---

[1] Roy Porter and Dorothy Porter, *In Sickness and in Health The British Experience 1650–1850* (London, 1988); Dorothy Porter and Roy Porter, *Patient's Progress: Doctors and Doctoring in Eighteenth-Century England* (London, 1989). What is new about their work is their emphasis on the voice of the individual patient; particular groups or populations in society such as mothers, infants, adults, minors, the old etc., are all as such 'patients' and have, as groups, long been the concern of the social history of medicine.

changes in medical theory that occur during the seventeenth century (from a humoral to a chemical and/or mechanical view of the body) ideas such as the need for an uncrowded, spacious, clean, light environment remained constant and were informed by references to the Garden of Eden, by folk knowledge, tradition, personal experience and by newly developing demographic research. The chapter again indicates how the social history of medicine, once it forgets the categories of professional medicine, can capture a wide range not only of experience but of meanings.

The eighteenth century, the age of the Enlightenment saw a period of change, not as rapid as the century that followed but a clear quickening of pace. The success of the 'new science' of the seventeenth century, the science of Newton, influenced many other disciplines. The theories of medicine changed in line with these new developments. Medical theories were no longer based on the four humours of the Greeks but on chemistry and medicine. The human soul was abolished and the programme of reducing medicine to physics was underway; later, as the special nature of organic bodies was again brought to mind, the soul returned. Guenter Risse shows in his contribution, 'Medicine in the age of Enlightenment', that a sense of progress and of the perfectibility of society informed many Enlightenment developments in medicine. New medical theories and new systems of classifying disease replaced each other with startling rapidity, but despite the lack of effective cures the hope remained that progress in medical theory would have a practical pay off. Progress also took the form of an emphasis on a healthy life style and on personal hygiene based on the belief that illness was avoidable and that everyone could lead a healthy life, given a good enough education in medicine. The view that society could be medicalized was not new, there was a pervading interest in health from the Greeks onwards, but it was put on a more formal footing. In France, especially, the health of the poor became an object of scientific and medical interest and was researched by means of surveys. The medical regulation of life, by a system of 'medical police' was also mooted at this period.

Changes were afoot in the Enlightenment but the old structures of medicine only broke up in the nineteenth century. Many aspects of twentieth-century medicine had their origins in the nineteenth century. For instance, the rise of the hospital to a central position in medicine occurred after the French Revolution. Hospitals had existed since medieval times, founded for religious and charitable motives or by civic pride. In eighteenth-century Protestant England there were no longer church-run hospitals, but civic philanthropy established instead the voluntary hospitals.

As Lindsay Granshaw indicates in her chapter on 'The rise of the modern hospital in Britain' the voluntary hospitals were charitable institutions catering for the moderately poor, and in the nineteenth century they were joined by the workhouse infirmaries that housed the destitute. The hospitals, therefore, carried with them the stigma of charity until the twentieth century. The family home remained the place for the well-to-do to be ill. As the nineteenth century progressed the voluntary hospitals were increasingly run by medical men, rather than by lay governors, who saw hospital posts as essential to their careers. The reforms in medical education in both France and England required practical on-the-ward experience and teaching and this meant that hospitals came to dominate the medical world. Medical research was also centred on the hospital. That patients came from among the poor did not detract from the status of hospitals, rather it gave a boost to hospital research and increased the power of doctors in the doctor–patient relationship. In hospitals physicians and surgeons did not have to depend on the fees or the trade of the patients housed in them; there was less need to listen to the patient and to tailor treatment to the individual patient's requirements. The patients were poor, less articulate, less troublesome, and it was much easier to carry out research on them (especially statistically based research which required large numbers in one place – the hospital). Moreover, the advantage of the poor was that the large numbers of post-mortems that were carried out would elicit no complaints from influential families.

As the hospital became more important, so medicine itself changed. In the eighteenth century disease was defined in terms of the subjective feelings experienced by the patient. In the new hospital medicine of the early nineteenth century the subjective feelings of the patient became less important (this was perhaps made easier as the hospital patient was no longer the paymaster). Instead, the doctor tried to find a specific locus of disease, often hidden from the patient. The patient was starting to be seen objectively, as an object, rather than being listened to as a subject.

A particular event, the French Revolution, shaped the new hospital medicine. Some of the medical reforms of the Revolution had been foreshadowed in earlier eighteenth-century France. Although there was a medical market place and the medley of practitioners was similar to that in England, elite learned medicine, especially surgery, was more tightly regulated by the Crown. The relatively high status of surgeons

6

presages their great influence in the new type of medicine, 'hospital medicine' as historians have called it, which was created by the medical reforms of the Revolution.[2] The Revolution gave central importance to hospital training; state regulations prescribed in detail how in the hospitals physicians and surgeons were to be trained. The reforms merged physicians and surgeons together and gave priority to the surgeon's approach: traditionally practical, hospital-based.

Another facet of modern medicine which had its origin in the nineteenth century was the professionalization of medicine. In France, the state prescribed how the new medical profession should be structured and in the process gave it a legal basis for its existence. In early nineteenth-century England medical reform was also in the air, but here it was more in the hands of medical men themselves. The Apothecaries Act of 1815 attempted to regulate the training of the 'regular' practitioners, but as Irvine Loudon points out it did not do away with the large numbers of medical corporations, nor did it provide 'one portal of entry' to the medical profession (something that the 1858 Medical Act also failed to accomplish). In his chapter on 'Medical practitioners 1750–1850 and the period of medical reform in Britain' Loudon argues that much of the medical reform was initiated by medical men rather than by the government.

His focus is on the general practitioner, one of the mainstays of modern medicine who perhaps had his origin around 1750. This was a time when incomes for medical practitioners were increasing. However, by the end of the century competition from the dispensing druggist, who began to sell medicine to the public rather than wholesale and to offer medical advice, impoverished many 'regulars' or general practitioners (often surgeon–apothecaries). The cry went up for a system of medical regulation that would exclude quacks (though the dispensing druggists were selling the same medicines as the regulars). As Loudon traces the medical politics of the time it is clear that cries for scientific medicine, for better medical education, more rigorous examinations, all had their altruistic side but were also mixed with financial and social considerations. The general practitioners failed to gain higher status and financial rewards, despite their attempts to reform medicine. Instead, hospitals and consultants dominated medicine as did the old corporations

[2] On this see Toby Gelfand, *Professionalising Modern Medicine. Paris Surgeons and Medical Science and Institutions in the 18th Century* (Westport, CT, 1980); Matthew Ramsey, *Professional and Popular Medicine in France, 1770–1830. The World of Medical Practice* (Cambridge, 1988); Erwin H. Ackerknecht, *Medicine at the Paris Hospital 1794–1848* (Baltimore, 1967); Michel Foucault, *The Birth of the Clinic* (London, 1973).

like the royal colleges, and the universities. In nineteenth-century novels the GP became a loveable character, but in the world of medicine he remained a lowly figure. This, despite the fact that the reforms had at first been initiated by GPs and had increased the general status of medicine. Indeed, medicine became fully professional. The Medical Act of 1858 gave a legal basis for the profession to control its own entry requirements, examinations and discipline, although unorthodox practice by practitioners not on the Medical Register was still allowed. The medical market place still continued, if on a diminished scale.

The state was also involved in the rise of public health medicine in the nineteenth century. As Katharine Park shows, in medieval and renaissance Europe, especially in Italy, states responded to repeated outbreaks of plague by instituting measures such as quarantine and by setting up magistracies, or health boards, with draconian powers over public health. The association of public health with government has been a long one. In the nineteenth century the health problems of large urbanized and industrialized populations, repeated outbreaks of cholera, and the developments of various social reform movements all directed attention to public health. Elizabeth Fee and Dorothy Porter in their chapter 'Public health, preventive medicine and professionalization: England and America in the nineteenth century' bring out the different meanings of public health in the first half of the century. For the French public health could ameliorate but not solve the problems of civilization. For Rudolf Virchow in Germany 'medicine was politics' and the right to health for the poor was part of political reform. In England, Edwin Chadwick thought that engineers held the key to public health for they could improve water supplies and sanitation. They, rather than medical men, were to be the agents of the public health reforms that the politicians were to direct. In England and on the continent public health was quickly dominated by medical men after the middle of the century. One of the great changes ushered in by public health was not only that the state controlled whole areas of life which before had been largely unregulated (conditions in the work place, hours of work, sanitary arrangements, water supplies, sale of food etc.), but also that the state came to know much more about the health of its inhabitants. Certain diseases became notifiable, surveys of health, illness and poverty were carried out, and industrial disease identified. This changed the way in which countries thought of themselves, and it also increased the 'medicalization' of society. One of the merits of Fee's and Porter's contribution is that it shows how, both in the United States and England, the bacteriological revolution initiated by Pasteur and Koch in the later nineteenth century affected public health medicine. In the United States public health had taken off later than in Europe and had been a largely voluntary reform movement in which lay people dominated. With the advent of bacteriology in the United States a much more specific approach to public health was introduced. Medical experts replaced lay people, and rather than trying to improve the living conditions of whole, undifferentiated, populations they targeted people into specific 'at-risk populations' whose living conditions could be changed in appropriate ways. The political significance of public health medicine as an agent of reform therefore declined. The hidden hand of public health, however, still regulates many of our everyday activities, and the public health doctor is still much more concerned with the health of the whole community, with preventing disease rather than treating individual ill patients which has been the traditional concern of medicine.

Before discussing bacteriology and the creation of scientific medicine, one other early-nineteenth-century development which still influences medicine today has to be considered. The asylum rose in the nineteenth century and fell in the next. It was an institution that illustrates the forces of medical reform and state power, and is perhaps a further example of how the patient was becoming more of an object and less of a person.

The history of madness is one of the growth areas of recent historical research. The influence here of Michel Foucault has been immense.[3] He substituted a pessimistic account of the history of madness for the triumphalist description of medical progress that had been the norm. The work of Porter, Scull and others has modified Foucault's conclusions in the light of detailed empirical data.[4] For instance, Porter argues that Foucault's 'great confinement' did not occur in large parts of Europe when the mad, because of the new economic rationality of the later seventeenth century, were supposed to have been incarcerated along with the unemployed, the vagabond, the old and infirm and other work-shy groups. Instead, in England the 'great confinement' occurred in the nineteenth century.

Roy Porter's chapter on 'Madness and its institutions' shows how the incarceration of the mad increased dramatically from around 10,000 in 1800 to 100,000 by the end of the century. Up to 1800 the family and

---

[3] Especially Michel Foucault, *Madness and Civilization: A History of Insanity in the Age of Reason* (London, 1971).
[4] For instance, Andrew Scull, *Museums of Madness* (London, 1979); Roy Porter, *Mind-Forg'd Manacles. A History of Madness in England from the Restoration to the Regency* (London, 1978); Anne Digby, *Madness, Morality and Medicine. A Study of the York Retreat* (Cambridge, 1985).

the private lunatic asylums had looked after the insane. Although often treated brutally and considered to have the status of animals, the insane were not always seen as hopeless cases in the eighteenth century. Humane treatment and ideas on 'managing' the insane out of their condition (Francis Willis tried to master George III by his eye, the force of his personality) mixed with barbarous conditions and handling. However, a series of scandals at the turn of the century helped to bring reform to bear on the treatment of the insane. Throughout Europe an optimistic new viewpoint prevailed: the insane, it was held, should be freed from their restraints and chains and be re-educated back to sanity. The new institutions that were established, such as the York Retreat, put the new approaches into practice. They acted as the models for the state-run asylums which began to proliferate. However, as the asylums grew ever larger and silted up with long-stay incurable cases, optimism gave way to pessimism, drug treatment replaced personal contact, the asylum came to be a place of dread. In the history of the relationship between the patient, medicine and the state the asylum represents a particularly depressing example of the failure of early promise.

In the second half of the nineteenth century the most significant change was the emergence of scientific medicine. This helped to increase the status of medicine, but it decreased the power of the patient in the doctor–patient relationship which had already been significantly weakened by hospital medicine. The discovery of the cell and of bacteria, the development of antiseptic techniques, the integration of chemistry with physiology, pathology and therapeutics meant that medicine could finally share with science its status as the most sure form of knowledge. Moreover, as Granshaw points out, scientific medicine gave added weight to the status and role of hospitals. Laboratories and the equipment for new techniques such as x-rays were housed in hospitals. As the twentieth century began the middle class as well as the poor had to go to hospital if they wanted to take advantage of the new scientific medicine. The hospital was slowly losing its association with poverty and with charity. The patient, it can also be argued, became more of an object; the accounts of his or her illness became even less important. Now chemical tests would decide what was wrong.[5]

A great demographic change occurred at the beginning of the

[5] Two influential articles on patient–doctor relationships have been written by N. Jewson, 'Medical knowledge and the Patronage System in Eighteenth-Century England', *Sociology*, 8 (1974), 369–85 and 'The Disappearance of the Sick Man From Medical Cosmology, 1770–1870', *Sociology*, 10 (1976), 225–44.

twentieth century. The great cause of death up to this period had been infectious diseases which produced especially large mortality rates in infants and children. The end of the nineteenth century saw a sharp decline in deaths from infectious diseases, so that in the first years of the twentieth century chronic diseases replaced acute diseases as the main cause of death. This 'epidemiological transition' has been credited to scientific medicine. Thomas McKeown argued in *Medicine in Modern Society* (1965) and elsewhere that most of the infectious diseases only became treatable with the discovery of the sulphonamides and antibiotics in the 1930s and 1940s. The reduction of mortality from infectious disease has to be seen, therefore, largely as the result of better diet (especially for tuberculosis), better sanitary conditions, water supplies and hygiene (one medical discovery, smallpox vaccination, did help to reduce the death rate from infectious disease). McKeown's general approach is still valid,[6] but Paul Weindling shows that the simple medical–social dichotomy is too crude. In his chapter 'From infectious to chronic disease: changing patterns of sickness in the nineteenth and twentieth centuries' he points out the complexities of the issue. The 'epidemiological transition' itself is not totally clear-cut, many chronic diseases in the pre-industrial period were probably undiagnosed or labelled as old age. Many of the causes of the transition are difficult to disentangle from each other. For instance, when antiseptic surgery began in the 1860s analogous social measures aimed at cleaning up the environment and improving the diet and living conditions of people were underway. Both social and medical measures could have increased the success rate of operations. Again, the scientific concept of immunology and of resistance to disease had social implications, for resistance could be raised by better diet etc.

Weindling points out that laboratory research could often be difficult to put into practice, but, as in the case of diphtheria immunization, scientific medicine became increasingly successful. At the same time hospitals were more strongly perceived as curative institutions and their influence was further increased.

The development of health services for particular groups of the population occurred at the same time as the growth in scientific medicine. Infant and maternal mortality was still very high in 1900. A

[6] A revision, but not a rejection, of McKeown's thesis can be found in Simon Szreter, 'The Importance of Social Intervention in Britain's Mortality Decline *c.* 1850–1914: A Re-interpretation of the Role of Public Health,' *Social History of Medicine*, 1 (1988), 1–37. For a more thorough critique of McKeown see Alex Mercer, *Disease, Mortality and Population in Transition* (Leicester, 1990).

combination of scientific knowledge, clinics and welfare services for mothers and babies, provided in England by local authorities, perhaps medicalized society further, but it certainly reduced the mortality rates. As Weindling argues the great alterations in the mortality regime of Europe have no simple causes but rather require sophisticated analysis and a sensitivity to their multiplicity.

At the time that scientific medicine was emerging health care was being extended to more of the population by the introduction of insurance schemes. Initially they were set up in the nineteenth century to benefit working men and were voluntary. As the twentieth century progressed they covered more and more of the population and became compulsory. In the end this created a great transformation in the expectations of medical care. Medical care, in the form of scientific medicine, came to be expected as a universal right, at least in the West. Jane Lewis charts this process in England in her chapter on 'Providers, "consumers", the state and the delivery of health-care services in twentieth-century Britain'. In 1911 the state took over the working men's insurance schemes, but women and children were not included. Generally, the voices of consumers had little effect on events; many social surveys and reports were commissioned but ignored. The state planning of health services concerned only politicians, administrators and doctors. After the founding of the National Health Service in 1948, which gave a universal right to medical care, there was still little real patient/ consumer influence on the shape of the service.

Moreover, rather than being a service which was founded on health and the prevention of disease as was hoped, the NHS increasingly centred upon sickness, a natural focus for most doctors. The dominance of hospitals and the independence of GPs was confirmed, public health medicine, which was based in local authorities, lost its control of municipal hospitals and much of its clinical work. Its loss of influence was an indication of the lower priority given to prevention.

The medical model of curative science-based medicine which has shaped most Western medical systems including the NHS has recently come under attack. Governments have begun to feel that the costs of health care are becoming too great. Lewis describes how the state has begun to attack the 'absolutist ethic of treatment' which guides doctors, whereby the needs of the patient rather than cost dictate treatment. In Britain and also in the United States, where private health insurance companies effectively shape the health-care system even after the introduction of Medicare and Medicaid, attempts have been made to 'manage' the system. The rhetoric of greater consumer participation (echoing criticisms of modern medicine) has been used to justify what, in effect, is the attempt to replace doctors by managers in the running of health services and to cut cost.

Criticisms of modern medicine abound. A list of these might include: 'hospitals are too impersonal', 'childbirth is no longer a natural but a technological process', 'doctors act like gods', 'dying has been medicalized and taken from its family setting'. At a level less orientated to the individual, medicine, especially scientific medicine, has been criticized for being concerned with treatment and not with prevention, for being unequally distributed in society, for influencing the health-care systems of Third World countries when simpler, more 'appropriate' medicine would better suit their needs. The list appears endless, and criticisms of medicine have certainly influenced the ways in which the social history of medicine has developed. This book will perhaps give a historical context to some of these criticisms. However, doctors have been criticized since classical times, after all in the end death, failure, is the outcome. Rather than being critical the book ends on a positive note with the exploration by Arthur Imhof of how demographic trends may have affected social behaviour. As he points out, the increase in the expectation of life was accompanied by the decline in religious belief. The solace of the after-life was needed less as people lived longer. However, our increased longevity is maintained at great cost and is often accompanied by the pain and debility of chronic illness. Despite these problems Imhof's overview of the centuries shows that things have improved, many children now live when before they would have died, old age is the norm not the exception. What the role of medicine has been in all this is a theme of this book.

But whether one is critical or positive about medicine, this book should show that medicine in all forms really was and is 'in society'.

Healers in the medical market place: towards a social history of Graeco-Roman medicine

VIVIAN NUTTON

Homeric Greece

The earliest literary record of classical Greece, the *Iliad* of Homer, provided the ancient doctor with both a paradigm of his success and a premonition of his failure. Among the Greek heroes who fought in the Trojan war were Podalirius and Machaon, the physician sons of Asclepius and Epione, who not only gave medical assistance but also took their places in the battle line. When Machaon was wounded by Paris' arrow in his right shoulder, Idomeneus ordered Nestor to remove him to safety in his chariot, for

> a doctor is worth many men put together,
> at extracting arrows and applying soothing ointments.

This quotation became a favourite among the Greeks, and its praise of the physician was further strengthened by the frequent omission of the qualification in the second line. It confirmed the doctor's own self-image as a man somehow raised above the majority by his skills, and could be supplemented by another passage from Homer's *Odyssey* which placed him among those whose fame could spread throughout the world.[1]

At the same time, although these healers might be on hand to treat wounds, they were by no means always successful. The great plague that afflicted the Greek army before Troy was not stayed by human power but by the divine intervention of Apollo, whose anger at the insult done to his priest had caused him to shoot his deadly arrows at the Greeks, 'so that the funeral pyres burnt incessantly'.[2] For such a divine cause, it was

---

[1] Homer, *Iliad*, Book XI, 514–15; *Odyssey*, Book XVII, 384–5, along with the diviner, the poet and the spear-maker.   [2] *Iliad*, Book I, 52.

necessary to have a divine solution; one must have recourse to a priest, diviner, augur or other religious official, and restore health to the nation by the therapy of expiation. In such a causal chain there is no place for a doctor working solely with non-religious means.

Even in Homer we can glimpse a further difficulty in identifying and pursuing the Greek doctor. Just as Machaon and Podalirius are depicted as fighting heroes, so other leaders display medical knowledge and even practical skill. When both the healers are away, Patroclus, under careful instruction from the wounded Eurypylus, stands in and removes an arrow from his thigh.[3] Patroclus had received his knowledge from Achilles, who had, in his turn, been instructed by Chiron the Centaur, traditionally the educator of the Greek heroes and often described as skilled in pharmacology.[4] Besides, the descriptions of wounds in both the *Iliad* and the *Odyssey* are largely technically accurate, which encouraged a nineteenth-century commentator to posit that Homer too was a military doctor after his fashion.[5] Yet the same author's speculation that there must have been several 'healers' among the Greeks and Trojans, while true in the sense that a knowledge of herbs and first aid was accessible to all, including, especially, the aristocratic leaders, is misleading in its implication that there must have been a specific group of men whose duty it was solely to treat the sick and wounded. There may have been, but all the evidence points to the general absence of such specialization. Some men might have had a widespread reputation for healing and made money by being summoned from afar to treat, presumably wealthy, patients, but their numbers will always have been few, and they are set on a par with the court prophet, poet or armourer. They were high-grade craftsmen, but craftsmen none the less.[6]

The Hippocratic Corpus in context

For our knowledge of Greek medicine and its physicians before the late fifth century BC, we are largely at the mercy of a combination of later legend and modern plausible speculation, and neither can be trusted entirely. Yet certain conflicting strands are discernible and it is historically

[3] *Iliad*, Book XI, 842–8.

[4] *Ibid.*, 831–2. In the celebrated series of miniatures in the sixth-century Vienna codex of Dioscorides, Österreichische Nationalbibliothek, cod. gr. 1, fol. 2, Chiron is depicted in the place of honour, and is surrounded by other great names of ancient pharmacology.

[5] H. Frölich, *Die Militärmedicin Homers* (Stuttgart, 1879), p. 65. Connoisseurs of the curious may enjoy Frölich's presentation of the statistics of battle injuries, pp. 58–9.

[6] Homer, *Odyssey*, Book XVII, 384–5. Cf. the similar list in Solon, *fr.* 13, 41–62 West.

wiser to accept these tensions than to posit any uniform development of medicine throughout the Greek world from Sicily to Naucratis in Egypt. The social forces at work in an expanding city like Athens were inevitably different from those affecting small towns like Abdera in Thrace or colonial settlements like Elea in Southern Italy.

The tradition of self-help in medicine must always have been strong, particularly in the countryside, although it appears infrequently in the literary sources. The Mycenean Greeks had a substantial number of native herbs at their disposal, as well as being able to take advantage of others brought from abroad.[7] An emphasis on natural herbal remedies can also be detected in the polemic delivered by the author of *The Art*, who is at pains to emphasise the necessity for medicine in the face of those who deny its validity and prefer themselves to follow nature's way.[8] Several of the tracts in the Hippocratic Corpus are apparently directed to the layman, to enable him to cure himself without needing a doctor.[9] These guides to health for the layman, which should be distinguished from tracts dedicated to lay *cognoscenti*, continued to be produced, especially by writers on pharmacology, and the distinguished later physician, Rufus of Ephesus (*c.* AD 110), encapsulated all his teachings in a large work entitled *The Layman*, which survives today only in fragmentary quotations.[10] This popular tradition of self-help, reinforced by the frequent absence of any medical expert, of whatever level of proficiency, provides one constant boundary against which to set the art of medicine in antiquity.

At the other extreme can be placed the medical clans, keeping their own drugs and therapies within the family, and enjoying within the community recognition as local medicine men. The literary tradition lays particular stress on the Asclepiadae, the descendents of Asclepius, the legendary founder of medicine and, later, a healing god, and historians have often been content to follow the bias of these sources. There is a certain degree of truth in them, for the family of the great Hippocrates, himself an Asclepiad, can be traced on Cos directly for four more generations, is still recognizable as a closed medical association about

[7] For Mycenean drugs, see C. W. Shelmerdine, *The Perfume Industry of Mycenean Pylos* (Gothenburg, 1985).   [8] [Hippocrates], *Art*, 8–9.

[9] [Hippocrates] *Ancient Medicine* 2; *Airs, Waters, Places*; *Breaths*. For the 'openness' of much of Greek medicine, cf. G. E. R. Lloyd, *Magic, Reason and Experience* (Cambridge, 1979), pp. 228–9.

[10] Cf. the *Euporista* (*Home remedies*) ascribed to Dioscorides (*fl.* AD 60), and the work of a similar title by Galen. For Rufus' book, see the fragments preserved by Rhazes and available in Latin in the Daremberg-Ruelle edition of Rufus of Ephesus. The fact that this tradition of self-help can be traced back to classical Greece is enough to caution against the traditional dichotomy between a physician-dependent Greece and a self-reliant Rome.

275 BC, and has its last known medical representative in C. Stertinius Xenophon, doctor to the Roman emperors Claudius and Nero (*fl.* AD 55).[11]

Yet Galen's pleasant tale of three separate groups of Asclepiads, on Cos, Cnidos and Rhodes, in whom alone resided all medical knowledge, bears all the hallmarks of a late literary fiction, and should not be relied upon.[12] The tradition may be fittingly compared with that of the *pholarchoi* of Elea (or Velia), whose known representatives are called Oulis and who claim descent of some sort from Parmenides, the Ouliad, philosopher and doctor (*fl.* 470 BC).[13] This rare family name, which seems to come from S.W. Asia Minor, derives from one of the cult titles of Apollo, Oulios, 'the healer'. Whether the bearers of this name were in origin healers is doubtful; the evidence is against it for the historical period, when, equally, the name Asclepiades is not confined either to one family or to healers.

The great migrations of the Greek colonial movements to Southern Italy, to Sicily and the Black Sea region from the eighth-century onwards and, perhaps still more, the growth in the sixth century of Athens and the wealthy cities of the coast of western Asia Minor, helped to break down some of the old ties of clan and class. The Greek doctor now could travel much further, although to what extent he was open to non-Greek influence is a matter for considerable debate. There are no recognizable traces of Babylonian medicine among the Greek medical writers, and not all have concurred with Steuer and Saunders in linking the medicine of Cnidos with an Egyptian theory that ascribes all disease to putrefying residues.[14] The notion of itself is not so unusual as to be the discovery of any single group, and the plurality of Greek ideas on causation found in the Hippocratic Corpus shows that the early Greek medical writers were capable of such innovation in their theory.[15]

[11] S. M. Sherwin-White, *Ancient Cos* (Göttingen, 1978), pp. 256–63, 283–5.

[12] F. Rosenthal, 'An Ancient Commentary on the Hippocratic Oath', *Bulletin of the History of Medicine* 30 (1956), 58, 80; W. D. Smith, 'Galen on Coans v. Cnidians', *ibid.*, 47 (1973), 569–85; I. M. Lonie, 'Cos versus Cnidus and the Historians', *History of Science*, 16 (1978), 42–75, 77–92.

[13] V. Nutton, 'Velia and the School of Salerno', *Medical History*, 15 (1971), 1–11, offers an English summary of the evidence, although perhaps drawing too definite a line between philosophy and medicine. G. Pugliese Carratelli, 'Ancora di Parmenide e della scuola medica di Velia', *La Parola del Passato*, 40 (1985), 34–8, stresses the intellectual traditions of Velia, whereas S. Musitelli, 'Ancora sui φώλαρχοι di Velia', *ibid.* 35 (1980), 241–55, emphasizes the religious nature of the association and suggests that the title was, in some way, applied to a priest at a healing shrine. See also M. Fabbri, A. Trotta, *Una Scuola-Collegio di Età Augustea* (Rome, 1989).

[14] R. O. Steuer and J. B. de C. M. Saunders, *Ancient Egyptian and Cnidian Medicine* (Berkeley and Los Angeles, 1959).

[15] Lloyd, *Magic*, pp. 49–58, 230–4; A. Thivel, *Cnide et Cos?* (Paris, 1981), pp. 317–21, 366–7.

Egyptian doctors did have a reputation for excellence in the Persian Empire of the late sixth century BC; they had a distinct organization, as well as educational institutions; and the possibility of some influence, however small, cannot be excluded entirely.[16] The most obvious result of the Greek expansion around the Mediterranean lay in the new drugs available for therapy, coming both from the East via either Persia or Egypt and from the West, especially through the Phocaean colonies in Provence and Italy.

In such a mobile society, the intra-familial traditions of medicine gradually lost relevance, and were replaced by formal or informal instruction in medicine outside the family. The so-called Hippocratic *Oath* marks a point at which the doctor's obligations to his teacher, his patients and his art are sited outside the immediate family but within a context intended to be as like a family as possible. For the close ties of blood are substituted equally close intellectual ties, which, like true family relationships, cannot be expressed in monetary terms. Medicine is still seen as something holy, to be revealed only to the holy, to the initiate, and its secrets are to be kept within the small group.[17] But this quasi-familial phase could not last. One of the few facts known for certain about the great Hippocrates was that he was prepared to teach medicine for a fee to anyone who could afford it.[18] Public performances and treatments must also have served to transmit medical knowledge away from the immediate family.[19]

At the same time, the sixth century brings the first historical record of individual physicians. The beautiful statue of Sombrotidas, son of Mandrocles, from Megara Hyblaea in Sicily of *c.* 575 BC, and the very fine relief, now in Basle, of an unknown Greek doctor of *c.* 510 BC, which may have been carved in south-western Asia Minor near to Cos

[16] Herodotus, *Hist.* II, 84–5; III, 129; H. E. Sigerist, *A History of Medicine*, vol. I (Oxford, 1951), pp. 324–5. That such links went back a long way can be seen from the letters of Rameses II, published by E. Edel, *Ägyptische Ärzte und ägyptische Medizin am hethischen Kaiserhof* (Opladen, 1976). The Greek tradition, found in Clement of Alexandria, *Strom.* 1.16.75 and Suidas A.3217, that medicine was introduced into Greece by Apis 'before Io came to Egypt', can hardly predate 100 BC.

[17] See L. Edelstein, *The Hippocratic Oath* (Baltimore, 1943) = *Ancient Medicine* (Baltimore, 1967), pp. 3–63, although his suggestion of a Pythagorean origin for the *Oath* is unacceptable. Cf. also the *Law*, and the *Physician*, which have similar ethical presuppositions.

[18] Plato, *Prot.* 311 B–C, sees nothing unusual in the 'historical' Hippocrates teaching medicine for a fee. If this rare contemporary view of Hippocrates is correct – and I see no reason to doubt it – Hippocrates had already in his lifetime a reputation as a physician and as a teacher: *contra*, C. Lichtenthaeler, *Der Eid des Hippokrates* (Cologne, 1984), pp. 303–24, arguing for the *Oath's* authenticity.

[19] Lloyd, *Magic*, pp. 254–69, emphasises the public character of the Greek physician's activities, although there is no need to go along with his argument that this is also a consequence of Greek (or Athenian) democratic practice.

and Cnidos, both show the respect in which certain doctors were held or, indirectly, the wealth they could obtain.[20] Literary confirmation is available in Herodotus' description of the life of Democedes of Croton, who left Southern Italy to seek his fortune as a doctor on Aegina, and then moved to Athens, Samos and the Persian court *c.* 522 BC, where he owned a great house and ate daily with the king. He succeeded in escaping back to Croton, where, a wealthy and respected man, he married the daughter of the famous athlete Milo. Later civil war forced him to leave Croton yet again, with other defeated aristocrats, and he fled to Plataea in mainland Greece. His career exemplifies two types of doctor; the *Wanderarzt* and the civic physician.[21]

If Herodotus' account is reliable, Democedes is the earliest known civic physician by roughly a century, and his employment by Aegina and later Athens shows that even at this early stage the two cities, and possibly others like Miletus, had reached a high level of sophistication in their civic consciousness. Democedes had arrived full of hope but without instruments on Aegina, yet within six months he had built up such a reputation that he was offered 1 talent a year by the city to stay there. But there was competition for such a skilled operator, and, at the end of a year, he crossed the Saronic Gulf to serve at Athens, for a fee of 1 and two-thirds talents per annum. Yet even this city, which was expanding to a metropolis under the influence of the Peisistratids, could not keep him in the face of an even higher offer by Polycrates, tyrant of Samos. His move to Persia, however, was involuntary, in the train of slaves captured by King Darius.

At various times, then, Democedes served as a civic doctor, but there is nothing to suggest that this position required of him anything more than residence. In all the later documents referring to the appointment and activities of such practitioners, there is never any formal injunction on a doctor to treat the poor free of charge, although, of course, social pressures and individual inclination might well lead to such generosity.[22] There is a possibility that at Athens, in the heady days of the Periclean democracy of the middle and late fifth century BC, civic doctors gave

---

[20] E. Berger, *Das Basler Arztrelief* (Basle, 1970), pl. 162–3 (oddly misdating the statue to 480–470) and pl. 1.   [21] Herodotus, *Hist.* III, 131–8.

[22] L. Cohn-Haft, *The Public Physicians of Ancient Greece* (Northampton, Mass., 1956); A. R. Hands, *Charities and Social Aid* (London, 1968), pp. 136–41; V. Nutton, 'Continuity or Rediscovery? The City Physician in Classical Antiquity and Mediaeval Italy', in A. W. Russell (ed.), *The Town and State Physician in Europe* (Wolfenbüttel, 1981), pp. 11–17. (repr. in V. Nutton, *From Democedes to Harvey* (London, 1988) The 'case notes' in *Epidemics* show doctors treating patients from all classes, although they might well tailor their remedies to the ability of their patient to pay.

free treatment to citizens or to the poor citizens alone, but doubtful quotations from the comic poet Aristophanes are scarcely solid evidence, and the procedure for such distinctions is hard to imagine.[23]

Plato in his *Gorgias* alleges that in his day doctors were chosen for public service after they had addressed the public Assembly of Athens, and often more from their rhetorical than their professional skills.[24] This public contest of words may have had its lesser counterpart in demonstrations and multiple consultations, on which medical authors show a decided ambivalence. It is good to seek other advice in doubtful cases, but unseemly wrangling does not benefit the patient and harms the cause of medicine as a whole.[25] But the Greek doctor could not avoid being caught up in public confrontation, either with a patient, an audience, or fellow practitioners, and, as G. E. R. Lloyd has suggested, it may be precisely the need for the doctor to explain and defend himself in front of others that led to the peculiar stress in Greek medicine on logic and consistency of argument.[26] Thus in many texts we find an emphasis on the use of analogies drawn from the world around them whose self-consistency serves also to validate the explanations for which they are used. The position of the arm in archery justifies a type of splint and bandaging; the various crafts provide examples of activities that parallel those posited for the human body; the kidneys work like cupping glasses, attracting fluid to themselves.[27] The early anatomical descriptions, given by Syennesis of Cyrene and Diogenes of Sinope (*fl.* 440 BC), are schematic, logical constructs, in sharp contrast to the practical, detailed and generally accurate accounts of surface anatomy in the Hippocratic Corpus.[28] The emphasis is on the effectiveness of the medical data in convincing an audience rather than on any rigorous examination of the truth of the data itself.[29]

[23] Nutton, 'Continuity', p. 12; L. Gil and R. Alfageme, 'La figura del médico en la comedia Atica', *Cuadernos de Filologia Clásica*, 3 (1972), 40, 51–53. A. G. Woodhead, 'The State Health Service in Ancient Greece', *Cambridge Historical Journal*, 10 (1952), 237–9, argues for free medical care for citizens, but his authority is a very late scholiast (*c.* AD 400 or later), whose knowledge of Athenian life eight centuries before is unlikely to have been better than our own.

[24] Plato, *Gorgias* 455 B; cf. Xenophon, *Mem.* 4.2.5.   [25] [Hippocrates], *Precepts* 8–9.

[26] Lloyd, *Magic*, pp. 86–98.

[27] [Hippocrates], *Fract.* II; *Reg.* I, 12–24; *Ancient medicine* 22.

[28] C. R. S. Harris, *The Heart and the Vascular System in Ancient Greek Medicine* (Oxford, 1973), pp. 20–8. V. Di Benedetto, *Il medico e la malattia* (Turin, 1986), pp. 225–47, counsels against underestimating the anatomical knowledge of fifth-century healers.

[29] I. M. Lonie, *The Hippocratic Treatises 'On Generation', 'On the Nature of the Child', 'Diseases IV'* (Berlin, 1981), pp. 72–86. It should perhaps here be mentioned that there were severe technological restraints on investigating the human body: no microscopes, few instruments, and rudimentary antiseptics and anaesthetics.

This openness and accessibility of medicine in the fifth and fourth centuries BC, not only in its argumentation but also in its vocabulary – for a purely medical technical vocabulary, neologisms and all, we must wait another century[30] – , enabled it to draw on the lively debates of the so-called Pre-Socratic philosophers. Controversy over the precise extent of mutual influence should not be allowed to obscure the crucial point,[31] the fluidity of the boundaries between medicine and philosophy. The author of *Ancient Medicine* vehemently attacks philosophers for introducing vague suppositions into medicine, yet he is himself equally guilty in that respect.[32] Celsus writing over four centuries later praised Hippocrates for being the first to separate medicine from philosophy, but both the meaning of this encomium and the evidence on which it is based are questionable.[33] Whatever view is taken, the separation did not last long, for Plato's *Timaeus*, in particular, was a synthesis of medical and philosophical learning.[34]

The Pre-Socratic philosophers, even if they did not entirely create the concepts and ideas found in the Hippocratic Corpus, at any rate developed them in their own lively debates and enabled some doctors to draw on them to form the framework for their own theoretical expositions. This was not surprising, given the proximity of the questions discussed by both groups. 'What is man?' 'What is he made of?', 'How does he operate?', could be answered by both parties, and their answers could be mutually influential. The arguments of Parmenides and the Eleatic philosophers effectively ended the earlier search for a single primal element out of which all things came, and focused attention on the need to explain the stability and, at the same

---

[30] A. Parry, 'The Language of Thucydides' Description of the Plague', *Bulletin of the Institute of Classical Studies* 16 (1969), 106–18. Galen in the second century AD often inveighs against those who invented new technical terms where ordinary words sufficed, e.g. x.423–6 κ.

[31] Contrast J. Burnet, *Early Greek Philosophy*, 4th edn (Oxford, 1945, but originally 1914), p. 201, with Edelstein, *Ancient Medicine*, pp. 349–66. An isolated protest against Edelstein's very influential view is J. Longrigg, 'Philosophy and Medicine, Some Early Interactions', *Harvard Studies in Classical Philology*, 67 (1963), 147–75.

[32] Lloyd, *Magic*, pp. 135, 146–9; *Science, Folklore and Ideology* (Cambridge, 1983), pp. 86–94; *The Revolutions of Wisdom* (Berkeley, Los Angeles and London, 1987).

[33] Celsus, *De medicina*, Pr. 8. The difficulties of interpreting this statement were elegantly summarized by L. S. King, 'Hippocrates and Philosophy', *Journal of the History of Medicine*, 18 (1963), 77–8. P. Mudry, *La préface du De medicina de Celse* (Rome, 1982), pp. 63–5, argues that Celsus thought of Hippocrates as the creator of a discipline of medicine as distinct from that of philosophy, but this formulation still seems to me to lack a basis in actuality.

[34] G. E. R. Lloyd, 'Plato as a Natural Scientist', *Journal of Hellenic Studies*, 68 (1968), 78–92; other examples of the constant interrelation of philosopher and physician are given in his *Science*, pp. 94–110.

time, the capacity for change of the universe, and of man in particular.[35] Heraclitus' idea of a perpetual flux was taken up and used by writers of medical texts, who emphasised the precariousness of health and the ever-changing responses of the body to stimuli such as food and environment.[36] The idea of fluidity also had a medical counterpart in the doctrine of humours, bodily fluids, particularly bile and phlegm, and, later, blood and black bile, which were thought to cause illness through excess or deficiency. Another philosophical model adapted by doctors posited four basic elements, earth, air, fire and water, and derived everything from their proper mixture. Empedocles (*fl.* 440), whose medical interests were extensive, explained differences between substances like bone, blood and flesh, as deriving from the particular combination of their elements. Their existence and well-being depended on the preservation of this proper balance which was correlated by medical writers, like the author of *On the Nature of Man*, with four humours and, later, four primary qualities, hot, cold, wet and dry.[37] A variant of this is found in Anaxagoras' belief that everything had in itself a portion of everything else, and that individuality was determined by the predominance of particular portions. Since like was attracted to like, similarly balanced globules or seeds could come together to form larger uniform parts such as flesh or bone.[38] In contrast to Anaxagoras' derivation of diversity from the constitution of the ultimate molecule, the seed, his contemporary Democritus regarded all substance as homogeneous, and accounted for the apparently infinite variety of phenomena by mere differences of shape, size, position and arrangements of the basic building blocks, the indivisible atoms.[39]

It was philosophical speculation like this that enabled physicians to develop their own medical theories and in turn to influence the

[35] Convenient English discussions will be found in G. S. Kirk, J. E. Raven and M. Schofield, *The Presocratic Philosophers*, 2nd edn (Cambridge, 1983), pp. 214–79; and J. Barnes, *The Presocratic Philosophers*, vol. I (London, 1979), pp. 155–302.

[36] Kirk, Raven and Schofield, *Presocratic Philosophers*, pp. 181–212; Barnes, *Presocratic Philosophers*, I, pp. 57–81; C. H. Kahn, *The Art and Thought of Heraclitus* (Cambridge, 1979). This philosophical theory is most obviously used in the Hippocratic tract *Regimen*, cf. Thivel, *Cnide*, pp. 149–50, 271–5.

[37] Kirk, Raven and Schofield, *Presocratic Philosophers*, pp. 280–321; Thivel, *Cnide*, pp. 325–38, 369–84.

[38] Kirk, Raven and Schofield, *Presocratic Philosophers*, pp. 352–84; Barnes, *Presocratic Philosophers*, II, pp. 16–39; for the importance of Anaxagoras in Galen, see G. Strohmaier, *Galeni De partium homoeomerium differentia*, C(orpus) M(edicorum) G(raecorum) Suppl. Orient. 3 (Berlin, 1970).

[39] Kirk, Raven and Schofield, *Presocratic Philosophers*, pp. 402–33; Barnes, *Presocratic Philosophers*, II, pp. 40–75. Atomism, and Pythagoreanism to an even smaller extent, plays little part in classical Greek medicine of the fifth and fourth centuries BC, and only becomes influential with Asclepiades and his followers (and Plutarch's Democriteans) in the Roman period.

VIVIAN NUTTON

philosophers, and many of their arguments can be seen as an attempt either to use or to combat such ideas circulating in general debate. The result is often eclectic and *ad hoc*, and occasionally naive in the extreme, yet the vigour with which the cases are presented implies more than a tired restatement of long-held positions. Doctors and philosophers are having to think about basics, and to respond to contemporary objections and propositions from their competitors, their patients and their audience.

The obvious eclecticism of the treatises in the Hippocratic Corpus is a further argument against seeing early Greek medicine purely as a dichotomy between Cos and Cnidos, later joined by an 'Italian' or 'Sicilian' school.[40] Some texts do exhibit close links, but most borrow from a variety of current theories whose precise origins and affiliations are unknown. Besides, the geographical closeness of Cos and Cnidos is a further argument in favour of some mutual influence, and if the intellectual world of the late fifth century was in no way rigidly compartmentalized, there is no reason to suppose that medicine was too.[41] Evidence for medical schools at this period depends entirely upon late reconstructions and on a touching belief in the validity of 'school traditions', for there is, as yet, no evidence, literary, epigraphic or archaeological, for the existence of places or buildings where medical instruction was carried on, or for students flocking to particular areas to be taught by distinguished masters of medicine. True, Cos had a reputation for its doctors and Hippocrates taught medicine for a fee, but the doctors on Cos are all apparently natives, perhaps taught by relatives, and occasional instruction from an individual on his travels is somewhat different from the traditions of a permanent school.[42] Nineteenth-century scholarship created ancient medical schools in the image of contemporary institutions, without considering the social differences between the centuries.

[40] Although Thivel, *Cnide*, provides a comprehensive demolition of the Cos/Cnidos theory, he still believes in an Ionian and an Italian 'school'; cf. also Di Benedetto, *Il medico*, pp. 70–96.

[41] In all likelihood, a physician would have a pupil or an apprentice living with him in his house. Although some treatises in the Hippocratic Corpus hang closely together, it is doubtful whether all, or even most, came from an institutional library of the fourth century BC, still less that this was the library of the medical school of Cos, cf. W. D. Smith, *The Hippocratic Tradition* (Ithaca and London, 1979), p. 39.

[42] Sherwin-White, *Cos*, pp. 265–74; J. Benedum, 'Inscriptions grecques de Cos relatives à des médecins hippocratiques et Cos Astypalaia', in M. D. Grmek (ed.), *Hippocratica* (Paris, 1980), pp. 35–43. Of the doctors there mentioned, only one, Onasandros is possibly a non-Coan, but the inscription itself has never been fully published, and its assumed date, c. 200 BC, makes it dangerous evidence on which to base a reconstruction of medical life two centuries earlier. Onasandros is expressly mentioned as having had pupils.

24

We should also be careful about laying too much stress on the signs of incipient medical specialization, particularly surgery and gynaecology. The doctor in the Hippocratic Corpus had to be a generalist in the small communities in which he found himself, yet there is clear evidence of a hierarchy of preferred treatments ranging in order of safety, from diet through drugs to surgery. The latter was obviously attended with considerable risk to the patient, even if circumstances were favourable and the operation performed by a skilled and experienced hand, and, if the patient died, the shadow of incompetence could easily fall on the operator.[43] 'Killed by the hands of the doctor' is an understandable reproach from the relatives of the dead, and a reputation as a murderer, however unjustified, would not enhance a doctor's career. It is for this reason, and also for the related ethical desire to abstain from causing unnecessary harm, that we find some authors in the Hippocratic Corpus leaving certain operations to those more skilled in the art.[44] The treatment of war wounds should, by rights, be entrusted only to a man experienced in warfare: and the Hippocratic *Oath* expressly leaves surgery, even cutting for the stone, to those who are experienced workers in it.[45] This does not constitute a total rejection of surgery, but is a sober recognition of its value only if performed by those with long practice at it. Cutting for the stone, although painful, could be carried out, like trepanation, with a good chance of success, and where, as in Athens and some of the larger Greek cities of Asia Minor, there were both sufficient patients and sufficient doctors, it was entirely open to a physician to entrust such cases to another more skilled than he. The *Oath* is, once again, to be seen in the context of a small group of physicians, working alongside lithotomists, midwives and laymen to promote health. Male doctors wrote about women's complaints and assisted at births, although female nurses and wise women would have officiated far more often; while, in turn, women could equally, if rarely, practise medicine, especially if they belonged to a medical family.[46] Plato even

---

[43] Edelstein, *Ancient Medicine*, pp. 87–110; Di Benedetto, *Il medico*, pp. 161–80.

[44] V. Nutton, 'The Perils of Patriotism; Pliny and Roman Medicine', in F. Greenaway and R. French (eds.), *Science in the Early Roman Empire: Pliny the Elder, his sources and influence* (London, 1986), pp. 36–7 (repr. in Nutton, *From Democedes to Harvey*).

[45] [Hippocrates], *Doctor* 14; *Oath* 5, with Edelstein's discussion, *Ancient Medicine*, pp. 26–30. For ancient surgery in general, see G. Majno, *The Healing Hand* (Cambridge, MA, 1975).

[46] The great variety of healers is emphasised by H. Pleket, 'Arts en maatschappij in het oude Griekenland. De sociale status van de arts', *Tijdschrift voor Geschiedenis*, 96 (1983), 325–47; for female practitioners, cf. A. Krug, *Heilkunst und Heilkult. Medizin in der Antike* (Munich, 1984), pp. 195–7; Lloyd, *Science*, pp. 58–86. Cf. also H. F. J. Horstmanshoff, 'The Ancient Physician: Craftsman or Scientist,' *Journal of the History of Medicine*, 45 (1990), 176–97.

suggests that there could be slave-doctors who treated slaves, as well as a range of medical men of varying degrees of competence.[47] It is in this social situation of competition or cooperation between healers that we should locate the formation of the first ethical codes and writings in the Hippocratic Corpus. While they do impart words of advice that continue to be normative today – the confidentiality of the doctor–patient relationship, and strong condemnation of any abuse of the doctor's medical privileges for private or personal satisfaction – it is impossible to state how far they were then regarded as possessing permanent and universal utility.[48] Certainly there is no suggestion that at this stage any of these texts, even the *Oath*, was held up as an unimpeachable standard to which all doctors must conform or else cease to practice.[49] There are, it is true, hints of demarcation disputes between healers, and, as Edelstein insisted, the Hippocratic physician used prognosis, not just as a guide to medical treatment, but also for propaganda purposes, to proclaim his own merits and to forestall the loss of a reputation, should things go wrong. An appropriate ethic could also serve to enhance his standing in a society where, in the absence of licensing and, for the most part, any public medical appointments, reputation and sound experience counted for almost all.[50] Even when there was competition and a public choice of physicians, as in Periclean Athens, for certain official positions for the fleet and possibly also as civic doctors, the choice might not always be made on properly medical grounds, so it was alleged, but could be determined solely by the doctor's skills as orator and showman.[51] Moralizing treatises like *Precepts* and *Decorum*, which can be dated on stylistic and philosophical grounds to the later Hellenistic period, confirm the subordination of a universalist ethic to one more ostensibly devoted to the practical success of the physician. The benefits to the patient are balanced by advice to the physician to act in a way that is socially acceptable as well as moral.

[47] F. Kudlien, *Die Sklaven in der griechischen Medizin* (Wiesbaden, 1968); R. Joly, 'Esclaves et médecins dans la Grèce antique', *Sudhoffs Archiv*, 53 (1969), 1–14.

[48] Edelstein, *Ancient Medicine*, pp. 319–48.

[49] Knowledge of the ethical rules of the Oath is presupposed by Scribonius Largus, *fl.* 50 AD, in the preface to his *Compositiones*, but the fragments of Galen's commentary on the *Oath*, see Rosenthal, *Commentary*, say nothing that indicates that Galen thought the Oath was (or indeed ought to be) taken by every physician.

[50] Edelstein, *Ancient Medicine*, pp. 65–85; Nutton, *Pliny*; and 'Murders and Miracles: Lay Attitudes Towards Medicine in Classical Antiquity', in R. Porter (ed.), *Patients and Practitioners* (Cambridge, 1985), pp. 23–53 (repr. in Nutton, *From Democedes to Harvey*).

[51] Above, note 24; cf. also F. Kudlien, 'Schaustellerei und Heilmittelvertrieb in der Antike', *Gesnerus*, 40 (1983), 91–8.

Precepts 3–13 is full of practical hints to the intending doctor on how to make the best impression in a whole variety of situations so that he can gain professional success. Haggling over a fee before a cure is to be avoided for the possible worry it may cause the patient (and the consequent reduction of chances of success). A judicious waiving of fees might, in fact, bring in more paying customers: 'for where there is love of man, there is also love of the art'. Professional quarrels should be hidden from the patient, although proper consultation is advisable; and if one is to give a medical lecture to a lay audience, one should avoid irrelevant poetic quotation or the tedious definitions, flowery language and invocations to the gods offered by the 'later learner'. All these might give the incompetent doctor away, and, in the end, reduce his chances of a select and wealthy clientele.[52]

The Hellenistic East

Precepts is one of the latest books in the Hippocratic Corpus, perhaps composed in the first century BC or even later, and fits well with the picture given by the epigraphic and literary sources of the activities of contemporary physicians. The conquests of Alexander the Great and their consolidation by his successors, the Hellenistic kings, brought Greek ideas and institutions to the borders of India and the sands of Libya. The ruling classes accepted Hellenization as the price for a continuance of their local domination, and a veneer of Greek language and culture emphasised the unity of the new civilization, and, increasingly, penetrated non-Greek societies. The precepts of Apollo at Delphi could be announced by a wandering philosopher to the citizens of a Greek settlement in Afghanistan, and the gymnasium, part club and part academy, became an essential feature of even the smallest of cities.[53] From Istros on the Black Sea to Seleucia and Perge in Southern Turkey doctors can be found delivering public lectures and performing demonstrations in the theatre or gymnasium, although later descriptions of their flashy instruments and verbal fireworks might suggest that their audiences were as likely to be bewildered as enlightened, and that a desire for a spectacle might be at least as compelling as a thirst for medical knowledge.[54] There is increasing evidence for the employment of civic

---

[52] H. M. Koelbing, *Arzt und Patient in der antiken Welt* (Zurich, 1976), pp. 120–31; D. Gourevitch, *Le triangle hippocratique dans le monde greco-romain; le malade, sa maladie et son médecin* (Rome, 1984).

[53] L. Robert, 'Inscriptions grècques nouvelles de la Bactriane', *Comptes rendues Ac. Inscr.* (1968), 442–54.   [54] Nutton, 'Murders', p. 37; M. Vegetti, *Il coltello e lo stilo* (Milan, 1979).

doctors, some expressly requested from Cos, others recognized after some service within the community, and even for a reappointment, in an emergency, of a doctor who had earlier resigned or been dismissed from his post.[55] In all this the choice was made by the council, no longer an institution involving the whole citizen body, but one increasingly confined to its upper strata, those with sufficient wealth and culture. It is to impress these people, from whom a doctor could expect preferment and wealth, that the late Hippocratic tracts on medical conduct were written. The choice of free treatment for the poor and needy was the doctor's own, but the abnegation of fees, so ostentatiously recorded on some honorary decrees, also attests a level of prosperity, almost certainly from land, on the part of some doctors that would enable them to exist without this professional income.[56] An investment in generosity might also pay off later in access to wealthy patients.

The transfer of the city states of classical Greece to the broader geographical setting of the Hellenistic world brought other changes to the social background of Greek medicine. The vigorous intellectual and political life of Periclean Athens had ended with the defeat of Athens by Sparta in 404 BC, and with it too, if the comic poet Aristophanes can be trusted, went payment for civic doctors, at least temporarily.[57] Democratic participatory politics was replaced by a progressive *embourgeoisement* and the rise of professional politicians; the openness of medical authors to a whole range of exciting influences was succeeded gradually by the formation of sects and school-doctrines: philosophers withdrew from the market place to the porch or the garden.

But all was not decline, even if historians of both politics, literature and science have tended to see it as such. The sheer size of the Hellenistic world, and of cities like Antioch, Pergamum and, in particular, Alexandria, brought advantages too. The development of specialization, particularly in surgery, cannot be divorced from the existence of centres of population sufficiently large to support a doctor who practised only a limited number of medical skills.[58] Knowledge of foreign herbs, plants

[55] Sherwin-White, *Cos*, p. 178, translates the decree for the doctor who acted in an emergency; for civic physicians, see above, n. 22.
[56] Cohn-Haft, *Public Physicians*, pp. 32–45. The 'stipend' of a public physician was more in the nature of a retainer. Few towns in antiquity were large enough to support a healer, let alone a specialist, whose income derived solely from the practice of medicine; hence the necessity for the doctor to travel in search of patients, or to have some additional source of income.
[57] Aristophanes, *Plutus* 408 (a play put on in 388 BC).
[58] M. Michler, *Das Spezialisierungsproblem und die antike Chirurgie* (Berne, Stuttgart and Vienna, 1969).

and drugs also grew substantially, encouraged by the conquests of Alexander which enabled the followers of Aristotle, particularly Theophrastus (*c.* 370–288/5 BC) to inspect and describe many rare or novel specimens. But how far or when these new drugs entered medicine is hard to determine in the almost total absence of pharmaceutical literature before the Roman period, and recent studies of the spice trade with India, Arabia and Africa have not contributed much towards a solution.[59] A citation in Theophrastus only indicates that a plant was known, not the extent of its use.

The interests of Aristotle (384–322 BC) in medicine and science mark a major shift in the development of Greek medicine towards a consolidation of knowledge and its extension by means of systematic research, particularly in anatomy and pharmacology. Early courts, like those of Macedon, Persia and the Sicilian tyrants, had been centres of culture, fostering, in particular, poets and dramatists, but although a few court doctors are named, they are isolated and transitory figures whose contributions to medical learning are negligible. The institutionalizing of Platonic philosophy in the Academy and Aristotle's creation of his Lyceum provided a framework for continuity, and Aristotle's own biological researches, which he had made while at the court of the tyrant of Assos in western Turkey, could be extended and built on by a generation of pupils at Athens. The example of Aristotle and Alexander was followed by the various successor kings, who vied with each other in the promotion of culture. Although poets and historians are the most prominent among the favoured literati, doctors and scientists also were encouraged to attach themselves to one centre or other, and their work could be considered a practical symbol of princely munificence.[60]

The development of anatomy has long been associated with the new order of the Hellenistic monarchs, although the exact relationship between the two is unclear. The descriptions of the internal organs of the human body in the early texts of the Hippocratic Corpus are rarely based on direct observation, and such knowledge was amassed largely empirically and by chance. But Aristotle's investigations of animal

---

[59] A. G. Morton, *History of Botanical Science* (London, 1981), pp. 27–57, offers a brief account of Theophrastus; cf. also Lloyd, *Science*, pp. 119–35. The drug trade with the East is studied at length by M. Raschke, 'New Studies in Roman Commerce with the East', in H. Temporini (ed.), *Aufstieg und Niedergang der römischen Welt*, vol. IX, part 2 (Berlin, 1978), pp. 650–76.

[60] On Aristotle, see A. G. Preus, *Science and Philosophy in Aristotle's Biological Works* (New York, 1975); Lloyd, *Science*, pp. 18–26. J. N. Longrigg, 'Superlative Achievement and Comparative Neglect: Alexandrian Medical Science and Modern Historical Research', *History of Science*, 19 (1981), 155–200, offers a detailed bibliographical survey.

anatomy seem to have encouraged others to carry out systematic enquiry at Athens and elsewhere with royal encouragement. The first known text specifically devoted to anatomies is by one of his pupils, Diocles of Carystus, who settled at the court of Antigonus of Macedon c. 320 BC, and it was followed by the famous researches of Herophilus and Erasistratus at Alexandria. But two qualifications must be made before accepting royal patronage as the essential element in the development of anatomy.[61] The text On the Heart,[62] which shows an understanding of some of the anatomical structures of the heart, cannot be linked with any known centre, and might indicate a broader interest in anatomy independent of a court. Secondly, as Edelstein argued, the growing acceptance of a Platonic separation of soul and body may have led to a general lessening of hostility towards the cutting open of a corpse, since, on this philosophical theory, the body was no more than a shell for a personality which migrated at death.[63] But how far this belief penetrated downwards into society is uncertain, and Galen may well be right in his supposition that royal involvement or protection was essential for the systematic investigation of human body by dissection, let alone by vivisection.[64] The tradition that links Herophilus and Erasistratus (fl. 280 BC) with the vivisection of condemned criminals is a strong one, and can be paralleled with tales in Galen of the later exploits in pharmacology of Attalus III, of Pergamum (170–133 BC) and Mithridates VI of Pontus (120–63 BC). For both Galen and the pro-anatomical tradition recorded in Celsus, it was the fact that the criminals had lost their own humanity by their crimes that in part justified their experimental treatment like animals, and, for this, royal permission and protection were essential.[65]

At the same time by assembling, whether by deliberate policy or not, many scientists and intellectuals in one city, and even in one place, a

---

[61] On Diocles as an anatomist and zoologist, see W. Jaeger, Diokles von Karystos (Berlin, 1938), pp. 154–80.

[62] I. M. Lonie, 'The Paradoxical Text "On the heart"', Medical History, 17 (1973), 1–15, 136–53.

[63] Edenstein, Ancient Medicine, pp. 247–301. Doubts on this thesis have been expressed by F. Kudien, 'Antike Anatomie und menschlicher Leichnam', Hermes, 96 (1969), 78–94.

[64] Galen, XIV.2 K. His silence about the possible vivisection experiments of the Alexandrian is notorious. Cf. for a similar argument, Celsus, De medicina, Pr. 23.

[65] For modern discussions of the arguments involved, note P. M. Fraser, Ptolemaic Alexandria, I, (Oxford, 1972), pp. 348–51; J. Scarborough, 'Celsus on Human Vivisection at Alexandria', Clio Medica, 11 (1976), 25–38; G. E. R. Lloyd, Science and Morality in Greco-Roman Antiquity (Cambridge, 1985), pp. 3–10. It might also be argued that, to the eyes of a conquering Greek, in the metropolis of Alexandria, an Egyptian peasant was little more than an animal, and hence his corpse could be treated like that of a dog. See now the masterly discussion by H. von Staden, Herophilus. The Art of Medicine in Early Alexandria (Cambridge, 1989).

Museum, 'a shrine of the Muses', the Hellenistic kings fostered an environment congenial to intellectual activity and cooperation.[66] The mechanistic physiological doctrines of Erasistratus cannot be understood without reference to the theories of his physicist contemporary Strato of Lampsacus or the later mechanical models of Philo, Ctesibius and Hero.[67] When Ptolemy VIII broke up the intellectual circles of Alexandria, including the 'bird-cage' of the Muses, he filled the cities and islands with exiled grammarians, musicians, philosophers, doctors and other craftsmen. The Museum itself, however, was more of a club than a teaching institution. Herophilus seems to have taught his pupils within his house, and no text expressly connects any student with the Museum. Indeed, the only direct references to medical teaching at Alexandria make no mention of the Museum. Philo Judaeus (*fl.* AD 40), himself an Alexandrian, talks of public lectures in the city, open to all, while the leading Alexandrian doctor of the AD 330s, Magnus of Nisibis, was provided with a public lecture room by the city.[68] Yet the presence of famous doctors in Alexandria, whether at the Museum or not, must have attracted there many aspiring medical students, and the size of the city, together with its intellectual institutions, gave it a reputation, particularly for anatomy, that lasted until the end of classical antiquity and beyond.

The Alexandrian Library also exercised a decisive influence on medicine. According to Galen, it was here that the Hippocratic Corpus was assembled, and the tale of forgery and deliberate false ascription that he tells provides a convincing explanation for the heterogeneity of the writings contained within it.[69] Hippocrates was a great name, for whom it was necessary to invent writings in sufficient numbers to justify his reputation. The library, which continued a tradition of compilation and classification that can be seen in the Aristotelian Meno's *History of Medicine* (*c.* 330 BC), enabled the doctors of Alexandria to develop, if not to create, a tradition of medical philosophy and commentary on

[66] Fraser, *Ptolemaic Alexandria*, is fundamental; our knowledge of lesser courts is, alas, almost non-existent as far as concerns medicine and science.

[67] Harris, *The Heart*, pp. 195–233; but note the caution expressed by W. D. Smith, 'Erasistratus' Dietetic Medicine', *Bulletin of the History of Medicine*, 56 (1982), 398–409.

[68] Philo, 1.199 Manguey; Eunapius, *Vitae phil.* 530 Wright. Cf. also V. Nutton, 'Museums and Medical Schools in Classical Antiquity', *History of Education*, 4 (1975), 3–15. For a brief survey of the fortunes of Alexandria in later antiquity, see V. Nutton, 'Ammianus and Alexandria', *Clio Medica*, 7 (1972), 165–75. John Duffy, 'Byzantine Medicine in the Sixth and Seventh Centuries: Aspects of Teaching and Practice', *Dumbarton Oaks Papers*, 38 (1984), 21–3, offers an introduction to the teaching methods of Alexandria in the last years of Roman rule.

[69] Smith, *Hippocratic Tradition*, pp. 199–201.

Hippocrates.[70] The Hippocratic *lexica* ultimately go back to those written in Alexandria in the third century BC, and the earliest surviving commentary on Hippocrates, by Apollonius of Citium (*fl.* 90 BC), is the product of a long line of Alexandrian exegesis. The prestige of Alexandrian scholarship also helped to ensure the primacy of Hippocratic medicine, and in part to fix the terms for subsequent debate on the historical Hippocrates.[71]

Although the doctors of Alexandria had potentially an opportunity to draw upon another tradition of medicine, that of the native Egyptians, there is no evidence that they did so. The Greek medical papyri show no influence from Egyptian beliefs, whereas the later demotic papyri reveal traces of Greek learning.[72] Egyptian specialties like clystering still continued to have their adherents and professionals; in one papyrus an apprentice clysterer is promised an income for life.[73] Only in the organization of doctors in rural Egypt can one find traces of continuity between the Pharaonic and Hellenistic periods, and even there it is likely that the Hellenistic public doctors' liability to provide free treatment extended only to state employees on state business. There was no *universal* system of free health care for the great majority of the population.[74]

Greek medical theory seems to have been insulated from the medical systems of the non-Greek lands over which it spread. Yet alongside the writings of a Heraclides of Tarentum or an Apollonius can be set the medico-magical writings of a Bolus of Mende, or an Ostanes. The transmission of these writings in the Greek world offered an alternative to the Hippocratic tradition, existing alongside rather than directly competing with it. This magical medicine, particularly associated with Persia and Egypt, is always present as one boundary for 'orthodox' medical practice.[75] More sophisticated authors, like the Roman Pliny, could rail against the nonsense of the magicians, and Galen could rationalize his use of techniques derived from folk medicine and magic,

[70] *Ibid.*, pp. 199–222; Fraser, *Ptolemaic Alexandria*, I, pp. 365–69.
[71] Apollonius of Citium, *fl.* 80 BC. The best edition of his *Commentary on Hippocrates' On joints* is by Kollesch and Kudlien, CMG 11.1.1. (Berlin, 1965). V. Langholf, 'Kallimachos, Komödie und hippokratische Frage', *Medizinhistorisches Journal*, 21 (1986), 3–30, argues that not only did Callimachus know *De flatibus*, but agreed with Meno in ascribing it to the great Coan physician.
[72] Egyptian influence on Greek anatomy, although widely believed in, is succinctly rejected by Longrigg, 'Superlative Achievement', p. 164.
[73] F. Kudlien, *Der griechische Arzt im Zeitalter des Hellenismus* (Wiesbaden, 1979), 65–72.
[74] *Ibid.*, pp. 18–64; Nutton, 'Continuity', pp. 21–23.
[75] G. Luck, *Arcana mundi* (Baltimore and London, 1985), offers a useful sample of magical medical documents. Note also H. G. Benz, et al., *Greek Magical Papyri*, I (*Chicago*, 1985).

but both of them knew and recorded these traditions for others to use.[76]
It is impossible also to tell, at this distance in time, exactly why any
individual doctor or patient accepted or rejected any specific piece of
magic, for the distinction between magic and medicine, between high
culture and popular belief, is fluid.

A similar description can be given of the relationship in the Greek
world between religion and medicine. The two coexisted happily, and,
as Edelstein argued, it was only the Methodist doctors, whose medicine
was based on an Epicurean philosophy that rejected the gods and divine
intervention, that denied the possibility of divine healing.[77] The author
of *The Sacred Disease* (c. 420 BC) was not opposed to gods in his denial of
the divine status of epilepsy; he accepted *all* diseases as divine since they
were all part of a god-created universe.[78] The significance of dreams was
accepted by Herophilus and Galen (129–c. 199 or after 212), whose own
career and even aspects of whose practice were determined by
instructions from the god Asclepius.[79] Two areas of medicine in
particular were associated with a divine cause and a religious therapy,
plague and chronic disease. In both of these, the doctor's inability to do
more with the armamentarium at his disposal than provide temporary
palliatives may have influenced sufferers to turn to divine healing, but
this is by no means the whole story. If a community was suddenly struck
down with illness, something more was required as an explanation than
a mere imbalance of an individual's humours, or even a change of
climate. Thucydides reports how in the plague of Athens (430–427 BC)
there were supplications in the temples, and citation of an oracle to prove
divine wrath, in addition to a straightforwardly medical response to the
disease. All were futile, in his opinion.[80] Others certainly disagreed, for
Pausanias records that the plague was ended by Apollo the turner-away

[76] P. Green, 'Prolegomena to a Study of Magic and Superstition in the Elder Pliny' (Diss.,
Cambridge, 1954); for Galen, cf. XII.207 K.

[77] Edelstein, *Ancient Medicine*, pp. 205–46. This is not to say that some physicians did not feel that
there were areas of healing for which religious therapy was inappropriate or where their own
techniques would be more effective.

[78] [Hippocrates], *Sacred Disease* 1.10–12; cf. Lloyd, *Magic*, pp. 10–15.

[79] P. H. Schrijvers, 'La classification des rêves selon Hérophile', *Mnemosyne*, 30 (1977), 13–27; S.
M. Oberhelman, 'Galen, On Diagnosis from Dreams', *Journal of the History of Medicine*, 38 (1983),
36–47; S. R. F. Price, 'The Future of Dreams: from Freud to Artemidorus', *Past and Present*, 113
(1986), 3–37. The Hippocratic *Regimen*, IV, is devoted entirely to a medical interpretation of dreams.

[80] J. C. F. Poole and A. J. Holladay, 'Thucydides and the Plague of Athens', *Classical Quarterly*,
29 (1979), 282–300; J. N. Longrigg, 'The Great Plague of Athens', *History of Science*, 18 (1980),
209–25. More recent attempts at identification of the disease (as glanders, tulaeraemia, toxic shock
syndrome or the result of arsenic poisoning) all seem to me unconvincing, and open to the same
objections as described by the three authors cited. See now, favouring smallpox, R. Sallares, *The
Ecology of Ancient Greece* (London, 1991).

of evil, and the successful ending of the contemporary plague at Phigalia in the Peloponnese was marked by the building of the great temple at Bassae to Apollo.[81] It was Apollo, with his various local cult titles, who was the chief healing god of Greece in the sixth century BC, but he was gradually superseded by Asclepius. The fourth century BC saw a great boom in temple-building to Asclepius, perhaps not equalled until the second century AD. The great shrine of Epidaurus, the early temple at Cos, and the main Asclepieion at Athens, all date from this period, and hymns of praise to Asclepius and Apollo circulated around the Greek world. The shrines were filled with sufferers from all social classes, although most appear to be of humble origin. Their cures were recorded on tablets on the Asclepieion's walls, and from them it can be seen that most came with chronic disorders, many, in modern parlance, of a psychosomatic type. The patient usually spent only one or two nights incubating, i.e. sleeping within the sacred precinct, before he saw a dream or a vision of the god appearing to cure him. The priest of Asclepius then interpreted the vision, where necessary, and prescribed treatment, although in several cases the patient found himself instantly cured.[82] Doctors as such played no part, certainly in the Hellenistic period, in these shrines, but there was no opposition to temple medicine. Indeed, in the Roman period, doctors were frequently found among the benefactors of healing shrines and temples.[83] Conversely, in the accounts of these divine cures, references to the failures of doctors are almost mute, by comparison with the frequent denunciation of medical incompetence in Christian lives of the saints. God and man could work together, and only the Methodists attempted to remove God from medicine.

The Methodists, a sect which flourished in the Graeco-Roman world from the first century BC for at least five centuries, present certain features which typify the development of medicine and its relationship to society in the late Hellenistic world.[84] They were a sect, a group of doctors with definite school doctrines and school traditions, who took their origins from Themison and Thessalus of Tralles, or, as some said,

---

[81] R. Parker, *Miasma* (Oxford, 1983), pp. 207–79; Nutton, 'Murders', pp. 45–8.

[82] The testimonia are set out in E. and L. Edelstein, *Asclepius* (Baltimore, 1945).

[83] Pugliese Carratelli, 'Parmenide', pp. 37–8, draws attention to the existence of an 'iatrom(antis)' alongside physicians at Velia.

[84] G. Rubinstein, 'The Methodist Method' (Diss., Cambridge, 1985), offers a detailed critique of earlier views on Methodism. An attempt at a synthesis of one aspect of Methodism is provided by M. Frede, 'The Method of the So-called Methodical School of Medicine', in J. Barnes (ed.), *Science and Speculation* (Cambridge, 1982), pp. 1–23.

from Asclepiades of Bithynia (*fl. c.* 92 BC).[85] This crystallizing of medicine into schools is characteristic of Hellenistic philosophy and medicine. Parallel to the Stoics, the Academy and the Epicureans in philosophy can be set the Empirics, the Erasistrateans, the Methodists and the Dogmatists, to be joined later by the Pneumatists. But it may be doubted how far these sects could exercise any tight doctrinal control, and different areas and individuals could always exhibit their own brand of medicine of a particular sect. The Methodists are on this reconstruction but one group among the Asclepiadeans.[86]

Roman medicine

The Hellenistic sects also are a product of the bookish culture of the time, and their divisions are based far more often on philosophical presuppositions than on any practical therapy.[87] The medical practitioners of Latin-speaking Italy in the Hellenistic age were unlikely to have contributed anything to current debate in the Greek World, for the Roman medical tradition as expounded by Cato the Elder and, long after him, by Pliny the Elder (*fl.* AD 75), was one of domestic, practical medicine, marked by a strong chauvinism. The effete philosopher was contrasted with the sturdy, self-sufficient Roman farmer. Modern historians have been content to accept these stereotypes at their face value, and to date the arrival of Greek medicine in Rome precisely to 219 BC, when Archagathus came from the Peloponnese and was given citizenship and a surgery at public expense at a main crossroads. His subsequent failure, according to Pliny, reflected on his art and fellow practitioners, and gave the Romans a healthy distrust of interfering, chattering Greeks. The truth, I suggest, was somewhat different. It is important first to remember that very little Latin literature, save for some comedies of Plautus and Terence, survives to us from the period before Cato (*fl.* 180 BC) and that it is not until the first century BC that our sources become sufficiently numerous to allow any satisfactory generalizations about the development of Roman society except in the

[85] J. T. Vallance, *The Lost Theory of Asclepiades of Bithynia* (Oxford, 1990), supersedes previous discussions of this controversial figure. Its final chapter suggests how 'Asclepiadeanism' could be easily transformed into Methodism.

[86] K. Deichgräber, *Die griechische Empirikerschule*, 2nd edn (Berlin and Zurich, 1965), is a detailed study of one Hellenistic sect. One would like to know more of the 'Democriteans' mentioned by Plutarch, *Symp.* VIII.9.

[87] H. von Staden, 'Hairesis and heresy: the case of the *haireseis iatrikai*', in B. F. Meyer and E. P. Sanders (eds.), *Jewish and Christian Self-definition*, III (London, 1982), pp. 76–100; O. Temkin, *The Double Face of Janus* (Baltimore, 1977), pp. 137–53, provides some context.

broadest terms. Thus for any descriptions of the part played by doctors and healers in early Roman society we are at the mercy of one author, Cato, whose avowed hostility to Greece and things Greek was at least in part a facade designed to win political favour, or of the scattered testimony of later writers of varying worth. The failure of medical historians to examine these documents critically and to fit them into a proper social context has resulted in a one-sided and often implausible reconstruction of events.[88]

Roman medicine is an ambiguous description. It may be defined by a geographical area, Rome and Latium; by a historical event, the conquest of the Italian peninsula by the legions of Rome; or by a linguistic feature, writings in Latin; and the shift from one definition to another has caused problems and misunderstandings. Cato talks solely of Rome and Latium; historians generally combine this with a linguistic criterion. Yet all three aspects need to be considered to gain a proper appreciation of the complexities of the subject.

By the middle of the third century BC, the Latin-speaking citizens of Rome had conquered the whole of the Italian peninsula south of the Po, and had a foothold on Sicily. They had incorporated in their state various linguistic and political groupings, including the Etruscans to the north, the Oscan-speaking Samnites to the south and east, and the Greek cities of the coasts of Southern Italy. Of Etruscan medicine little can be said, although that has not prevented considerable discussion about the meaning of the artificial liver for divination discovered at Piacenza. Archaeological evidence also suggests some skill in surgery, but one should be careful before positing a medical literature in Etruscan on the evidence of inscriptions in Latin and Etruscan from Perugia recording two doctors.[89] Evidence for the medicine practised in the Samnite Apennines comes only from a much later period, yet it offers a plausible reconstruction. In Galen's day, the Marsi were famous for their skills in the use of herbs and drugs, and particularly for their knowledge of snakes. They provided the best herbs and venoms for the Roman market, and their reputation was empire-wide.[90] Cato's idea of a solely domestic

---

[88] The most critical assessment of Cato is by A. E. Astin, *Cato the Censor* (Oxford, 1978). J. Scarborough, *Roman Medicine* (London, 1969), is most unreliable. Better is R. Jackson, *Doctors and Diseases in the Roman Empire* (London, 1988).

[89] H. J. von Schumann, 'Didaktisches Anschauungsmaterial der Haruspices', *Deutsches Ärzteblatt*, 79 (1982), 79–83: *Corpus Inscriptionum Etruscarum* 3731–2; W. V. Harris, *Rome in Etruria and Umbria* (Oxford, 1971), pp. 4–31, sets out the evidence for the survival of Etruscan literary documents.

[90] V. Nutton, 'The Drug Trade in Antiquity', *Journal of the Royal Society of Medicine*, 78 (1985), 138–45 (repr. in *From Democedes to Harvey*).

medicine is also plausible at least for Latium, if not for Rome of the third century BC. Substantial village communities were few, and on the isolated upland farms, the owner would have had to fend very much for himself. The combination of chants, charms, and local herbal remedies, including notoriously the cabbage, resembles the domestic medicine of sixteenth-century England, where some recipes could be applied equally to people and animals.[91] But these chants and charms differ in their use in one significant way from the religious medicine of early Greece: the power to act resides in the chants, not in the individual, for it makes no difference whether a drug or a charm is given by a doctor, a priest, a head of the household or a slave told to go and cure a horse.

This practical medicine, consisting largely of collections of recipes devised empirically, seems to have had little or no theoretical basis, and in this differs markedly from the medicine of the Greeks of the South.[92] Here were Greek cities, with Greek institutions, and with traditions of theoretical debates on medicine that went back to the fifth century. The Ouliadai at Elea, the Pythagoreans at Croton, Locri, and Tarentum, to say nothing of the successors of the so-called 'Sicilian school' of medicine, all flourished in Southern Italy, and the most celebrated of the Empirics of the first century BC, Heraclides, was born, and may have spent most of his life, at Tarentum.[93] Rome had had commercial and cultural links with the Greek cities for centuries and the third century BC reveals an increasing Hellenization of Rome. The story of the introduction of the Asclepius cult, first to Latium and then to Rome itself in 291 BC, demonstrates both cultural ties and the gradual spread of Greek influence.[94] The arrival of the Laconian surgeon Archagathus in Rome marks the culmination of this process in medicine, for here we find the Roman senate acting as a Greek city in inviting a distinguished doctor to come and providing him with privileges.[95] The invitation does not preclude the existence of doctors in Rome, even of Greek doctors, for both Pliny and the later Greek historian Dionysius can be interpreted to show their presence, and Archagathus' departure from Rome may be due at least as much to the expiry of his contract and his reluctance to

---

[91] W. H. S. Jones, 'Ancient Roman Folk Medicine', *Journal of the History of Medicine*, 12 (1957), 459–72; U. Capitani, 'Celso, Scribonio Largo e Plinio il Vecchio', *Maia* n.s. 2 (1972), 120–40. It should be stressed that such 'domestic medicine' was equally a feature of Greek rural communities, and the stereotype of the Roman farmer was not so far different from his Greek counterpart in the diseases he faced and in the means at his disposal to counteract them.

[92] It is hard to fit Roman remedies into the standard Greek schema of cure by contraries.

[93] Deichgräber, *Die griechische Empirkerschule*, pp. 172–202.

[94] Testimonia in Edelstein, *Asclepius*, I, pp. 431–52.

[95] Nutton, 'Murders', pp. 42–3; 'Patriotism', pp. 38–40.

remain in what, to a Greek, was still the backwoods as to calamitous failure and Roman distaste for the Greeks.

The physician in the Roman Empire

Archagathus was a surgeon, and hence one should not imagine a straightforward confrontation of Greek theory with Roman practicality. But the absence of a theoretical component from Roman domestic medicine was increasingly likely to offend these men of wealth who were experiencing for themselves the delights of Greek culture and philosophy and whose cultural outlook was becoming hellenized. For them Greek physicians were necessary, as much for ostentation as for practical value, and senators like Cicero and Pansa (fl. 50 BC) could speak of their personal physicians in the same words as their friends.[96] Greek doctors, too, were becoming more common in Rome as a result of Rome's conquest of the East in the last two centuries BC and through the increasing pull of the great metropolis. Some Greeks came of their own volition, but others came as prisoners of war or as slaves.[97] Like all foreigners, they were not Roman citizens, and were hence subject to legal constraints and disabilities. Even an ex-slave with Roman citizenship still had to perform certain obligations of service to his ex-master, although lawyers ruled it unfair for the master to be ill and requiring his attentions all the time. Not surprisingly, the social position of the doctor in Rome was substantially different from that in the bourgeois Greek East, even after the grant by Julius Caesar c. 45 BC, confirmed by his successor, Augustus, of Roman citizenship to all foreign doctors practising in Rome. This was, indeed, a privilege but its magnitude was only visible back home, where Roman citizenship was rare and confined to the upper classes, and there is little evidence for doctors returning from Rome with their newly acquired citizenship.[98] In the city of Rome itself, citizenship was the norm, and although possession of it reduced one's legal and fiscal liabilities, it may also have brought with it some, admittedly very rudimentary, form of supervision by a lay magistrate.

[96] Nutton, 'Murders', p. 32. For the background of increasing Hellenisation, see E. D. Rawson, *Intellectual Life in the Late Roman Republic* (London, 1985).

[97] J. H. Phillips, 'The Emergence of the Greek Medical Profession in the Roman Republic', *Trans. Stud. Coll. Phys. Philadelphia*, ser. 5, 2 (1980), 267–75; F. Kudlien, *Die Stellung des Arztes in der römischen Gesellschaft* (Stuttgart, 1986), pp. 92–118.

[98] Kudlien, *Stellung*, pp. 46–70; Nutton, 'Murders', p. 29, with references to a new Ephesian inscription which records a grant (or a regranting) of some forms of tax immunity by the triumvirs, c. 42 BC, to all doctors within the Roman Empire.

Table 1. *The civil status of doctors as recorded on inscriptions prior to AD 300*

Century		First	Second	Third
I	Citizen	15 (13)	57 (29)	27 (15)
II	Citizen, without indication of family*a*			
	A: Greek name	17	36	16
	B: non-Greek name	3 (1)	9 (8)	6 (2)
III	Freedman	92 (3)	72 (8)	6 (1)
IV	Slave	40	12 (1)	3
V	Foreign, non-citizen	9	16 (5)	6 (3)
		176 (17)	202 (51)	64 (21)

Notes: *a* This may indicate a new citizen, but the omission of family or freedman status might be accidental. Bracketed numbers refer to doctors of non-Greek origin.

How far he would be able to check an immigrant's credentials is, however, dubious, and it may be that a simple assertion of one's own competence and intent was enough.

The relatively low status of doctors in the western half of the Roman Empire can best be demonstrated from a study of inscriptions referring to doctors and dating from before AD 300.[99] Such epigraphic evidence for the late Republic is almost entirely absent, although the literary records confirm the same pattern – immigrants, slaves, freedmen, and, in the countryside, travelling drug-sellers of dubious expertise. The relevant inscriptions are tabulated in table 1.

In other words, in the first century, 80 per cent of all doctors recorded on inscriptions lacked full citizen rights in law, in the second, 50 per cent, and even in the third, when citizenship was extended to all inhabitants of the Roman world, 25 per cent. This figure for the low civil status of doctors in the Western world is likely to be generally accurate, especially as the bias of this sort of evidence is towards an over-representation of the wealthier sectors of society.[100]

[99] V. Nutton, 'The Medical Profession in the Roman Empire' (Diss., Cambridge, 1970); the list of statuses is based on the list of inscriptions given by H. Gummerus, *Der Ärztestand im römischen Reiche nach den römischen Welt* (Helsinki, 1932), with later additions.

[100] It should perhaps be stressed that, in following, for the most part, Gummerus' dating, the figure for non-citizens in the third century may be too high. Kudlien, *Stellung*, pp. 211–12, objects to the 'chance' character of the epigraphic (and, indeed, literary) evidence, and warns against too

One can see also from this a general trend towards the employment of citizen doctors, particularly apparent in the great drop in the percentage of freedmen doctors between the second and third centuries. Too much, however, should not be made of this, especially as there is a reduction in the number of great slave households belonging to the emperors and senators for which much epigraphic information survives from before 68 AD. More significant may be the apparent persistence well into the third century of slave and freedmen doctors, a fact perhaps confirmed by the presence in the Roman law codes of the sixth century AD of detailed enactments and prices for slave doctors. Undoubtedly many masters saw a way to make money by training their slaves in medicine before sending them out as agents to treat the sick. Their training need not have been long and certainly would not have satisfied the fastidious Galen, who lost no time in attacking Thessalus of Tralles (fl. 60 AD) for his claim to teach his brand of Methodist doctrine to anyone within six months.[101] Even Celsus (fl. 45 AD), who was far less hostile to the followers of Asclepiades than Galen, comments unfavourably on their judgement of cases simply from their gross 'common conditions', which could be easily learned and which did not require either the delicate diagnostic technique or long experience of the Hippocratic practitioner in treating individual idiosyncrasies.[102] A Roman emperor, either Domitian in 93–4 AD or, more likely Trajan in AD 108–9, even seems to have intervened in this dispute in an attempt to restrict the teaching of medicine to slaves for the sake of making money, but, even so, the medical training of slaves went on happily, and there are many later references to 'slaves' of physicians.[103]

A second point which emerges clearly from the epigraphic statistics is that the overwhelming majority of those who call themselves doctors came from the hellenistic East, almost 90 per cent in the first century, 75 per cent in the second and 66 per cent in the third. Only in the inscriptions of Roman Africa do non-Greek doctors equal Greeks, while, by contrast in Rome itself only 7 per cent of the named doctors show a non-Greek origin. Again, this impression is confirmed by literary

great reliance on these statistics. But, while admitting some force in these criticisms, I would still argue for the 'objective' character of the inscriptions as opposed to much of the literary evidence Kudlien prefers. Furthermore, legal status is only one of the parameters involved in a study of the healer's social status; but it is possible to determine this with far greater accuracy than to tabulate and assess literary comments about patients' reactions to their physicians. Gourevitch, *Le triangle hippocratique*, provides an exhaustive survey of such evidence, but the banal conclusion to be drawn from it is that good doctors (however defined) were, on the whole, more highly regarded than bad.

[101] Nutton, 'Patriotism', p. 41, with references.   [102] Celsus, *De med.*, I, pr. 65.
[103] *Fontes Iuris Romani*, I, 77.

sources. A doctor from Phrygia is martyred in Lyons, Galen inveighs against his colleagues who flee to a successful practice in Rome to escape obloquy in their native Greek towns, and the literary stereotype of the doctor is of a Greek.[104] Even if not everybody shared Pliny's violent antipathy to Greek doctors, 'who make experiments at the cost of our lives, and can commit homicide with complete impunity', there was in Roman society a considerable prejudice against immigrant, hungry Greeks, selling their culture at Romans' expense.

It comes as no surprise to find in the period of the early Roman Empire a substantial dichotomy between the social position of doctors in the two halves of the Empire. While no doctor becomes a member of the Senate of Rome, whatever his origins, and only a few, usually imperial physicians, act as imperial equestrian procurators, there is a marked difference at the next level of society, the provincial and local gentry.[105] Only one doctor, C. Iulius Q.f. Rogatianus, from Sufetula in Africa, is recorded as holding a municipal office in the West, and only a few memorials suggest even moderate wealth.[106] Western doctors play little part in the associations of freedmen – only twelve officials in a religious cult of emperor-worship organised by freedmen doctors are recorded as *seviri Augustales* – and the ostentatious P. Decimus P. Merula Eros, *medicus clinicus chirurgus ocularius*, who paid 2,000 sestertii (HS) for the office of *sevir*, and gave 30,000 HS for statues at the temple of Hercules at Assisi, and 37,000 HS for paving roads, and who left 800,000 HS, is unusual in his wealth outside the ranks of the imperial physicians. He suffered for his ambition too: the 50,000 HS he gave for his freedom was far in excess of the contemporary norm of 2,000 HS.[107] A doctor at

[104] Galen, XIV.620–24 K. = CMG V.8,1, pp. 90–3, with my commentary *ad loc*. It is, of course, impossible to determine whether all the bearers of Greek names were themselves Greek, cf. French restaurateurs and Italian hairdressers in England, but their existence shows at worst a readiness to believe in a Greek-dominated trade.

[105] For the difficulties of assessing social status, cf. H. W. Pleket, 'Sociale stratificatie en sociale mobiliteit in de Romeinse Keizertijd', *Tijdschrift voor Geschiedenis*, 74 (1971), 215–51. This dichotomy, on which I insisted in *Medical Profession*, p. 67, is denied by Kudlien, *Stellung*, pp. 36–9, who concludes, p. 215, that the 'social prestige' of the doctor, in both East and West was 'all in all, considerably high'. But his evidence in no way bears out this conviction, except for imperial physicians, and his citation, p. 36, of Cohn-Haft as evidence for municipal office in the West is fallacious, for with the exception mentioned in the next note, and the *seviri*, that evidence is drawn entirely from the Greek half of the Empire. Granted that more inscriptions survive from the municipalities of the East than the West, the pattern of medical involvement is still very different. Considerations of the size, quality and type of grave or monument reveal little obvious sign of great wealth among Western doctors, although there are exceptions.

[106] *Inscriptiones Latinae Selectae* 7796.

[107] Nutton, *Medical Profession*, p. 67; for Merula, *ILS* 5369, 7812. Kudlien, *Stellung*, p. 35, doubts whether all these *seviri* were, in fact, freedmen, but, even if he is right, his hesitations apply only to one inscription, *Corpus inscriptionum latinarum*, XI.5412.

Sassina was elected patron of a Guild, but the presence of doctors in burial clubs at Tibur, Larinum, and Aquileia, attests poverty rather than wealth.[108] This is not to say that long residence in a community could not bring its rewards. At Beneventum in the second century, the son of a Greek citizen-immigrant (possibly a doctor) became a civic doctor and made enough money to rank as a knight. He was rich but not entirely respectable: his son was, becoming a local magistrate and expending his paternal wealth on bounties to his fellow citizens.[109]

This is in sharp contrast to the picture of the social position of doctors provided by inscriptions from the Roman East. Here the doctor is frequently a prosperous member of local provincial society, and if not as wealthy as a great magnate like Polemo or Herodes Atticus, at least on speaking terms with them. Galen's father and Galen himself associated with senators and magistrates, although Nicon's zeal for culture might indicate that he was one of the despised 'late-learners'; and a civic doctor of Synnada in Phrygia married his daughter into the highest provincial nobility.[110] By contrast with the West and Rome, where mobility and immigration appear normal, the East shows families with deep roots in medicine and their locality – the Philalethae of Men Karou, the Statilii of Heraclea, the Acilii of Claudiopolis, while at Thyateira at least three generations and four members of Moschianos' family were civic doctors.[111] One finds more gifts and benefactions to the local populace, greater participation in public rites, and a generally higher level of wealth.[112] One should not exaggerate this, for there were certain backwoods areas where no self-respecting doctor would go and practise

[108] CIL XIV.3550; IX.740 (but the restoration is doubtful); Gummerus, Ärztestand, n. 292.

[109] CIL IX.1655, 1971. My argument is not that doctors could not make money, but that, by comparison with the Greek East, the amount was less and the opportunities for equestrian status reduced.

[110] Monumenta Asiae Minoria Antiquae, VI.373. For an example from Thessalonica, see Nutton, Medical Profession, p. 74. Kudlien, Stellung, pp. 84–6, argues that Galen was a peregrinus, i.e. a non-Roman citizen. But given his father's wealth and connections, this seems implausible, and the fact that Galen is never given a Roman name is no strong argument against. The case of Plutarch, whose Roman nomen, Mestrius, is known only from an inscription, provides a telling counter-example.

[111] Nutton, Medical Profession, pp. 71, 76.

[112] Ibid., pp. 69–80. Although in this section I have taken serious issue with Kudlien, Stellung, this book opens up many possibilities for further work, and is the most detailed attempt so far made to answer the question of the position of the doctor in Roman society. Its general concentration on the healer in (generally) Rome and Italy has robbed its readers of a detailed comparison with the contemporary Greek East (which also tends to be left out of studies of Greek physicians as being 'Roman'). But, in both method and sophistication, Kudlien's book marks an improvement over what has gone before, even if its limitations may be inevitable, given the fragility of the evidence at our disposal. In 'Der ärztliche Beruf in Staat und Gesellschaft der Antike', Jahrbuch des Instituts für Geschichte der Medizin der Robert Bosch Stiftung, 7 (1988), 41–73, Kudlien offers a wider perspective on the question of the social status of doctors.

unless forced to, like the unlucky Philistion, a medical friend of Galen's from Pergamum.[113] But it was always possible for a man to make a good living and name for himself in the East without coming to Rome. There is no evidence that the elegant M. Modius Asiaticus, champion of a medical method, ever moved far from Smyrna, and Ephesus in the second century AD served as the medical nodal point for a wide area of Asia Minor. It had its own Museum, its own association of doctors, and an annual series of medical contents divided into four sections, and the distinguished physician, Rufus of Ephesus, seems to have spent all his active life there.[114] His contemporary, Soranus, however, did visit Rome, but only after practising for a time at Ephesus.[115]

It is, of course, possible to argue that the difference in public profile between the doctors of East and West is less of a historical fact than a reflection of the bias of the epigraphical sources towards the civic prosperity of Asia Minor in the golden age of the Antonines. Wealth led to the erection of inscriptions of all kinds, which reveal the life of the local township in greater clarity and detail than the correspondingly fewer Latin inscriptions do for, say, Como, Naples, or Tarragona. An absence of data, then, need not indicate an absence of doctors, and the situation in Gaul might resemble that in Egypt rather than that in Asia Minor. In the peasant communities of the Nile Valley, to judge from Greek papyri, the doctor was never a man of outstanding wealth. His income was rarely derived solely from medicine, for he had his own plot of land, and his brother might as easily be a woodcarver as a teacher. Yet he was among the local elite: he was literate: he was among the wealthiest in the community, though he was rarely a Roman citizen (of the ninety-seven doctors recorded on papyri before AD 212 the date of Caracalla's grant of universal citizenship, no more than twenty-seven, and possibly only fifteen are citizens), and he enjoyed certain legal privileges and exemptions which gave him an edge over his fellow peasants.[116]

That some Western doctors lived in a similar social situation to those

---

[113] Galen, CMG v.10.1.1, pp. 401–2.

[114] J. Benedum, 'Markos Modios Asiatikos', *Medizinhistorisches Journal*, 13 (1978), 307–9; J. Ilberg, 'Rufus von Ephesos, ein griechischer Arzt in trajanischer Zeit', *Abhandlungen der Sächsischen Akademie der Wissenschaft, phil.-hist. Kl.* (1930). The researches of Manfred Ullmann have resulted in the discovery or identification of several treatises by Rufus that are not to be found in the standard edition of Rufus by C. Daremberg and C.-E. Ruelle (Paris, 1879).

[115] Soranus, *Gyn.*, II.44, unless this is information derived from hearsay.

[116] Nutton, *Medical Profession*, pp. 87–104: cf. E. Boswinkel, 'La médecine et les médecins dans les papyrus grecs', *Eos*, 41 (1956), 181–90. See also the lists of Egyptian healers in H. Harrauer, *Corpus Papyrorum Archeducis Raineri*, vol. XIII (Vienna, 1987), pp. 89–100.

of Egypt is highly probable, although there is little evidence to go on. But two considerations militate against a facile overall identification of East and West. The first is that, outside Rome, with one exception, the prosperous areas of Italy, Provence and Spain, although they show an occasional wealthy individual with a passionate amateur interest in medicine, reveal only low-status doctors. The exception is Marseilles, but Marseilles was an anomaly, a Greek city in Southern France, proud of its Hellenic heritage and different in culture and outlook from Lyons or Arles.

Secondly, there is a crucial division between the two halves of the Roman world in the early and middle Empire which has an important influence on the social status of its doctors. Unlike the East, the West had few large urban centres where doctors could earn a living largely or even entirely by practice. If, as Galen believed, specialists could only flourish in the great metropolis like Alexandria and Rome, physicians needed a relatively prosperous community around them, or land, if they were to remain for long in any one place.[117] As immigrants, the Greek doctors often lacked access to land, and hence through lack of sufficient payments had to be constantly on the move. There were, of course, travelling physicians in the East, but they explain their wanderings as an educational experience rather than an economic necessity. For Galen, the doctor's place is in the town, and the peasant comes to him. In Gaul, as the so-called oculists' stamps and the archaeological finds of instruments make clear, the doctor travelled around to meet his patients in the rural areas.[118] The absence of roots and of a suitable clientele to allow permanent residence is a major factor in the doctor's failure in the West to play an obvious role in his society. This could be, and indeed to some extent was, cured by the passage of time and the growth of Western municipalities. Ausonius' professors at Bordeaux in the fourth century are little different from those described at Alexandria by his Greek contemporary Eunapius.[119] Similarly, the gradual disappearance of the

---

[117] Galen, CMG, Suppl. Or. II.29. Cf. G. Baader, 'Spezialärzte in der Spätatike', *Medizin-historisches Journal*, 2 (1967), 231–8, whose evidence suggests that the growth of the metropolis at the expense of small towns in late antiquity may have encouraged the growth of specialization.

[118] V. Nutton, 'Roman Oculists', *Epigraphica*, 34 (1972), 16–29; H. Lieb, 'Nachträge zu den römischen Augenärzten und den Collyria', *Zeitschrift für Papyrologie und Epigraphik*, 43 (1981), 207–15; G. C. Boon, 'Potters, Oculists and Eye-Troubles', *Britannia*, 14 (1983), 1–12. For the instrument sets, see E. Künzl, *Medizinische Instrumente aus Sepulkralfunden der römischen Kaiserzeit* (Bonn, 1982). The instruments of the so-called Gallo-Roman oculists differ little from those recently published by R. Jackson, 'A Set of Roman Medical Instruments from Italy', *Britannia*, 17 (1986), 119–67.

[119] Ausonius, *Parent.* 1; *De profess.*; Eunapius, *Vit. phil.*, 528–39 Wright. In the sixth century, medical teaching at Ravenna seems to have been modelled on (if not deliberately cribbed from)

great slave households and of slave and freedman doctors, together with the universal grant of Roman citizenship by Caracalla in 212 AD, will have reduced the most obvious status difference between doctors in the two areas.

Two other factors may have helped to improve the image of the doctors in the West, one cultural, the other political. Under the Roman Empire Greek culture enjoyed a remarkable renaissance. Its propagators, the sophists, journeyed all over the Roman world, and performed before enthusiastic audiences. A knowledge of Greek became a mark of culture in any Roman and in the second century a Roman emperor, Marcus Aurelius, wrote his *Meditations* in Greek, while another, Hadrian, received the dedication of a complete edition of the works of Hippocrates.[120] At the same time, the leading citizens of the Greek-speaking world came increasingly to participate in the government and control the Empire. Plutarch might bewail the loss of talent from the provinces to the centre, and emperors legislate to ensure, they hoped, that Eastern cities were not impoverished by the departure of their wealthiest men for life in Rome, but the process of Hellenization was, on the whole, welcomed. It provided an outlet for the Greek upper classes, a new source of patronage for the Greek litterati, and a cultural bond to tie together the Roman Empire. The recent find of a stylishly learned inscription of a Greek doctor in Chester exemplifies the success of this movement.[121]

If the Romans were becoming Hellenized, the transformation of their constitution from republic to monarchy brought further advantage to those physicians in close proximity to the autocrat himself, the emperor. Greek in origin, occasionally former slaves, they gained wealth, recognition and possibly influence. Artorius Asclepiades of Smyrna, doctor to Augustus, received honours from Athens and Smyrna; the freedman Antonius Musa, for curing Augustus in 23 BC by a daring technique of cold baths, was rewarded with money, a gold ring (the mark of a free man), a statue, and tax immunity for himself and his fellow practitioners (solely in Rome?); Tiberius Claudius Menecrates, *fl.* AD 40, doctor to the emperors, founder of a medical sect of logical,

Alexandria, cf. Temkin, *Double Face of Janus*, pp. 178–97; Agnellus of Ravenna, *Lectures on Galen's On sects* (Buffalo, 1981). [120] Galen, CMG v.9.1, p. 13 = XV.21 K.

[121] V. Nutton, 'A Greek Doctor at Chester', *Journal of the Chester Archeological Society* (1970), 7–13 = *Bulletin Epigraphique* (1970), n. 667. Hence Galen is rightly studied in the context of the Greek literary revival by G. W. Bowersock, *Greek Sophists in the Roman Empire* (Oxford, 1969), pp. 59–75, and by B. P. Reardon, *Courants littéraires grecs des IIe et IIIe siècles après J.C.* (Paris, 1971), pp. 47–63.

'obvious' medicine, and prolific author, was honoured with formal decrees by famous cities.[122] His contemporary, Tiberius Claudius Tyrannus, continued his medical activities on returning to his home city of Magnesia on the Maeander, and was granted tax exemption for himself and the surgeries he set up in the town's territory.[123] Their prominence and assumed influence may in part explain Pliny's contempt for the leading doctors of the day in Rome, for their fads in astrological or hydropathic medicine, for their wealth and for their moral failings. Did not Eudemus and Valens commit their adulteries even with members of the imperial family?[124]

The reputation of Caius Stertinius Xenophon is similarly suspect for his involvement in the alleged poisoning of Claudius in AD 54. A Coan doctor, descended, he claimed, from the two healing gods, Asclepius and Hercules, he combined administrative duties for the emperors, from at least Caligula to Nero, with a medical practice. Already a member of the wealthy local family on Cos, he amassed an immense fortune. His practice in Rome, he alleged, brought him in 600,000 HS a year (the top administrative posts of the Empire were paid only 200,000 HS), and in recompense Claudius doubled his salary as an imperial doctor from the previous 250,000 HS to 500,000 HS. Along with his equally wealthy brother, he rebuilt much of Naples; he restored the shrine and library at the Asclepieion of Cos; and, on his retirement to Cos, he held, ostentatiously, many local civic and religious offices. He owned a large house on the Caelian hill in Rome, a very aristocratic area, and at his death he left, together with his brother, an immense fortune of 3,000,000 HS. His wealth and proximity to the emperor brought other benefits – citizenship for various members of his family, and freedom from imperial taxation for his native island.[125] Later imperial doctors show similar wealth. Statilius Criton (fl. 110), doctor and historian of Trajan's Dacian wars, held also a post as imperial procurator, and, on his

---

[122] *Inscriptiones graecae*, II².4116; *Corpus inscriptionum graecarum*, 3285 (but its authenticity has been suspected); Suetonius, *Aug.* 59, with Dio, *Hist.* LIII.30.: *IG* XIV.1759.

[123] *Inschriften von Magnesien* 113. The occurrence of the word 'ergasterion' on a Greek *defixio* referring to a 'group practice' in Southern Italy in the third century BC (*Suppl. Epigr. Graec.*, 30 (1980), 1175) suggests that it means here 'surgeries' rather than 'manufacturing establishments' (cf. *I. Magn.* 225).   [124] Pliny, *Hist. Nat.* XXIX.5.9–10.

[125] R. Herzog, 'Nikias und Xenophon von Kos', *Historische Zeitschrift*, 125 (1922), 189–247; Sherwin-White, *Cos*, pp. 149–52, 283–5; M. S. Kaplan, in his Harvard Ph.D. dissertation (1977) 'Greeks and the Imperial Court from Tiberius to Nero', which is known to me only from the summary in *Harvard Studies in Classical Philology*, 82 (1978), 353–5, discusses the careers of Xenophon and his family, and argues that the existence of his wealthy brother is the result of corruption in the text of Pliny.

retirement, was honoured for his civic services at Heraclea and at Ephesus.[126] His great-nephew (?) Attalus (*fl.* AD 160), doctor to Pius and Marcus Aurelius, gave a substantial amount of money to the association of young men at his home town of Heraclea.[127] Lucius Gellius Maximus, an imperial doctor at the beginning of the third century, was a government procurator as well as a lavish benefactor to Antioch in Pisidia.[128] At a lower level, Caius Calpurnius Asclepiades of Prusa gained citizenship for himself, his parents and four brothers, and then served as one of the assessors of Roman magistrates in charge of the voting tablets.[129]

Doctors like these lived and worked on the fringes of Roman politics. Tacitus claims that Tiberius' doctor, Charicles, used to offer him much political as well as medical advice. The surgeon Alcon, wealthy and disreputable, protected senators involved in the assassination of Caligula in AD 41, while Galen records the nervousness of senators under Commodus in the 180s who confided in him their fear of being murdered by the emperor.[130] His remedy is typical of the man: one should use tact and keep the consultation confidential. But not even Galen, for all Marcus Aurelius' praise of him, became a member of the senate. He and his confrères were certainly wealthy enough, but the highest office they achieved was that of a procurator.[131] It was the next generation that could enjoy the fruits of their fathers' activities. The son of Gellius Maximus entered the senate, became a legionary commander, raised an unsuccessful revolt in AD 219, and paid for it with his life. The contemporary historian, Cassius Dio, himself an Eastern provincial, tartly remarked that things had come to a pretty pass when the son of a doctor could aspire to the Empire.[132]

Court doctors were men of wealth, and this may have helped their fellow practitioners to gain greater status. But one should not exaggerate this, for there is a tendency for these grandees to separate themselves from their less successful and humbler colleagues. Galen's views on

---

[126] J. Scarborough, 'Criton, Physician to Trajan: Historian and Pharmacist', in J. W. Eadie, and J. Ober (eds.), *The Craft of the Ancient Historian: Essays in Honor of Chester G. Starr* (Lanham, MD, 1985), pp. 387–405.

[127] J. Benedum, 'Statilios Attalos: ein Beitrag zur medizinhistorischen Numismatik der Antike', *Medizinhistorisches Journal* 6 (1971), 264–77.

[128] V. Nutton, 'L. Gellius Maximus, Physician and Procurator', *Classical Quarterly*, n.s. 21 (1971), 262–72. [129] *ILS* 7789.

[130] Tacitus, *Ann.*, VI.50.3; Josephus, *Ant. Jud.*, XIX.1.20; Galen, CMG V.10.2.2, pp. 483–4.

[131] Kudlien, *Stellung*, p. 3, rightly remarks that the financial qualification for an equestrian procuratorship was the same as that for the senate, and that the wealth amassed by imperial personal physicians was frequently immense.

[132] Dio Cassius, *Hist.*, LXXX.7.1–3, with the article mentioned in n. 128.

contemporary doctors in Rome are as vitriolic and as contemptuous as those of Pliny's, and the later legal enactments, which favour court physicians, reveal the lower groups engaged in a constant struggle to maintain even their traditional privileges.[133] They are craftsmen, even if high-grade craftsmen, and certainly not gentlemen in the eyes of the law.

Whether developments within medical theory and practice helped the doctor to gain social advancement is impossible to say. Methodist doctrine, by its simplistic emphasis on common conditions and its avowed treatment of symptoms rather than causes, gained many followers, but also the contempt of Celsus and Galen. Surgical technique, to judge from the pseudo-Galenic *Introduction*, became exceedingly sophisticated and possibly more effective, and the revival of animal anatomy about AD 120 and Galen's own anatomical researches led to important new discoveries about the workings of the body.[134] Yet literary sources stress fine flashy instruments and the charlatanesque patter, and the surgeon is depicted as even more to be feared than death. To die at the hands of the doctors was apparently no empty metaphor.[135]

It may perhaps be significant that when Galen wishes to press the claims of medicine and to enhance the profession of medicine, he does so less by appealing to its efficacy than by transforming it into something different, into philosophy.[136] Both in his *Exhortation* and still more so in *The Best Doctor is also a Philosopher*, he emphasised that medicine leads to an understanding of the workings of the universe, that it can be explained philosophically, and that, since all parts of virtue are conjoined and, as Plato taught, all virtue is knowledge, then the doctor will be fearless, temperate, incorruptible, in short, a paragon of excellence. Galen prided himself on his own philosophical skills and on his close friendship with the Aristotelians in Rome, and it might be suspected that, as with the list of moral accomplishments he gave in his commentary on *Epidemics VI*, his ideal practitioner is merely himself writ large.[137] But there is a striving among other crafts for respectability by a similar

[133] Nutton, 'Two Notes on Immunities: *Digest* 27, 1, 6, 10 and 11', *Journal of Roman Studies*, 61 (1971), 52–63; 'Continuity', pp. 15–23 (repr. in Nutton, *From Democedes to Harvey*).

[134] L Toledo-Pereyra, 'Galen's Contribution to Surgery', *Journal of the History of Medicine* 28, (1973), 357–75, but all his evidence, after n. 53, refers to the pseudo-Galenic *Introduction*; a good guide to Galenic anatomy is given by M. T. May in the *Introduction* to her translation of Galen's *On the Usefulness of the Parts of the Body* (Ithaca, 1968).

[135] Nutton, 'Patriotism', pp. 34–6, with references.

[136] Temkin, *Double Face of Janus*, pp. 137–53. But it should also be remembered that several philosophical accomplishments, notably the ability to think logically, were of direct relevance to medical practice.

[137] Galen, *Quod opt. med.*: 1.53–63 K.; CMG v.10.2.2, pp. 202–7, with the detailed commentary by K. Deichgräber, *Medicus gratiosus* (Wiesbaden, 1970).

association with philosophy, which is regarded as the mark of a truly free man. Vitruvius in his preface to his work *On Architecture*, and Quintilian in his *Training of the Orator* make at least a nod in the direction of, in particular, moral philosophy. The truth is revealed by the arch-satirist Lucian. He describes an art that puts philosophy into practice, that by its activities introduces the mind to the deepest speculations and that makes of its possessor a model of virtue – the noble art of the pantomime dancer.[138]

Hospitals and healing shrines

The gradual move from largely non-citizen to largely citizen doctors in the Roman Empire is perhaps best explained as a reflection of general trends within Roman society – a reduction in numbers of slaves, the broadening (and cheapening as a status symbol) of Roman citizenship, and the gradual cultural penetration of Greeks and Greek ideas. At the same time, the special needs of Roman society led to the creation of new types of medical institution, in particular of hospitals. As far as is known, hospitals, in the sense of places where the sick could reside for long periods under medical supervision, were unknown to the Greeks. The shrines of Asclepius provided, by their incubation rooms, places where sufferers could stay for treatment, but few remained for more than one night. Even Aelius Aristides, whose orations reveal his dependence for treatment on Asclepius, was not a permanent resident at the shrine of Pergamum, and many of its rich habitués would have lived in the houses that abutted on to it on three sides rather than sleeping all the time in the small cubicles of the incubation building.[139] The Hippocratic physician would also have had room in his house for treating the sick who could not be treated in their own homes, or who lived too far away for adequate supervision. They were always a small minority. The same situation is true for the Roman world. Galen generally visited his patients' houses and, very often, with the patient's servants as assistants and nurses. Sick slaves were dumped at the Temple of Asclepius on the Tiber Island in Rome for the god to cure them. Although there were

---

[138] Vitruvius, *De archit.* 1.1ff.; Quintilian, *Inst. orat.*, 1.1; Onasander, *Strat.* 1–2; Lucian, *De salt.* 35.81. The fact that this is a common *topos* need not mean that it was not thought, in some way, to validate and reinforce the specific art, perhaps in the same way as the Roman theory of the 'liberal arts'. But it should also be remembered that, according to the law codes, city councils, when choosing a civic doctor, had to have regard to his morality as much as to his skill, and that the doctor's own morality was often the sole guarantee of his competent performance.

[139] For Asclepieia, see Edelstein, *Asclepius*. And for Aristides, an older contemporary of Galen, see his *Hieroi Logoi*.

complex arrangements made for the medical well-being of visitors to great festivals, including the attendance of doctors, and although there were permanent guesthouses for pilgrims and travellers, this did not extend to the creation at public expense of hospitals to receive the sick and weary. Although the Jewish Talmud might recommend among the necessities for the good life the presence of a surgeon and a circumcizer, paid for by the Jewish community, and although the Christians were respected for their charitable concern for the sick and poor in their church (and were to extend this to the population at large), pagan concepts of a public duty towards the sick were largely negative. It was not the job of the town council to intervene in what was an individual or at most a family concern. It was the job of a head of the family or a patron to succour his dependents.[140]

That this was so is clear from the two types of hospitals created in the Roman world. They were not for the general public but for two restricted groups, slaves and the army. Our evidence for slave hospitals, as Georg Harig has argued, comes first from the great slave and freedmen households of the early Roman emperors, and later from the writings of Celsus and Columella, who associate the hospital with the dependent workers on great landed estates.[141] A hospital for the household of Augustus, with its special squads of slaves and freemen doctors, would not have been open to the public, and, certainly, no man of wealth would have seen dead (or alive) in a *valetudinarium* alongside his slaves. Even on an estate, although the social composition of patients might have been broader than in Rome, the treatment and supervision by the bailiff's wife, with or without a doctor, would have been rough and ready. Celsus notes that in these great hospitals one could only attend to gross common symptoms, in what he saw as a travesty of the proper method of medicine.[142] From all this we may deduce that these slave hospitals existed at least as much for the convenience of their owners as for the welfare of the slaves, and that their creation was an extension of Catonian *Hausvatermedizin* and was brought about largely by the decline in the number of slaves introduced into the Roman world

---

[140] For the Jewish, see Nutton, 'Continuity', p. 23 (based on *Sanhedrin*, 17B). Ancient ideas on charity are discussed by Hands, *Charities*. T. S. Miller, *The Birth of the Hospital in the Byzantine Empire* (Baltimore, 1985), pp. 37–49, discusses the pagan evidence for 'hospitals', and his survey of the evidence for hospitals in late antiquity, from the fourth century until the reign of Justinian in the sixth, is the most complete known to me. But his book is marred by serious errors, of fact and perspective, see my review in *Medical History*, 30 (1986), 218–21.

[141] G. Harig, 'Zum Problem "Krankenhaus" in der Antike', *Klio*, 53 (1971), 179–95.

[142] Celsus, *De med.*, Pr. 65.

in the first century BC. When slaves were cheap, their lives were almost worthless; when they became harder to come by, or, as in the imperial household, were taught specific, useful skills, greater thought was given to their physical well-being.

Similarly, it was new developments in military practice that occasioned the creation of military hospitals. In classical Greece and republican Rome, although doctors might attend the troops (and certainly their general), since most campaigns were short and citizen armies regularly disbanded, there was no need for permanent hospitals even for the wounded. They were treated either in their own tents or left behind in a friendly (or at least conquered) town.[143] This was still the case in the Roman civil wars of Julius Caesar, and, even in the Roman Empire, frontier garrisons in the Eastern provinces, at a fort like Dura Europus, seem to have mingled with the local population and may have been attended to in the traditional manner. But the conquests of Augustus brought something new – long, hard campaigns by professional soldiers in areas where not only were the natives unfriendly but also there were no suitable civilian settlements for sick troops to rest in. Hence, for purely military reasons, the massive, permanent base fortresses like Xanten or Bonn in Germany or, later, Inchtuthil in Scotland, and even smaller forts for frontier defence, were all provided with 'hospitals'.[144] They were not field hospitals in a modern sense – even forts like Fendoch or Housesteads were not close to the scene of the fighting, and the legionary hospitals at York, Chester and Gloucester, or Lambaesis in Africa, were many miles from even the frontier.[145] On campaign the wounded were treated on the spot, by their unit's doctors and bandagers; for recuperation and possible surgery, they would then go back to a base hospital. By contrast with the hospital at the siege camp at Hod Hill in south-western England, which shows provision for an expected casualty rate of up to 25 per cent, the legionary hospitals could take little more than 10 per cent of available troops, even at Bonn or

---

[143] Caesar, *Bellum civ.*, III.78, 87, 101.

[144] L. F. Pitts and J. K. S. St Joseph, *Inchtuthil: The Roman Legionary Fortress* (London, 1985); for Germany, D. Jetter, *Geschichte des Hospitals: I, Westdeutschland von den Anfängen bis 1850* (Wiesbaden, 1966), provides detailed plans and descriptions. The most recent military hospital to be excavated is at Novae (Bulgaria), see L. Press, 'Valetudinarium at Novae', in *Studien zu den Militärgrenzen Roms* (Stuttgart, 1986), pp. 529–35.

[145] A. Johnson, *Roman Forts of the First and Second Centuries AD in Britain and the German Provinces* (London, 1983), pp. 157–64, offers an accessible discussion, but envisages the fort hospitals as taking 'undoubtedly the more severe cases' in need of 'more specialist care'. Given the distance of York or Chester from Hadrian's Wall, let alone any campaigning, such cases would have died long before reaching hospital.

Neuss, where they abutted onto the Rhine frontier. These hospitals developed a sophisticated plan, from the quasi-tents of Haltern on the Lippe (c. AD 9), to the magnificent buildings of Neuss and Inchtuthil (AD 83–7), and were serviced by doctors, bandagers, and even trainee doctors. The army could, it seems, provide experience and instruction, and an army doctor, however trained, could be assured of a respectable position as a doctor in civil life.[146]

The boundaries of competence

Military hospitals were for the troops, not for the civilians, who had to make do with every assistance they could find. Not surprisingly, it varied in competence and accessibility according to where one happened to be and what one could afford. Galen claims never to have charged a fee (although he gladly received payment for his services), but, as his opponents bitterly noted, this was because his great inherited wealth freed him from the sordid constraints of having to earn his money from medicine.[147] In a big city like Rome or Antioch, one could find specialists, oculists, ear surgeons and so on; in the countryside, one had to rely on passing strangers, with possibly doubtful knowledge, or on one's own resources.[148] The tradition of self-help and household medicine remained strong. Pliny praised the centenarian Antonius Castor, pottering in his garden for his herbs, and the emperor Tiberius' solicitude for his men on a military campaign extended to treating them within his own tent.[149] Domestic medicine provides one boundary for medical activity; the other is given by the specialists and the doctors who received official recognition from a town council, particularly after the financial restrictions imposed by the emperor Antonius Pius (c. AD 150).

[146] Scarborough, *Roman Medicine*, pp. 66–75, is largely fanciful. Better are V. Nutton, 'Medicine and the Roman Army: a Further Consideration', *Medical History* 13, (1969), 260–70; R. W. Davies, 'The Medici of the Roman Armed Forces', *Epigraphische Studien*, 8 (1969), 83–99; 'Some More Military Medici', *ibid.*, 9 (1972), 1–12; 'The Roman Military Medical Service', *Saalburg Jahrbuch*, 27 (1970), 84–104.

[147] Galen, x.561 K. (wealth); CMG v,8,1, p. 116 with comm. ad loc. (fees). Good introductions to Galen are by Lloyd, *Greek Science after Aristotle* (London, 1973), pp. 136–53) and by O. Temkin, *Galenism* (Ithaca, 1973). W. D. Smith, *Hippocratic Tradition* is, despite its title, devoted largely to Galen.

[148] Whether the breakdown of the organization of towns and cities in the western half of the late Roman Empire was responsible for the survival of several books of 'self-help' medicine from this period is an open question, cf. K. D. Fischer, 'Anweisungen zur Selbstmedikation von Laien in der Spätantike', *Proceedings of the 1986 International Conference on the History of Medicine, Düsseldorf* (Düsseldorf, 1988), pp. 867–74.

[149] Pliny, *Hist. Nat.* xxv.5.9–10; Velleius Paterculus, *Hist.*, II.114–2.

For at least thirty years before Pius, if not from that of the triumvirs, two centuries earlier, all doctors had enjoyed immunity from local taxation, possibly simply on their own attestation before a magistrate. But immunities, however attractive, had to be paid for by someone, and the prudent Pius, in his concern for civic finances in general, restricted the benefits of tax immunity to ten, seven or five doctors, depending on the size and importance of the town. The choice of doctors was left to the unfettered judgement of the council, concerned only with the candidates' morals and ability, and free from the pressure of a governor with a protégé. Only constant good performance guaranteed the continuation of immunity, but no record exists of any doctor being deprived of his privileges, and a slightly earlier Egyptian papyrus shows a doctor whose competence was bitterly disputed still being allowed his immunity just on his own claim to be a doctor. A town council was composed of laymen – for judgement by fellow professionals we must wait until Valentinian's regulations for Rome in AD 368 – but they may well have been able to make a reasonable guess at a practitioner's ability from his testimonials and, still more, his demeanour and treatments once he resided among them. But we cannot be sure that their expectations and definitions of medical competence were the same as ours, and in some communities, the bird in the hand, however bedraggled, might be preferable to any number of unknown birds in the bush.[150]

Between the civic doctor and self-help came a great variety of healers – circuit doctors going round the countryside from a home base in a market town, wise women, magicians, druggists, faith healers and quacks.[151] Galen tells how he had a quack doctor arrested after he had claimed to cure toothache by a treatment taught him by Galen himself, but which was no more than a clever conjuring trick.[152] The Roman lawyer Ulpian (*fl.* AD 210) attempted to lay down who was a proper medical practitioner entitled to sue for fees. He accepted midwives at any rate 'who apparently displayed a knowledge of medicine', as well as specialists in the treatment of ears, fistulae and teeth. He drew the line at those who practised incantations, imprecations, and exorcisms – for those were not types of medicine, even though some claimed to have

---

[150] V. Nutton, 'Archiatri and the Medical Profession in Antiquity', *Papers of the British School, Rome*, 45 (1977), 198–226; 'Continuity', pp. 9–23.

[151] D. W. Amundsen, 'Images of the Physicians in Classical Times', *Journal of Popular Culture*, 11 (1977), 643–55; F. Kudlien, 'Schaustellerei und Heilmittelvertrieb in der Antike', *Gesnerus*, 11 (1983), 91–8; Nutton, 'The Drug Trade'; 'Murders', pp. 29–38.

[152] M. Meyerhof, 'Autobiographische Bruchstücke Galens aus arabischen Quellen', *Sudhoffs Archiv*, 22 (1929), 83.

derived benefit from them.[153] The conflict between what the educated lawyer perceived as medicine and what the man in the street saw as relieving his suffering is here patent, and shows the difficulty of generalizing about the medical profession in Rome.

Even if we restrict our gaze to female doctors and midwives, the differences are still great. Some women were trained in medicine by a father, husband or patron, and were even consulted with respect for their learning by Galen.[154] Soranus' injunctions on the education of the midwife demand a paragon of virtue, intelligence, energy and patience, to say nothing of her long fingers and soft hands.[155] How many midwives came even close to this ideal is as futile to determine as the number of true Galenic doctors. At the other extreme, a woman could break off from serving behind the bar of an inn to go and attend a birth, and reappear later before her impatient customers with her hands still wet from washing off the blood.[156] In cases like this, competence and experience may have been a better test than theoretical knowledge.

The education of a doctor varied equally widely. A doctor might learn his trade as an apprentice to a town doctor or, like Galen, travel to famous centres of medical instruction, like Smyrna, or, in particular, Alexandria 'the foundation of health for all men'. Galen is scathing about some of his lecturers, who were even more obscure and irrelevant than their proof texts, but Alexandria had its own cachet, and even Galen praised the (animal) anatomies of Marinus. In the fifth and sixth centuries, the medical curriculum of Alexandria, which emphasized commentary on set Galenic or Hippocratic texts, contributed to the growth of Galenism and became the model for later educational establishments.[157] But no medical education was compulsory; Phaedrus' cobbler just turned from his last to practising medicine, and the tradition that the great Asclepiades formerly taught rhetoric is not *ipso facto* implausible. Galen, whose first medical appointment, to the gladiators at Pergamum, was not until he was twenty-eight, is unusual in the length and range of his education. The *Introduction* ascribed to Soranus

---

[153] Ulpian, *Digest*, 50.13.3. For religious healing in late antiquity, cf. Nutton, 'Murders', pp. 46–50; 'From Galen to Alexander: Aspects of Medicine and Medical Practice in Late Antiquity', *Dumbarton Oaks Papers*, 38 (1984), 5–9; G. Vikan, 'Art, Medicine and Magic in Early Byzantium', *ibid.*, 65–86.   [154] Galen, CMG v.8.1, p. 110, with comm. ad loc.

[155] Soranus, *Gyn.*, 1.3–4.

[156] Eunapius, *Vit. phil.* 21. The role of the female physician is discussed by Helen King in 'Agnodike and the profession of medicine', *Proceedings of the Cambridge Philological Society*, 32 (1987), 53–77.

[157] Smith, *Hippocratic Tradition*, pp. 62–74, describes Galen's training in detail; for late antiquity, see the references cited above, n. 67.

recommends beginning one's medical education at the age of fifteen, and inscriptions and papyri record doctors who died at the age of eighteen or nineteen. A low age for beginning practice is far more likely than that most people followed the advice and example of Galen and amassed a great deal of book knowledge before ever coming near a patient.[158]

Even if a competent doctor was accessible or one managed to consult a Galen at long distance by letter, successful treatment was by no means assured. The medical texts, both in the Methodist and Hippocratic traditions, stress the importance of nursing and of letting nature take its guiding course. Indeed, since most conditions cure themselves in time, this was perhaps the most sensible and effective advice.[159] Hence, the doctor must take responsibility for the competence of nurses and other attendants on the patient. Surgery was dangerous, and drugs were liable to abuse and adulteration. Doctors were expected to make up their own prescriptions, but in addition there were certain drug specialists as well as practitioners of folk or magical remedies. The list of authors of drug recipes recorded by Galen ranges from doctors who participated in a long tradition of pharmacological learning, as with the doctors at Tarsus, to Flavius the boxer, Achilles the vet, Diogas the trainer, Orion the currier, Pharnaces the rootcutter and sundry men from the wilds of Phrygia, Egypt and Crete, not forgetting Axius, doctor in the British fleet.[160]

Magical medicine was always around, particularly, it was said, in Egypt, and the boundary between meteorological and astrological

---

[158] Phaedrus, 1.14; Pliny, *Hist. Nat.*, XXVI.12–20; [Soranus], *Introd.*, 244–5 Rose; for Galen, see n. 156.

[159] This survey has deliberately omitted any discussion of the prevalent diseases of antiquity, and their causes and their treatments, for, for much of this period, we are dependent on very dubious sources, which may be interpreted in many different ways. Hence it would be unwise, at this stage in our knowledge of ancient medicine, to enter into large hypotheses about how far disease and illness were culturally determined (although this is a topic not without interest in the light of Lloyd, *Magic*). There are few diseases that are clinically as clear through the ages as epilepsy, the subject of a celebrated book by Temkin, *The Falling Sickness*, 2nd edn (Baltimore, 1971), and the findings of palaeopathologists and palaeobotanists are still highly speculative. One sober assessment of the diseases of antiquity is M. D. Grmek, *Les maladies à l'aube de la civilisation occidentale* (Paris, 1983), translated as *Diseases in the Ancient Greek World* (Baltimore and London, 1989); see also Jackson, *Doctors and Diseases* and Sallares, *Ecology*. The relationship between diseases and their social environment in antiquity needs further study, particularly in the light of the recent work of Peter Garnsey on famine, e.g. 'Famine in Rome', in P. Garnsey and C. R. Whittaker (eds.), *Trade and Famine in Classical Antiquity* (Cambridge, 1983), pp. 56–65. Determining the efficacy of proposed remedies is hazardous, given the problems of identifying both ancient diseases and ancient drugs, as well as the assumption that ancient physicians diagnosed correctly, and used the appropriate herb in good condition. Hence, I find the arguments of J. M. Riddle, *Dioscorides on Pharmacy on Medicine* (Austin, 1985), overly sanguine, although others may disagree.

[160] Nutton, 'The Drug Trade', p. 145.

medicine was easily crossed. Most of our medical authors, when they notice folk or magical remedies, do so only to warn against them or to rationalize them. The activities of bird-diviners, prophets, astrologers and number mystics are poohpoohed by Galen – the carved jasper stone laid on the pylorus in stomach ache, as recommended by King Nechepso, works perfectly well without being carved.[161] Yet Pamphilus and Xenocrates, whose books, according to Galen, were full of superstition, sorcery, incantations and Egyptian mumbo-jumbo, were famous for their learning, and their works were read and copied for generations.[162] Pliny, in his diatribe against Persian magicians, unwittingly provided ample propaganda for the techniques and cures he opposed.[163] Scribonius Largus (*fl.* AD 50), who doubted the value of the additional injunction of Ambrosius of Puteoli to compound a drug against the stone only with a wooden pestle and when not wearing an iron ring, and who rejected the Cretan remedy of a piece of Hyena skin for rabies, refused to employ the liver of a dead gladiator in curing epilepsy, for this fell 'outside the claims of medicine'. But this remedy continued to be copied down, if not used, for generations, and was accepted five hundred years later, without comment, by Alexander of Tralles as a sound remedy from Marsinus the Thracian.[164] Our literary texts play down magical and folk healing: the papyri and the long survival of many such remedies reveal that for many people such treatments had some value and, possibly, were all that was accessible.[165] Unlike religious healing, which was not on the whole opposed by doctors, magic was regarded by some physicians as dangerous and non-medical, yet both continued to exist and indeed to flourish. The success of Galen's contemporary Alexander in setting up his own cult of

[161] Galen, XII.207 K.; cf. M. Wellmann, 'Beiträge zur Geschichte der Medizin im Altertum', *Hermes*, 65 (1930), 322–31.

[162] M. Wellman, 'Xenokrates aus Aphrodisias', *Hermes*, 42 (1907), 614–30; idem, *Markellos von Side als Arzt und die Koiraniden des Hermes Trismegistos* (Leipzig, 1934). Xenocrates of Aphrodisias must not be confused with another medico-magical author, Xenocrates of Ephesus, for whom see M. Ullmann, 'Das Steinbuch des Xenokrates von Ephesos', *Medizinhistorisches Journal*, 7 (1972), 49–64; and 'Neues zum Steinbuch des Xenokrates', *ibid.*, 8 (1973), 59–76.

[163] Green, *Magic in Pliny*, is fundamental. The perspective of the collective volume on Pliny, edited by French and Greenaway, would have been improved by a survey of magic.

[164] Scribonius Largus, *Compositiones*, 152; 172; 17 (and cf. 13); Alexander, 1.15; see also Temkin, *Falling Sickness*, pp. 22–7.

[165] Hence the definition of what is medical and what is magical is very fluid, and the more obvious presence of so-called magical or sympathetic remedies in later writers may not represent the 'capture' of medicine by magic, but rather the absence of such authors as Galen and Aretaeus, whose use of such remedies is less overt or explained in different ways. Cf. also J. Röhr, *Der okkulte Kraftbegriff im Altertum* (Leipzig, 1923), pp. 97–133, for an overlap between magical and medical explanations of the workings of drugs.

Asclepius at Abonuteichos is attested by archaeological and literary sources, and it defied the well-merited score of Lucian.[166] The Christian church found it necessary to repeat in its rules for discipline that instruction or baptism was not to be given to bird-diviners, magi, astrologers, soothsayers, conjurors and makers of phylacteries. Nonetheless, so the dubious *Augustan History* claimed, in Egypt every Jewish and Christian priest was an astrologer, a soothsayer or a medical trainer.[167]

Conclusion

The study of the social history of medicine in Greece and Rome shows, above all, the pitfalls of wide generalization. One can pick out certain epochs and associate various trends in medical theory or practice with them. The vigorous medical-cum-philosophical debates of the early Hippocratic writings may owe much to the open, combative society of Athens and the Aegean in the middle and late fifth century BC; the benevolent patronage of the Hellenistic monarchs may have furthered research into anatomy and pharmacology; and the systematizing genius of Galen may be compared with the contemporary achievements of Ptolemy in astronomy or, at a much lower scientific level, with the compilations of Plutarch, Athenaeus, and that *Reader's Digest* columnist of antiquity, Aelian.[168] Yet the precise relationship between ancient society and its medicine is impossible to determine. Did the knowledge of the limited means at their disposal lead doctors to recommend nonintervention in doubtful cases, or was it to preserve their own reputation? Was it the lack of definitive aetiologies that fostered the custom of multiple consultations? Was the success of Methodist medicine in Rome due to its simplistic theory, its practicality, or to a gradual acceptance of things Greek? And, perhaps the most difficult question of all, did Greek medicine triumph over early Roman patriarchal medicine from its own merits or simply as a result of long-term forces of familiarity, social change, and, to a certain extent, cultural snobbery?

To raise these questions is perhaps to reveal their insolubility. Yet the

---

[166] Lucian, *Alexander*, with L. Robert, *A travers l'Asie Mineure* (Paris, Athens, 1980), pp. 392–421.

[167] *Traditio apostolica*, 16; Hist. Aug., *Vitr Saturnini* 8. Cf. Nutton, 'Murders', pp. 48–50.

[168] Undoubtedly, as Bowersock, *Sophists*, and Reardon, *Courants*, have shown, the success of Galen as a literary figure owed much to the literary revival of the Greek world of his day, and, equally, to the great prosperity of the Greek provinces of Asia Minor at that time. But whether the economic chaos of the later third century was responsible for the growth of Galenism and the concentration (in our surviving texts) on summarizing, rather than extending, existing knowledge (which is by no means a characteristic of late antiquity but seems to have been a common feature of medicine throughout Hellenistic and Roman antiquity), remains a matter for controversy.

idea of a straightforward march of medical progress by a medical profession composed entirely of Hippocrates, Herophilus, Galen and their like, which is the impression given by older textbooks, is even more false. The doctor's position in society affects his medical practice, and vice-versa, and more recent research has sought to consider various strata within the medical profession in their relationship with contemporary society.[169] The result is inevitably fragmentary, for we do not have Roman public opinion polls or a medical register, and many hypotheses are at best tentative. Tales of distinguished medical heroes or failures often reveal more about the bias of their sources than about historical facts, and medical historians have only recently begun to approach the ancient evidence with due historical scepticism.[170] The time for the grand synthesis is not yet; indeed, given the state of the evidence for several long periods of time, such a synthesis may never come to pass. But to the social and medical historian, the new picture of the medical history of classical antiquity may continue for a long while yet to attract and allure, for, like the kaleidoscope, it can in its own way express the workings of change. Athens was not Alexandria, Rome was not Pergamum, the republican world of Cato was not the benevolent, hellenized autocracy of Marcus Aurelius; and Galen was no Fadianus Bubbal, a *medicus* buried at Caesarea in Mauretania, aged sixty-two, and depicted on his tomb with his rough tunic, book and cleaver.[171]

---

[169] Notably by Kudlien, *Der griechische Arzt*; *Stellung*; 'Schaustellerei'; 'Jüdische Ärzte im römischen Reich', *Medizinhistorisches Journal*, 20 (1985), 36–57; and Nutton, 'Archiatri'; 'Continuity'; 'Murders'; and 'Patriotism'.

[170] Cf. my strictures at 'Murders', p. 24. Although scholars like Gourevitch, *Le triangle hippocratique*, have brought to prominence many neglected texts, the interpretation given to them still rests ultimately on the preconceptions of eighteenth-century or earlier historians, whose definition of physician more closely resembles that of our own day than that of antiquity. It was the merit of Lloyd, *Science*, and *Magic*, to break away from this traditional schema.

[171] P. Gauckler, *Le Musée de Cherchel* (Paris, 1895), pl. III, n. 2. Contrast the elegant portrait of Galen in the Vienna Dioscorides, Vienna gr. 1, fol. 3.

Medicine and society in medieval Europe, 500–1500

KATHARINE PARK

The hallmarks of medieval medical care were its variety and its intensity. Our own society boasts a relatively small (although growing) range of both medical institutions and publicly recognized medical practitioners, narrowly defined, similarly trained, and socially homogeneous. Medieval society, on the other hand, like many present-day traditional societies, looked to a much broader set of healers and strategies to care for its precarious health.[1] In part this situation reflected much higher levels of illness than we are used to – levels that sprang from extensive poverty and unhealthy living conditions as much or more than the limits of medieval therapeutics. In part it reflected the variety of medieval society itself. A millenium separated the Europeans of 1500 from their counterparts in 500, and that millenium encompassed changes arguably far more radical than those of the five centuries that separate us from them. Furthermore, Europe was much more diverse then than now, when advances in transportation and communication and other social shifts have acted to homogenize institutions and to break down cultural and linguistic barriers between nations, between city and countryside, between rich and poor.

For these reasons, historians have tended to describe medieval medicine as a dense set of discrete forms of theory and practice tenuously related – if related at all – whose principles frequently contradicted one another and whose practitioners rarely overlapped: physic and surgery, academic medicine and empirical medicine, rational medicine and

---

[1] Cf. Margaret Pelling and Charles Webster, 'Medical Practitioners', in Charles Webster (ed.), *Health, Medicine and Mortality in the Sixteenth Century* (Cambridge, 1979), p. 235. For a general survey of European medicine in this period, see Nancy G. Siraisi, *Medieval and Early Renaissance Medicine: An Introduction to Knowledge and Practice* (Chicago, 1990).

magical medicine, men's medicine and women's medicine, religious medicine and secular medicine, medicine of the rich and medicine of the poor. Such a view is at best exaggerated. It is increasingly apparent that medieval medicine, for all its diversity, formed a cultural unity. Academic writers incorporated the occult properties of plants and minerals into their pharmacology. 'Popular' vernacular treatises were almost all translated from the Latin. Physicians cooperated with surgeons and midwives. Men treated women and women, men. Institutions such as hospitals and municipal doctors offered high-quality medical care to the poor of both city and countryside. And few people appealed to saints before consulting their local lay practitioner.

We cannot understand this complicated social world without considering it whole, including some kinds of health care – faith healing, for example, nursing, or midwifery – that no longer form part of our own more narrowly defined professional medicine. To do so would yield a picture both incoherent and incomplete. Many of my conclusions are tentative; the social history of medieval medicine is a recent and undeveloped field, sources are sparse, especially for the early period, and the variety and breadth of the topic make generalization difficult. I have adopted both a topical and a chronological approach; beginning with a brief account of the special health conditions that shaped medieval medicine, I go on to characterize the social response to those conditions, which I have divided into two main periods: the early medieval period, from roughly 500 to 1050, and the high and late medieval period, from roughly 1050 to 1500. My aim throughout is to trace the gradual growth in medieval society of a complicated and sophisticated medical order. During the later period, I will argue, medicine began to emerge as an autonomous area of expertise, located in an increasingly well defined and differentiated body of practitioners, and in specialized medical institutions newly evolved to organize their practice and draw upon that expertise.

A universe of disease

Jacques Le Goff has described the European Middle Ages as 'a universe of hunger'.[2] It was also, and for many of the same reasons, a universe of disease. Like hunger, illness was arbitrary and inescapable, tied to the caprices of nature. Like hunger, it was serious, frequent, and preoccupying. Much of medieval writing – private letters as well as

---

[2] Jacques Le Goff, *La civilisation de l'occident médiéval* (Paris, 1964), p. 290, and in general pp. 290–303; translated as *Medieval Civilisation, 400–1500*, trans. Julia Barrow (Cambridge, MA, 1989), pp. 229–44.

religious and literary texts – reveals an obsession with illness, and medieval saints, mirrors of contemporary anxieties and aspirations, appear above all as healers of the sick.

Medieval men and women considered themselves old at forty-five. Although their possible life span was the same as ours, their average life span seems to have hovered between thirty and thirty-five years, dropping to as low as eighteen or twenty years during the half-century after the advent of plague in 1348; this corresponds to a death rate two to four times our own.[3] These are of course aggregate figures. Life expectancy was lower in the city than in the countryside and lower for the poor than for the rich, reflecting crowding, malnutrition and material deprivation. It was lower for females than for males, reflecting the dangers of pregnancy and childbed. At risk above all were children, especially infants, whose fragility dominated and drove these high mortality rates; from 15 to 30 per cent (even higher in some periods and areas) seem to have died before the age of one. The overwhelming cause of this premature mortality was disease. The high death rates indicate rates of illness that were truly staggering. The 'burden of sickness', as Paul Slacks calls it – the physical and psychological suffering it caused and the economic and social disruption – was far heavier than the burden of death.[4]

Various causes contributed to these high rates of illness. The technical inadequacies of medieval medicine were partly responsible; medieval doctors knew nothing of antibiotics, antisepsis, or immunization, and they lacked a clear idea of contagion. Far more important, however, were the living conditions of the time. Like many developing nations, pre-industrial Europe was fundamentally poor and its meager wealth extraordinarily unequally distributed. The great majority of the urban and rural population lived at the level of bare subsistence, lacking adequate housing, clothing, fuel, and especially food and drink.[5] Their diet was deficient in both quantity and quality, and many lived in conditions of periodic famine and chronic malnutrition, particularly toward the end of the thirteenth century, when western Europe began

[3] Summaries of recent research in J. C. Russell, 'Population in Europe, 500–1500', in Carlo M. Cipolla (ed.), *The Fontana Economic History of Europe*, 6 vols. in 9 (London, 1972–76), 1: *The Middle Ages*, esp. pp. 41–50, and Carlo M. Cipolla, *Before the Industrial Revolution: European Society and Economy 1000–1700*, ch. 5; see also associated bibliographies. On old age, David Herlihy, 'Vieillir à Florence au Quattrocento', *Annales: Economies, sociétés, civilisations*, 24 (1969), 1338–9.

[4] Paul Slack, *The Impact of Plague in Tudor and Stuart England* (London, 1985), p. 176.

[5] Cipolla, *Before the Industrial Revolution*, chs. 1–3; Maria Serena Mazzi, *Salute e società nel Medioevo* (Florence, 1978), pp. 5–26. See in general Thomas McKeown, *The Role of Medicine: Dream, Mirage or Nemesis* (Princeton, NJ, 1979), esp. chs. 2, 8.

to suffer from relative overpopulation.[6] The low level of collective and personal hygiene also contributed to disease, particularly in the cities, where sewer systems were inadequate and water supplies often polluted by animal and human waste. Most houses were poorly heated, poorly ventilated, and extraordinarily crowded. Soap was expensive, when available at all, and domestic and human parasites flourished – not only rats, fleas and lice, but also a whole host of micro-organisms and worms. These conditions fostered an exuberantly varied world of disease. Demographers and historians of medicine have tended to concentrate on the more dramatic and exotic episodes in the history of medieval illness, the successive epidemics of plague, leprosy, and St Anthony's fire (now identified as gangrenous ergotism) that swept through Europe after 1050.[7] But other infections, both endemic and epidemic, took a heavy toll in lives and health: influenza, for example, tuberculosis, malaria, typhus, and the great killers, especially of children, smallpox, dysentery, and other forms of diarrhoea.[8] The dangers of pregnancy and childbirth seem to have accounted for the shorter life expectancy of medieval women. Less prominent in a population dominated by the young but significant nonetheless were the diseases of old age: cancer, heart disease, circulatory problems, and gout.[9]

A few documents hint at an even broader experience of disease, shaped also by the non-lethal illnesses, both mental and physical, that tend not to capture the historian's imagination. In the first known list of diagnosed patients admitted to a European hospital, for example, the two largest categories – after those with fevers – suffered from skin diseases (rashes, boils, ulcers and sores) and trauma (wounds, fractures and bites).[10] Diseases of the teeth and eyes were also common, as well as

[6] Charles-M, de la Roncière, 'Pauvres et pauvreté à Florence au xive siècle', in Michel Mollat (ed.), Etudes sur l'histoire de la pauvreté (Moyen Age–XVIe siècle), 2 vols. (Paris, 1974), II, pp. 671–85; Fritz Curschmann, Hungersnöte im Mittelalter: Ein Beitrag zur deutschen Wirtschaftgeschichte des 8. bis 13. Jahrhunderts (Leipzig, 1900). On the complicated relations between nutrition and disease, see the discussion and references in Andrew B. Appleby, 'Nutrition and Disease: The Case of London, 1550–1750', Journal of Interdisciplinary History, 6 (1975), 1–2.
[7] E.g. Jean-Noel Biraben, Les hommes et la peste, 2 vols. (Paris, 1975–6), and the literature cited in Ann G. Carmichael, Plague and the Poor in Renaissance Florence (Cambridge, 1986), pp. 172–5; Peter Richards, The Medieval Leper and his Northern Heirs (Cambridge, 1977); Henri Chaumartin, Le mal des ardents et le feu de Saint Antoine (Paris, 1946).
[8] Carmichael, Plague and the Poor, chs. 1–3 and pp. 169–75 (bibliography). See in general William McNeill, Plagues and Peoples (New York, 1976), chs. 3–4.
[9] A. R. Burn, 'Hic breve vivitur: A Study of Expectation of Life in the Roman Empire', Past and Present, 4 (1953), 10–13; Vern Bullough and Cameron Campbell, 'Female Longevity and Diet in the Middle Ages', Speculum, 55 (1980), 317–25; Carmichael, Plague and the Poor, pp. 35–40.
[10] Bernice Trexler, 'Hospital Patients in Florence: San Paolo 1567–68', Bulletin of the History of Medicine, 48 (1974), 45–50.

hernia, to judge by the striking number of late medieval healers who specialized in those conditions, while the mentally ill figured prominently as subjects of both legal and medical concern. We must keep in mind, finally, the vast numbers of disabled who flocked to the healing shrines of medieval Europe. The deaf, the blind and the crippled – some congenital, some the victims of dietary deficiencies, infections, or accidents – were a standard feature of the social landscape.

Detailed study of the medieval experience of disease is in its infancy. We still know relatively little about the individual illnesses that shaped it and even less about how they interacted with one another.[11] The occasional skeletons exhumed from medieval graveyards illuminate mainly those diseases that leave traces in the bones and teeth – leprosy, caries, rickets, and the like – while the detailed death records kept by the public authorities of some northern Italian cities exist only from the late fourteenth century.[12] And even these, like the grim litanies of epidemics that mark early chronicles and the lists of miraculous cures kept at some shrines, require us to rely heavily on contemporary diagnoses. All of these sources are fragmentary and ambiguous, not least because it is often difficult to translate medieval medical terms and categories of illness into our own.[13]

For historians of medicine, however, as opposed to historians of disease, it is less important to identify the actual illnesses involved than to explore how individuals and societies responded to their experience of illness. Here the medieval sources are unambiguous. Despite the Christian cult of suffering, few European men and women accepted illness or still less sought it out, and those few were often set apart as saints. The vast majority, as far as we can tell, reacted vigorously against disease. They patronized private healers of all sorts, religious and secular, and during the later Middle Ages they began to develop complicated institutions – medical guilds and faculties, specialized hospitals, municipally subsidized medical practices, public health commissions – to prevent disease and to broaden access to medical care. Together with death and birth, hunger

[11] See the methodological comments in Mirko D. Grmek, 'Préliminaires d'une étude historique des maladies', *Annales: Economies, sociétés, civilisations*, 24 (1969), 1473–83, and in general his book, *Les maladies à l'aube de la civilisation occidentale* (Paris, 1983).
[12] Calvin Wells, *Bones, Bodies and Disease: Evidence of Disease and Abnormality in Early Man* (London, 1964); Carmichael, *Plague and the Poor*, esp. chs. 1–3; Alan S. Morrison, Julius Kirshner, and Anthony Molho, 'Epidemics in Renaissance Florence', *American Journal of Public Health*, 75 (1985), 528–35.
[13] See Guenter B. Risse, 'Epidemics and Medicine: the Influence of Disease on Medical Thought and Practice', *Bulletin of the History of Medicine*, 53 (1959), 519; Lester S. King, 'What is Disease?', *Philosophy of Science*, 21 (1954), 193–203.

and war, the experience of disease was one of the most fundamental features of medieval life, becoming a principal magnet not only for religious cult or literary expression, but also for intellectual reflection and social resources. It is to this that we owe the rich variety of medieval health care.

The early Middle Ages: religious and secular healing, 500–1050

In an eleventh-century hymn to St Pantaleon, Bishop Fulbert of Chartres described the relations between religious and secular healing:

As Christians we know that there are two kinds of medicine, one of earthly things, the other of heavenly things. They differ in both origin and efficacy. Through long experience, earthly doctors learn the powers of herbs and the like, which alter the condition of human bodies. But there has never been a doctor so experienced in this art that he has not found some illnesses difficult to cure and others absolutely incurable...The author of heavenly medicine, however, is Christ, who could heal the sick with a command and raise the dead from the grave.[14]

Fulbert distinguished, in other words, between the natural medicine of those who treated patients using the physical properties of objects like plants and stones, and the supernatural healing of Christ – and the apostles, saints and charismatics that succeeded him – who cured by a touch or a word.

In theory, the relation between these types of healing was problematic. From the patristic period on, Christian apologists had opposed the two, presenting faith healing as a competitor to secular medicine; disease sprang from the will of God, they argued, and only one with access to divine power could cure it. Except for polemicists and apologists, however, and those with an obvious interest in denigrating the competition to their own healing saints or shrines, most theologians and writers, like Fulbert, considered the two medicines complementary rather than mutually exclusive. Secular healing on natural principles had its own logic and utility, particularly for diseases of physical origin, but its practitioners were fallible; in intractible cases, or those rare instances where the disease sprang from sin, an appeal to supernatural forces was in order.[15]

[14] Fulbert, *Hymnus seu prosa de Sancto Pantaleone* (*Hymn to St Pantaleon*), in J. P. Migne (ed.), *Patrologiae latinae cursus completus*, 221 vols. (Paris, 1844–64), CXLI, col. 341.
[15] Vivian Nutton, 'Murders and Miracles: Lay Attitudes towards Medicine in Classical Antiquity', in Roy Porter (ed.), *Patients and Practitioners* (Cambridge, 1985), pp. 48–51; Darrel W. Amundsen 'Medicine and Faith in Early Christianity', *Bulletin of the History of Medicine*, 56 (1982),

In practice, this conciliatory attitude predominated. The consumers of health care, laity and clerics, rich and poor, saw the saint or holy man as 'one healer among many, prominent in the medical landscape of his area, but not, as a source of medicine or medical advice, wholly different from local physicians'.[16] Like their pagan predecessors, they appealed to many different kinds of healers – herbalists and midwives, exorcists and wise women, saints and doctors, lay specialists and monastic amateurs. These groups were not clearly differentiated; classically trained physicians might prescribe charms and incantations, while saints and charismatics could recommend medication or perform surgery.[17] Rather they coexisted and overlapped, as colleagues and as rivals, often sharing the same clientele and the same therapeutic techniques. Even the basic semantic distinctions between doctor and apothecary, physician and surgeon do not appear until the ninth or tenth century,[18] and it is only after about 1050 that we begin to see the process of formal stratification and exclusion, described in the next section, that led to the emergence of a relatively well defined medical profession.

In considering 'earthly' or naturalistic healing in the early Middle Ages, we must resist the common tendency to reduce it to 'monastic medicine', largely monopolized by monks and subordinated to religious values and concerns. This view reflects more the extreme scarcity of non-monastic sources for this period than the actual state of medical theory and practice. The western Roman Empire had disintegrated in the mid-fifth century under the military pressure of the Germanic tribes, but its social practices and intellectual traditions continued not only in the abbeys and cloisters of medieval Europe, but also in the shrunken remains of Roman cities presided over by Christian bishops and in the colourful courts of the new barbarian kings.

Although the importance of the monasteries in actual medical practice has been exaggerated, they did play an important part in preserving and

---

326–50; Stephen R. Ell, 'Concepts of Disease and the Physician in the Early Middle Ages', *Janus*, 65 (1978), 153–65; James Kroll and Bernard Bachrach, 'Sin and the Etiology of Disease in Pre-Crusade Europe', *Journal of the History of Medicine*, 41 (1986), 395–414.

[16] Peregrine Horden, 'Saints and Doctors in the Early Byzantine Empire: The Case of Theodore of Sykeon', in W. J. Sheils (ed.), *The Church and Healing: Papers Read at the Twentieth Summer Meeting and the Twenty-first Winter Meeting of the Ecclesiastical History Society* (Oxford, 1982), p. 13. See also Peter Brown, *The Cult of the Saints: Its Rise and Function in Latin Christianity* (Chicago, 1981), pp. 114–15; Ronald Finucane, *Miracles and Pilgrims: Popular Beliefs in Medieval England* (London, 1977), pp. 59–68.

[17] Examples in Aline Rousselle, 'Du sanctuaire au thaumaturge: La guérison en Gaule au IVe siècle', *Annales: Economies, sociétés, civilisations*, 31 (1976), 1090–104.

[18] Loren C. MacKinney, *Early Medieval Medicine with Special Reference to France and Chartres* (Baltimore, 1937), pp. 131–2.

transmitting the classical texts that formed the nucleus of medicine as a learned discipline. Writing on medical theory, and to a lesser degree on therapeutics, was not the specialized field we think of today, but formed part of the general literary culture of the Greek and Roman world. As the knowledge of Greek declined in the last centuries of the western Empire, Latin writers began to translate and summarize in Latin those texts, including medical texts, they saw as central to their intellectual tradition. This labour of translation, compilation, and commentary was continued by medieval Christians.

The first centres of this activity, in the sixth and seventh centuries, were more or less formally organized groups of scholars and teachers of medicine in the cities of southern Gaul and northern Italy.[19] It was only in the years around 800, during the Carolingian revival, that monasteries emerged as the principal centres for the study and transmission of ancient medical texts, as monks began seriously to copy and collect classical medical works in Latin translation and to produce their own compendia and condensations of the material – antidotaries and herbals, treatises on midwifery, bloodletting, urine, and pulse. These works were modest in both number and scope. The best endowed monasteries, such as Gorze, Reichenau, and St Gall, possessed only eight or ten medical manuscripts, and many had only one.[20] Most of the new treatises were quite short and strongly derivative of their classical sources. Although they were decidedly practical in orientation, we do not know the extent to which their authors intended them for actual use. Some of the collections of medical recipes may have served in practice, but it is unlikely, for example, that the various gynaecological works from this period argue a flourishing monastic practice in midwifery.[21]

This somewhat notional approach to medical learning continued into the eleventh century, when the cathedral schools of northern France began to replace the monasteries as centres of intellectual culture. From the late tenth century on, masters in several of these schools – Rheims, Chartres, and apparently Poitiers and Amiens – taught medicine

---

[19] Gerhard Baader, 'Die Anfänge der medizinischen Ausbildung im Abendland bis 1100', in *La scuola nell'occidente latino dell'alto medioevo: settimane di studio del Centro italiano di studi sull'alto medioevo*, 19, 2 vols. (Spoleto, 1972), II, pp. 669–718. See in general Pierre Riché, *Education and Culture in the Barbarian West, Sixth through Eighth Centuries*, trans. John J. Contreni (Columbia, S.C., 1976).

[20] Augusto Beccaria, *I codici di medicina del periodo presalernitano, secoli IX, X e XI* (Rome, 1956), esp. pp. 70–4.

[21] See Monica Green, 'The Transmission of Ancient Theories of Female Physiology and Disease through the Early Middle Ages' (unpublished Ph.D. dissertation, Princeton University, 1985), esp. pp. 172–3 and ch. 4.

alongside the liberal arts to an audience that seems to have included some laymen as well as monks and secular clerics.[22] Yet the apparent disjunction between the literary tradition in medicine and medical practice continued; there is no evidence that the medical scholar Richer of Rheims practised, even in the amateur fashion of his contemporary bishop Fulbert of Chartres, author of the hymn to St Pantaleon. The main exceptions to this pattern appear in southern Italy, at Salerno, which had been a centre for the lay study of empirical medicine as early as the mid-tenth century, and to some degree in Anglo-Saxon England. By the middle of the eleventh century, Salerno, in cooperation with the great Benedictine monastery at Montecassino, had also begun to emerge as a centre of theoretical learning based on Greek and Roman medical sources.[23]

If we can turn from medicine as an intellectual discipline in the early Middle Ages to medicine as a system of practice, however, we find a much broader and more heterogeneous world. References to doctors and other 'earthly' healers exist in the written records for virtually every level of society, although the sources are often extremely sketchy. Among the best documented medical practitioners in this period were the doctors attached to the courts of particular bishops and above all of the Germanic kings that laid claim to the various territories of the dismembered western Empire. From the sixth century on, for example, the Frankish monarchs regularly employed doctors to attend them and their families. (This exalted position was sometimes a mixed blessing; the last wish of Austrechild, wife of King Guntram, was for the execution of her two physicians. 'When my friends grieve for me,' she is reported to have said, 'let their friends grieve for them too.')[24] The list of the Frankish royal doctors in this period reveals the remarkable variety of medical practice. They included among many others a Greek doctor, Anthimus, trained in Constantinople, who wrote a learned treatise on foods for King Theodoric I of Austrasia; the humbly born Marileif, previously director of the royal mills, whose 'brothers, cousins and other relations had been employed in the royal kitchens and bakery';[25]

---

[22] MacKinney, *Early Medieval Medicine*, ch. 3, and 'Tenth-Century Medicine as seen in the *Historia* of Richer of Rheims', *Bulletin of the History of Medicine*, 2 (1934), 347–75.

[23] Paul O. Kristeller, 'The School of Salerno: Its Development and its Contribution to the History of Learning', *Bulletin of the History of Medicine*, 17 (1945), 143–59; G. Baader, 'Die Schule von Salerno', *Medizinhistorisches Journal*, 13 (1978), 124–45; M. L. Cameron, 'Sources of Medical Knowledge', *Anglo-Saxon England*, 11 (1983), 135–55; Stanley Rubin, *Medieval English Medicine* (New York, 1974), ch. 2.

[24] Gregory of Tours, *The History of the Franks*, v, 35, trans. Lewis Thorpe (Harmondsworth, 1974), p. 298.   [25] *Ibid.*, VII, 25, p. 407.

Zedechias the Jew, accused of poisoning his master, Charles the Bald; and two tenth-century rivals, the cleric Deroldus (later bishop of Amiens) and an anonymous Salernitan, 'unlearned in letters' but with a 'wide experience in practical affairs'.[26] They included, in other words, priests and laymen, nobles and commoners, men versed in classical theory and apprenticed empirics, Franks and foreigners, Christians and Jews.

Also relatively well documented were the medical practitioners associated with early medieval monasteries. Monastic medical practice seems to have been fairly limited in scope. Benedict had not envisaged his community as a source of medical care for the lay population – his *Rule* refers only to the treatment of the monks themselves – and his followers largely adopted this model.[27] Thus monastic documents refer to various abbots and monks as doctors (*medici*) or describe them as caring for themselves and their brothers or sisters. In some cases monastic doctors did venture outside their cloisters to treat the broader population, particularly the nobility, on whom the material welfare of the monasteries depended. According to his house chronicle, for example, Notker of St Gall (d. 975) 'poet, painter and doctor', visited not only the abbot and various monks of his own monastery, but also the bishop of Constance and a variety of lay people, including a neighbouring female recluse, a count feigning pregnancy, and Emperor Otto I.[28] But this practice was not formalized or institutionalized in any way, reflecting local initiatives on the part of individual abbots and monks rather than any general charitable program fundamental to medieval monasticism.

The sources are unfortunately scantiest – the word is laughably inadequate – for the most interesting and important type of medical practice: the activities of healers normally consulted by the villagers and townsfolk who represented the vast majority of the inhabitants of early medieval Europe. If the classical institution of the publicly salaried municipal doctor survived at all, it did so only into the sixth or possibly

[26] Richer of Rheims, *Historia*, II, 59, translated in MacKinney, 'Tenth-Century Medicine', p. 367. See in general André Finot, 'Les médecins des rois mérovingiens et carlovingiens', *Histoire des Sciences Médicales*, 4 (1970), 41–8; MacKinney, *Early Medieval Medicine*, ch. 2, passim; and the individual entries in Ernest Wickersheimer, *Dictionnaire biographique des médecins en France au Moyen Age*, 2nd edn, ed. Guy Beaujouan, 2 vols. (Geneva, 1979), and Danielle Jacquart, *Supplément* (Geneva, 1979).

[27] Anne F. Dawtry, 'The *Methodus Medendi* and the Benedictine Order in Anglo-Norman England', in Sheils, *The Church and Healing*, pp. 25–30. See in general E. Patzelt, 'Moines-médecins', in *Etudes de civilisation médiévale, IXe–XIIe siècles: Mélanges offerts à Edmond-René Labande* (Poitiers, 1974), pp. 577–88.

[28] Johannes Duft, *Notker der Arzt: Klostermedizin und Mönchsarzt im frühmittelalterlichen St Gallen* (St Gall, 1972), pp. 39–50, 56–8.

the seventh century in certain cities of northern Italy and southern Gaul.[29] In other areas and during the rest of the period, the population at large was served by a variety of local practitioners, almost all of whom would have learned healing not as an intellectual discipline but as a practical craft. Some were monks from local monasteries or members of the secular clergy, but the majority were laymen and women. We catch occasional glimpses of them – primarily the literate or well-to-do exceptions – when they witness wills, join monastic orders, treat religious dignitaries, or catch the attention of the local clergy, like the woman Gregory of Tours described as healing sores with a combination of saliva, fruit leaves, and the sign of the cross.[30] (This last example confirms the obvious, that women worked as healers and certainly as midwives, even though, obscure and illiterate, they do not appear by name in the surviving records.) Except for these few references to individuals, however, we must make do with more general evidence – the provisions concerning doctors and their fees in the various law codes of the Germanic tribes[31] and, above all, the predictable references to incompetent and money-grubbing doctors that are a leitmotiv of the accounts of miraculous healing discussed below.

As a result, we know very little about the actual practice of these men and women – or indeed of their clerical counterparts. Their activities were varied; as the early ninth-century bishop Halitgarius of Cambrai wrote in his *Book of Penance*, 'doctors compound various medicines to treat wounds, disease, tumors, corruption, weak sight, fractures, and burns'.[32] Their therapeutic approaches included not only the three classical naturalistic techniques of medication (mainly herbal), diet (control of food, drink, exercise and the like) and surgery (bleeding, for example, cautery, lancing, and setting bones), but also magical devices

[29] Vivian Nutton, 'Continuity or Rediscovery? The City Physician in Classical Antiquity and Mediaeval Italy', in Andrew W. Russell (ed.), *The Town and State Physician in Europe from the Middle Ages to the Enlightenment* (Wolfenbüttel, 1981), pp. 14–21, 24–5; MacKinney, *Early Medieval Medicine*, pp. 72–3.

[30] Gregory of Tours, *Liber in gloria confessorum* (*Book on the Glory of the Confessors*), ch. 24, in *Scriptores rerum merovingicarum*, 7 vols. (Hanover, 1884–85), I/I, p. 313; cited in MacKinney, *Early Medieval Medicine*, p. 175, n. 132. Documentation on individual healers appears in C. H. Talbot and E. A. Hammond, *The Medical Practitioners in Medieval England: A Biographical Register* (London, 1965), and in Wickersheimer, *Dictionnaire*, and Jacquart, *Supplément*.

[31] See Amundsen, 'Visigothic Medical Legislation', *Bulletin of the History of Medicine*, 40 (1971), 553–69; Gerhard Baader 'Gesellschaft, Wirtschaft und ärztlicher Stand im frühen und hohen Mittelalter', *Medizinhistorisches Journal*, 14 (1979), 180, nn. 26–7, and MacKinney, *Early Medieval Medicine*, nn. 62, 128.

[32] Halitgarius of Cambrai, *Liber poenitentialis*, in Migne, *Patrologiae*, CV, cols. 706–7; cited in MacKinney, *Early Medieval Medicine*, n. 159.

such as charms and invocations, and minor Christian rituals. (Halitgarius considered it legitimate, for example to use the sign of the cross and the Lord's Prayer when collecting herbs, but not 'incantations and other superstitions'.)[33] This mixture of naturalistic and magical elements already characterized much of late Roman medicine, as we can see from the compilation (c. 400) of Marcellus Empiricus; later lists of remedies, such as the famous Anglo-Saxon *Leechbook of Bald* (c. 900), drew on Marcellus and other classical authors, enriching them with practices drawn from Germanic folklore.[34]

There is little textual evidence of specialized practice during the early Middle Ages, although this certainly existed; Gregory of Tours' female healer, who treated sores with the colourful poultices described above, cannot have been exceptional. Only in the tenth and eleventh centuries does a rudimentary vocabulary begin to emerge for distinguishing between different kinds of practitioners: physicians, surgeons, herbalists, bleeders, and appliers of leeches.[35] But even as late as the eleventh century, the practice of an illustrious doctor such as Eudes the Seneschal might embrace horses and birds as well as humans.[36] In general, then, the contours of the body of early medieval healers and medical practitioners were fluid, its members relatively undifferentiated, and its clientele varied. Doctors became monks and monks, doctors. Lay healers treated the religious and religious, the laity. Magic played a part in the natural medicine of both rich and poor. From the twelfth century on, the rise of formal standards for training and apprenticeship, and later of set medical curricula for universities and set procedures for licensing, produced a much more exclusive model for the discipline and the profession. Before then, however, what little we know of the healers who worked in courts, monasteries, and villages points to an inclusive system of medicine, where a variety of practitioners – clerical and lay, male and female, literate and illiterate – and a variety of approaches to healing coexisted in loose relationships of cooperation and competition.

One final aspect of 'earthly' medicine in this period deserves mention: institutions that received the sick and provided them with nursing and

---

[33] Halitgarius, *De poenitentia*, IV, 26, in Migne, *Patrologiae*, CV, col. 686.

[34] Rousselle 'Du sanctuaire au thaumaturge', pp. 1089–1094; Marcellus Empiricus, *De medicamentis liber*, ed. M. Niedermann (Leipzig, 1916); *Leechbook of Bald*, in O. Cockayne (ed. and trans.), *Leechdoms, Wortcunning and Starcraft of Early England*, 3 vols. (London, 1864–66), II; see Talbot, 'Notes on Anglo-Saxon Medicine', *Medical History*, 9 (1965), pp. 156–69.

[35] Jole Agrimi and Chiara Crisciani, *Medicina del corpo e medicina dell'anima: Note sul sapere del medico fino all'inizio del secolo XIII* (Milan, 1978), p. 62, n. 31.

[36] Wickersheimer, *Dictionnaire*, I, p. 144.

medical treatment. Very few of these were hospitals in anything approaching the modern sense. Only the monastic infirmaries isolated the sick from the healthy, and we know very little about how even they operated in the early Middle Ages. The idealized plan of St Gall (about 820) shows an elaborate complex, with housing for doctors and patients, along with a separate kitchen, baths, dispensary, herb garden, and room for bloodletting, but there is no evidence that it was ever built; not until the mid-eleventh century can we begin to trace in detail the construction of actual infirmaries in abbeys such as Cluny.[37] More common were the urban hospices (*xenodochia*) of Spain, Italy, and southern Gaul, that received the sick together with other needy elements of the lay population, notably widows, orphans, travellers, and the aged. An inheritance of the Christian Roman Empire, most offered only general nursing. A few, however, such as the guesthouse of Bishop Masona of Merida, employed doctors who, in the words of Paul the Deacon, 'searched the whole town and when they found a sick person, whether slave or free, Christian or Jew, carried him back to the hospital, laid him in a bed made up with mattress and sheets, prepared him delicate and abundant foods, and eventually, with the will of God, restored him to his former health'.[38] From the ninth century on, however, the monasteries assumed a central role in the care of the poor, and monastic hospitals became the main institutions serving the needy and the sick, particularly in northern Europe. Abbot Othmar of St Gall, for example, founded both a poor house and a hospital for lepers outside his cloister in the years around 830.[39]

The few leprosaria that existed before 1050 should not, however, be classified as hospitals, or indeed as medical institutions at all. From the fifth century on, bishops, abbots, and private individuals founded special houses for lepers, and by the twelfth century – the high-water mark of public concern with leprosy – about half of all new hospitals were of this kind.[40] But such institutions were charitable rather than therapeutic in intention. As early as the sixth century, a few communities had begun to pass laws requiring the expulsion of lepers, while others limited their

[37] Dieter Jetter, 'Klosterhospitäler: St Gallen, Cluny, Escorial', *Archiv für Geschichte der Medizin*, 62 (1978), 313–31; John D. Thompson and Grace Goldin, *The Hospital: A Social and Architectural History* (New Haven, 1975), ch. 1.

[38] Paul the Deacon, *De vita patrum emeritensium*, ch. 9, in Migne, *Patrologiae*, LXXX, col. 139; cited in MacKinney, *Early Medieval Medicine*, n. 100. See in general *ibid.*, n. 140, and especially Egon Boshof, 'Armenfürsorge im Frühmittelalter: Xenodochium, matricula, hospitale pauperum', *Vierteljahrschrift für sozial- und Wirtschaftsgeschichte*, 71 (1984), 158–60.

[39] Duft, *Notker*, p. 15, and in general Boshof, 'Armenfürsorge', pp. 163–74.

[40] Charles A. Mercier, *Leper Houses and Mediaeval Hospitals* (London, 1915), p. 12.

movement or forced them to carry special signs, such as a horn, a bell or a clapper. (Early medieval medical theory did not concern itself with contagion, and medieval society did not in general isolate the sick; such measures aimed to set lepers apart as foci of moral and ritual defilement rather than as threats to public health.)[41] Thus the founders of early leprosaria intended to supply their beneficiaries, who had been deprived of home and livelihood, with food and shelter rather than medical care.

And what of the other sick, the chronically ill who, like lepers, could not be helped either by their society's medical practitioners or by time itself? They formed the principal clientele, it turns out, for Fulbert's second type of healing, the 'heavenly' medicine of Christ, mediated almost invariably through his successors and imitators, the saints. The cult of the saints as healers flourished throughout the entire Middle Ages, as it still does today. From the beginning it had taken over many rituals and practices from the wonderworkers and healing sanctuaries of late Roman paganism, but it added several features of its own: with a few exceptions (individuals such as Bernard of Clairvaux in the twelfth century, for example, or the English and French kings who treated scrofula by the 'royal touch') saints did most of their work after death, through direct contact with their relics – their physical remains – or with the tomb that sheltered them. The cult of the saints in the early Middle Ages was in fact a cult of shrines and relics, and most of the miracles performed there were miracles of healing.[42]

Monks and chroniclers associated with certain shrines kept meticulous records of their miracles, and from these we know what kinds of illnesses the saints cured. With few exceptions we find no trace of epidemic or acute infections, only congenital or chronic disease. From shrine to shrine and from century to century, the pattern is remarkably constant, at least among adults; cripples and paralytics comprised the single largest group of those healed (generally about 50 per cent of all cures), followed by the deaf, mute and blind (about 15 to 20 per cent) and by the mad or the possessed (about 10 per cent).[43] The others suffered from a variety

---

[41] Richards, *Medieval Leper*, pp. 48–9; Jean Imbert, *Les hôpitaux en droit canonique* (Paris, 1947), p. 105. References to early foundations and legislation in Ingrid Busse, *Der Siechkobel St Johannis vor Nürnberg (1234 bis 1807)* (Nuremberg, 1974), pp. 8–18.

[42] Finucane, *Miracles and Pilgrims*, pp. 17–34; Pierre-André Sigal, *L'homme et le miracle dans la France médiévale, XIe–XIIe siècle* (Paris, 1985); *idem*, 'Maladie, pèlerinage et guérison au XIIe siècle', *Annales: Economies, sociétés, civilisations*, 24 (1969), 1522–39; Rousselle, 'Du sanctuaire au thaumaturge'.

[43] Sigal, *L'homme et miracle*, ch. 5; Finucane, *Miracles and Pilgrims*, p. 146; Michel Rouche, 'Miracles, maladies et psychologie de la foi à l'époque carolingienne en Francie', in *Hagiographie, culture et sociétés, IVe–XIIe siècles: Actes du Colloque organisé à Nanterre et à Paris (2–5 mai 1979)* (Paris,

of illnesses: tumors and skin diseases, for example, sterility and complications of childbirth, malaria and other recurrent fevers, long-standing haemorrhages and non-healing abscesses and wounds. Lepers figured only rarely in the miracle lists, apparently because, especially on the Continent, they were not admitted into the sanctuaries and shrines.[44]

Why these diseases in particular? The biblical model was certainly important – these were precisely the kinds of conditions cured by Christ in the gospels – but this merely throws the question back to an earlier period. The deeper reason lies in the practical logic of illness, economics, and daily life. During most of the Middle Ages, healing was thought to require direct contact with the saint's relics, usually by touching them, drinking wine or water in which they had been dipped, sleeping next to the tomb, or eating dirt scraped from the site. This almost always involved a journey, a pilgrimage, and pilgrimages of any length were expensive, inconvenient, and time-consuming in a period when travel was difficult and dangerous, and when the average European was desperately poor. Thus we find only the chronically and stably ill on the roads, together with their companions and attendants. The acutely ill were much more likely to consult doctors or lay healers in their own towns or villages, and most had doubtless died or recovered before deciding to take to the road.

Medieval accounts of miraculous healing present in fact a clearly defined 'hierarchy of resort', in which saints and their relics stood alongside home remedies and local medical practitioners. The saints were in general a measure of desperation; only when the other two had failed was a pilgrimage in order. There were, of course, exceptions. Local doctors might refuse to take on a particularly difficult or dangerous case, or the earthly remedy might seem more terrible than the disease. (Two examples appear in the twelfth-century account of the miracles of St Fiacre: a man with a gangrenous foot, who wanted to avoid amputation, and a noblewoman who brought her young son to St Fiacre for bladder stones, 'knowing that St Fiacre could heal without pain'.)[45] In general, however, Christians tried doctors before resorting to a saint and often returned to them afterward if the pilgrimage itself failed to yield permanent improvement – a common outcome, since many of the cures

1981), pp. 322, 337. On the somewhat different pattern for children see Eleanora C. Gordon, 'Child Health in the Middle Ages as Seen in the Miracles of Five English Saints, AD 1150–1120', *Bulletin of the History of Medicine*, 60 (1986), 502–22.   [44] Rouche, 'Miracles', p. 323.

[45] *Miracula beati Fiacrii*, ch. 20, in Jacques Dubois, *Un sanctuaire monastique au Moyen Age: Saint-Fiacre-en-Brie* (Paris/Geneva, 1976), p. 127.

claimed by monastic scribes were in fact ambiguous (delayed, temporary, gradual, or incomplete) and relapses were not by any means unknown.[46]

These practices guaranteed competition between lay practitioners and the monks who acted as caretakers of healing shrines and profitted from their traffic – a situation that accounts for much of the negative press medieval doctors have received both from medieval clerics, who are our sole sources for many aspects of life in this period, and from the modern historians that rely on them. Monastic chroniclers and hagiographers in fact used doctors to account for those many instances in which a trip to the shrine failed to produce a cure; if the patient did not recover or suffered a relapse on returning home, he or she had doubtless consulted an earthly doctor, a telltale sign of lack of faith. In order to be cured, claimed one well-informed French peasant, it was necessary to reject doctors and look only to the saint.[47]

But faith healing did not appeal only to peasants; it attracted the chronically ill from all classes and all walks of life.[48] Early medieval practice remained quite stable until the early fourteenth century, when a dramatic shift occurred in the cult of the saints. From about 1300 on, an increasing number of miracles began to happen without direct contact with relics, mediated instead by an image of the saint in question or by a vision or prayer. Furthermore, Christians began to make pilgrimages only after the miracle they had request materialized, rather than before. ('Don't you know,' said a blind doctor to his wife, who had pressed him to travel from Marseilles to sleep on the tomb of Louis of Anjou, 'that the power of the saint can help me here just as well as there, and awake just as well as asleep? You don't know what you're talking about and it's clear you don't have faith in the saint.')[49] The reasons for this change in spirituality are complicated, but the implications for miraculous healing are clear: if saints could heal at a distance, then they could be invoked by sufferers of acute as well as chronic disease. Furthermore, they – or rather their custodians, who were responsible for their cult and lived off its proceeds – could begin to specialize without reducing the pool of potential patients to the point where it was no longer lucrative. Indeed specialization became a positive attraction for patients who wanted to feel that they had placed their illness in the most capable hands. Thus

---

[46] Finucane, *Miracles and Pilgrims*, pp. 69–82.

[47] Sigal, *L'homme et le miracle*, p. 139.   [48] Finucane, *Miracles and Pilgrims*, ch. 8.

[49] *Liber miraculorum sancti Ludovici episcopi*, in *Analecta franciscana*, VII (Quaracchi, 1951), p. 310; see in general André Vauchez, *La sainteté en Occident aux derniers siècles du Moyen Age d'après les procès de canonisation et les documents hagiographiques* (Rome, 1981), pp. 507–40.

many saints rapidly became identified with particular diseases: St Sebastian with plague, for example, St Mathurin with mental illness, St John with epilepsy, and St Maur with gout.[50] This phenomenon, which was rare in the early Middle Ages and embraced only epidemic conditions such as ergotism (St Anthony) and leprosy (St Lazarus), mirrors the general trend toward complication and specialization in all of high and late medieval medicine.

The high and later Middle Ages: medical institutions and medical practice, 1050–1500

The medical system of the early Middle Ages, as we have seen, was fluid and undifferentiated. The boundaries between the different kinds of healers remained blurred and indistinct. This fluidity echoed the lack of specialized medical institutions. The bodies that trained or employed experts in healing – the urban hospices of Mediterranean Europe, for example, the monasteries and courts – were not exclusively or even primarily medical in orientation; their medical functions were part of a much broader social and cultural life. This situation began to change in the late eleventh century, and the succeeding centuries saw two main developments: the growth of a more differentiated, stratified, and well-defined body of medical practitioners, with clear, if variable, standards and procedures for training, licensing, and practice (the process often referred to as nascent professionalization); and the emergence of specialized medical institutions such as medical faculties with set curricula, guilds and colleges for medical personnel, public doctors, and hospitals for the sick.

These changes formed part of the general transformation of western European society and culture in the years after 1050, a transformation that hinged on the revival of a commercial economy and an urban civilization for the first time since the disintegration of the Roman world.[51] This 'urban revolution' created a new social environment for the theory and practice of medicine. The growth of the population and its concentration in cities produced an increasing demand for medical services, and the relative prosperity of urban society made that demand effective. The result was an expanding market, both public and private, for medical services.[52] The new forms of medical organization had their

---

[50] Erik von Kraemer, *Les maladies désignées par le nom d'un saint* (Helsingfors, 1949).
[51] See Cipolla, *Before the Industrial Revolution*, chs. 1–8, and Cipolla (ed.), *Fontana Economic History*, I.   [52] See Cipolla, *Before the Industrial Revolution*, pp. 83–5.

roots in this same dynamic urban world, and they reflected a general tendency toward increasing institutional sophistication, specialization, and division of labour. Although we can see these developments in many different regions, they appeared first and most clearly in northern Italy, which remained in many ways a model for medical order and medical institutions throughout high and late medieval Europe.[53]

To begin with the medical practitioners themselves, the period after about 1050 witnessed two processes that were to transform the practice of medicine. The first was a series of moves to limit the number and variety of healers by excluding certain groups from legitimate medical practice; the second was a process of differentiation among the practitioners themselves. Indications of the former appear in the *Regimen of Health*, or *Flower of Medicine*, a long and influential poem produced at Salerno sometime after the middle of the thirteenth century. In a section called *Medicaster* the author inveighed against a colourful list of false doctors: 'The unlettered, the empiric, the Jew, the monk, the actor, the barber, the old woman – each pretends to be a doctor, as does the alchemist, the maker of cosmetics, the bathkeeper, the forger, the oculist. While they seek profit, the power of medicine suffers.'[54]

These were not merely the private grumblings of a discontented doctor; from the eleventh century on, religious and secular authorities moved to bar particular groups – including several mentioned above – from studying or practising certain kinds of medicine. These campaigns varied in their motives and their success. Most effective was the one to limit the medical role of the clergy, who had played such an important part in the theory and practice of early medieval medicine. Beginning in the 1130s, as part of the movement to reform the monastic orders and

[53] The following account relies heavily on several recent regional studies: for England, Edward J. Kealey, *Medieval Medicus: A Social History of Anglo-Norman Medicine* (Baltimore, 1981), and Talbot and Hammond, *Medical Practitioners*; for France, Jacquart, *Le milieu médical en France du XIIe au XVe siècle, en annexe 2e supplément au 'Dictionnaire' d'Ernest Wickersheimer* (Geneva, 1981); and for Italy, Katharine Park, *Doctors and Medicine in Early Renaissance Florence* (Princeton, 1985). Luis Garcia Ballester, Michael R. McVaugh and Agustin Rubio Vela, 'Medical Licensing and Learning in Fourteenth-Century Valencia', *Transactions of the American Philosophical Society*, 80 (1990) appeared too recently for me to consult. Another fundamental survey is Vern Bullough, *The Development of Medicine as a Profession: The Contribution of the Medieval University to Modern Medicine* (Basel/New York, 1966). I have also consulted Robert S. Gottfried, *Doctors and Medicine in Medieval England, 1340–1530* (Princeton, NJ, 1986), which should be used with care; see the critical essay review by Faye Marie Getz, 'Medieval English Medicine', *Bulletin of the History of Medicine*, 61 (1987), pp. 455–61.

[54] *Flos medicinae*, vv, 3472–6, in Salvatore de Renzi (ed.), *Collectio salernitana*, 5 vols. (Naples, 1852–9), v, p. 103: 'Fingit se Medicum quivis idiota, prophanus,/ Iudaeus, monachus, histrio, rasor, anus,/ Sicuti Alchemista Medicus fit aut Saponista,/ Aut balneator, falsarius aut oculista./ Hic dum lucra quaerit, virtus in arte perit.'

recall them to their original spiritual mission, various church councils issued a series of rulings prohibiting certain clerics from studying medicine 'for temporal gain', and later from performing surgery involving cutting or burning. These decrees produced a gradual but significant decline in the numbers of secular clergy and, especially, monks involved in practice both inside and outside the monasteries. By the mid-fourteenth century, most monasteries called in lay doctors to look after their members – a direct reversal of earlier practices, when monks had left their monasteries to care for the lay community.[55] These measures also ended the leading role played by monks in the study and diffusion of classical medical texts; from the thirteenth century on, that role was primarily assumed by scholars and teachers in the universities.

The church was less successful in its attempts to ban Jews from treating Christians. Beginning around 1100, prohibitions of Jewish practice appeared in canon law, reiterated by various ecclesiastical councils throughout the thirteenth and early fourteenth centuries. The prestige of Jewish doctors, however, and the growing demand for them by prominent individuals, including the popes themselves, undercut these bans, and Jews remained active in many parts of Europe until at least 1500.[56]

The impetus to exclude Jews and the clergy from medical practice was primarily religious and clerical, although these efforts were doubtless seconded by lay Christian doctors, who welcomed the opportunity to eliminate unwelcome competition. The case of female practitioners is more complicated. Some historians have argued that the high and later Middle Ages saw a successful campaign to eliminate women from the practice of medicine by prosecuting them for malpractice or unlicensed practice – the most notorious example being the trial of Jacqueline Felicie in 1322.[57] It seems, however, that the primary target of these cases was not women *per se*, but rather empirical and unlicensed practice in general, which happened to be the area in which women were the most

[55] Dawtry '*Methodus Medendi*', pp. 35–7; Jacquart, *Milieu médical*, pp. 150–9, 259. See Darrel W. Amundsen, 'Medieval Canon Law on Medical and Surgical Practice by the Clergy', *Bulletin of the History of Medicine*, 52 (1978), esp. pp. 28–38.

[56] Harry Friedenwald, *The Jews and Medicine: Essays*, 2 vols. (Baltimore, 1944), essays XIII, XIV, XLI, and XLII, esp. pp. 556–72; Joseph Shatzmiller, 'Notes sur les médecins juifs en Provence au Moyen Age', *Revue des Etudes Juives*, 28 (1969), 259–66; Jacquart, *Milieu médical*, pp. 160–7; Park, *Doctors and Medicine*, pp. 72–5; Siraisi, *Medieval and Early Renaissance Medicine*, pp. 29–31.

[57] John H. Benton, 'Trotula, Women's Problems, and the Professionalization of Medicine in the Middles Ages', *Bulletin of the History of Medicine*, 59 (1985), 30–53. On Jacqueline's trial see Pearl Kibre, 'The Faculty of Medicine at Paris, Charlatanism and Unlicensed Medical Practice in the Later Middle Ages', *Bulletin of the History of Medicine*, 27 (1953), pp. 8–12.

active. In other words the basic issue was training and licensing rather than gender, as doctors in the universities and guilds acted to exclude their socially and politically more marginal competitors; women, the most marginal group of all, were, as one writer has recently put it, 'caught in the crossfire'.[58]

The war over medical practice in the high and later Middle Ages centred on two disputed issues: what standards were appropriate for licensing and practice, and who was to establish and enforce them. The struggle was not unique to medicine. The same period saw the rise of guilds and other protective associations governing almost every urban occupation above the menial level, from carpentry to university teaching; all aimed to reduce competition by monopolizing and limiting access to their trades.[59] The conflict over medicine, however, was unusually intense because of the variety of approaches to healing and the social diversity of medieval healers – neither at issue, for example, among carpenters. The timing and results of this conflict were predictably mixed, varying from region to region and from city to city, but in general the principal types of practitioners ended by forming separate trade organizations (or occasionally separate subgroups within an umbrella guild) and setting their own standards. This worked to structure and stratify the world of medical practice, as socially and politically more powerful groups attempted, with varying success, to dominate and control lesser ones. Within the interstices of these conflicting groups, however, casual and unauthorised practitioners continued to flourish, sometimes to the pained dismay of the more established doctors.

By the middle of the thirteenth century, the battles over training and licensing had two main centres, universities and trade companies or guilds. The university (*studium generale*), which came to dominate European education in the thirteenth century, was the successor to the monastic and cathedral school; unlike the schools, it offered instruction in a wide range of subjects, an established curriculum, and a recognizable (if variable) set of degrees intended to guarantee a certain level of knowledge in the subject in question. Building on the intellectual legacy of the school of Salerno, medicine quickly became part of this system of higher education; by 1300 the universities of Bologna, Padua,

[58] Monica Green, 'Women's Medical Practice and Medical Care in Medieval Europe,' *Signs*, 14 (1989), 447.
[59] See Silvia L. Thrupp, 'The Gilds', in M. M. Postan and H. J. Habakkuk (eds.), *The Cambridge Economic History of Europe*, 7 vols. (Cambridge, 1941–78), III, ch. 5.

Montpellier, and Paris had emerged as the main centres of academic medical study, their curricula standardized and ratified in the early fourteenth century by the pope.[60]

The medical faculties based their claims to authority over all medical practice – including the activities of many people who had never owned a book, far less a university degree – on their contention that medicine in its highest form was not a mechanical skill, but an intellectual discipline, allied with philosophy and grounded in scientific and theoretical principles. (This does not mean, however, that medieval academic medicine was entirely a theoretical and bookish subject; medical professors, unlike the early medieval medical scholars, were invariably practising doctors, and they offered their students, particularly in the Italian universities, clinical training as well as exercise in disputation.)[61] The theoretical principles of medicine, like much of its practice, were grounded in the works of the Greek authors Galen and Hippocrates and of their Arabic followers, many of which had been translated into Latin, the language of the European scholarly community, beginning in the late eleventh century.[62] This enormous increase in medical learning, far beyond the limited texts of the early Middle Ages, fuelled the ambitions and self-confidence of academically trained doctors and buttressed their claims to dominate and regulate other practitioners.

For the most part, however, these claims remained wishful thinking. Except in Italy, where surgery became part of the university curriculum, academic medicine was limited to *physica*, the branch of medicine that based its therapeutics on diet and medication (thereby corresponding roughly to what we call internal medicine), and even in Italy only a tiny proportion of surgeons attended universities or received degrees.[63] Throughout most of Europe, university-trained doctors represented a

[60] See Bullough, *Development of Medicine*, chs. 3–4; Charles Talbot, 'Medical Education in the Middle Ages', in C. D. O'Malley (ed.), *The History of Medical Education* (Berkeley, 1970), pp. 73–87; Siraisi, *Medieval and Early Renaissance Medicine*, ch. 3.

[61] Luke Demaitre, 'Theory and Practice in Medical Education at the University of Montpellier in the Thirteenth and Fourteenth Centuries', *Journal of the History of Medicine*, 30 (1975), 103–23; Park, *Doctors and Medicine*, p. 61.

[62] Marie-Thérèse d'Alverny, 'Translations and Translators', in Robert L. Benson and Giles Constable (eds.), *Renaissance and Renewal in the Twelfth Century* (Cambridge, MA, 1982), esp. pp. 422–6, 453, and bibliography regarding medical translations on pp. 461–2. See also Agrimi and Crisciani, *Medicina del corpo*, pp. 24–36, and Nancy Siraisi, *Taddeo Alderotti and his Pupils: Two Generations of Italian Medical Learning* (Princeton, 1981), ch. 5. On academic medicine in general, Nancy Siraisi, 'Some Recent Work on Western European Medical Learning, ca. 1200–ca. 1500', *History of Universities*, 2 (1982), 226–38; Siraisi, *Medieval and Early Renaissance Medicine*, ch. 6.

[63] Tiziana Pesenti Marangon, '"Professores chirugie", "medici ciroici" et "barbitonsores" a Padova nell'età di Leonardo Buffi da Bertipaglia (+dopo il 1448)', *Quaderni per la storia dell'università di Padova*, 11 (1978), 1–38; Park, *Doctors and Medicine*, pp. 65–6.

small minority of medical practitioners, and their attempts to control practice met with scant success, except in university strongholds such as Bologna and Paris.[64] However, if the rise of medicine as a university discipline did not suffice to establish medicine as a learned profession, restricted to or dominated by those with academic training, it nonetheless changed the shape of the body of European healers, creating a professional elite of university-trained physicians, and establishing a growing gap between practitioners educated at the university and those trained outside.

In contrast to the relative social and professional homogeneity of academic physicians, this latter group was extraordinarily diverse. Even excluding casual healers – neighbours, friends, and family – it embraced a number of different kinds of practitioners: general surgeons, who treated wounds, sores, abscesses, fractures, and other external disorders of the skin and members; barbers or barber-surgeons, who in addition to shaving and cutting hair, performed minor operations, including bleeding and cupping, applying leeches, and pulling teeth; apothecaries, who sold various compound medicines as well as their ingredients and who offered medical advice on the side; empirics, who often specialized in treating a single surgical condition, such as fractures, cataracts, or hernias; and professional midwives, who appear in city records only in the thirteenth century.[65] While empirics and midwives were usually self-taught or informally trained by friends or family members, surgeons, barbers, and apothecaries normally underwent a formal apprenticeship, occasionally supplemented for surgeons, at least toward the end of the Middle Ages, by university lectures. In some places, midwives were licensed and regulated by the local church, although many, like many empirics, must have practised without authority. Surgeons, barbers, and apothecaries generally fell under the jurisdiction of their municipal 'college' or guild.

For most non-university-trained doctors, therefore – and for many academically educated physicians as well – the guild was the formal organization that licensed them, often after examining them for

[64] Kibre, 'The Faculty of Medicine'. Estimates of the proportion of university educated practitioners range from roughly a third, in late medieval Florence, to well under 10 per cent, in sixteenth-century England; see Park, *Doctors and Medicine*, p. 75, and Pelling and Webster, 'Medical Practitioners', pp. 188, 225.

[65] Michel Salvat, 'L'accouchement dans la littérature scientifique médiévale', in *L'enfant au Moyen Age* (*Sénéfiance*, 9) (Paris, 1980), pp. 92; Green, 'Women's Medical Practice'; Vern L. Bullough, 'Training of the Nonuniversity-Educated Medical Practitioners in the Later Middle Ages', *Journal of the History of Medicine*, 14 (1959), 446–58; Pelling and Webster, 'Medical Practitioners', pp. 175–80, 233–4.

competence, and regulated their practice. It is difficult to generalize about medical guilds in the later Middle Ages, given the extent to which conditions varied from city to city. In some, such as Florence, all medical practitioners, including physicians, matriculated in a single guild, which might embrace many other occupations; in others, such as Paris and London, each group had its own guild or other corporation.[66] In some cities, the various groups jockeyed for pre-eminence, while in others they coexisted in relative harmony. It is wrong, however, to project later conditions back on the earlier period and to assume that university-educated physicians necessarily succeeded in imposing their authority on other practitioners; except in a few university towns, the guild predominated over the medical faculty through at least the fifteenth century, and physicians often met with strong and effective resistance by barbers and surgeons, who significantly outnumbered them, and by apothecaries, who formed part of the merchant elite that dominated many municipal governments. Meanwhile, casual healers, midwives, and unlicensed practitioners continued their work in city and country-side, largely undisturbed by the political struggles of the medical elites.

By 1500, therefore, although far from homogeneous, the body of Europe's urban medical practitioners was more structured than during the early Middle Ages. Organized to some extent by medical speciality, it had had some success in edging out more marginal healers – clerics and, more recently, women and Jews – and constituting itself as largely lay, Christian, and (with the exception of midwives) male. (Practice in the countryside and smaller towns, as always, was more archaic in character.)[67] Throughout most of the high medieval period, the different types of practitioners identified only minimally with one another, despite clear bonds of solidarity within each group.

Over the course of the later Middle Ages, however, there are signs of an emergent professional culture shared by at least some of the various groups of practitioners. The culture of academic medicine, long the monopoly of the university educated, gradually found its way out into broader society; the medical faculties, even in northern Europe, began to offer occasional courses of lectures for surgeons and barbers, while Latin medical works were increasingly translated into the vernacular and disseminated through the new medium of printing, thus mediating

---

[66] Park, *Doctors and Medicine*, ch. 1; Jacquart, *Milieu médical*, p. 266; Gottfried, *Doctors and Medicine*, ch. 1.

[67] See, for example, James K. Mustain, 'A Rural Medical Practitioner in Fifteenth Century England', *Bulletin of the History of Medicine*, 46 (1972), 469–76.

between academic learning and more popular practice.[68] These changes formed part of a broader process of standardization in approaches to healing. As we have already seen, much of early medieval medicine, even in its most learned form, combined prayers and incantations with more naturalistic remedies. During the later Middle Ages, however, these methods were increasingly divorced, as officially recognized practitioners, incorporated in university and guild, made naturalism in healing one of the touchstones of their claims to monopoly and competence. (This did not exclude the use of occult and magical remedies, which fell within the natural realm and were often used by learned physicians.) In 1382, for example, Roger Clerk was prosecuted for malpractice after attempting to cure an old woman with a charm on parchment and several prayers; convicted as illiterate and an 'infidel', he was sentenced to be paraded through London with the offending parchment, two urinals, and a whetstone around his neck.[69] In this way, appeals to supernatural forces gradually became a hallmark of the illegitimate practitioner or the charlatan, at least in the eyes of city authorities.

This does not mean, of course, that doctors or their patients denied the efficacy of religious healing; like their predecessors, they continued to seek divine aid for illnesses that did not respond to normal treatment. Bernard Gordon's entry on scrofula, for example, which the divinely anointed French and English monarchs had long claimed to cure, clearly articulates this hierarchy of resort. The illustrious fourteenth-century professor advised his students to treat the condition first with diet and then with medication and surgery. Only if these methods did not succeed, he counselled, 'let us go to the kings'.[70] Like Bernard, however, most officially recognized doctors expected that God would channel his healing power not through a gaggle of self-styled healers but through his duly appointed ministers and through clearly recognizable saints, while their own medical cures drew entirely on physical remedies and natural causes.

Religious healers evidently continued to serve all levels of society in

---

[68] Linda E. Voigts, 'Medical Prose', in A. S. G. Edwards (ed.), *Middle English Prose* (New Brunswick, NJ, 1984), pp. 315–35; Paul Slack, 'Mirrors of Health and Treasures of Poor Men: The Uses of the Vernacular Medical Literature of Tudor England', in Webster (ed.), *Health, Medicine and Mortality*, ch. 7.

[69] Vern L. Bullough, 'The Term "Doctor"', *Journal of the History of Medicine*, 18 (1963), pp. 285–6.

[70] Luke Demaitre, *Doctor Bernard de Gordon: Professor and Practitioner* (Toronto, 1980), p. 149. See in general Park, *Doctors and Medicine*, pp. 48–52.

the high and later Middle Ages. This was less true of natural medicine. As late as the sixteenth century in London, for example, most inhabitants' 'contact with official medicine would have been limited to the lower echelons of the Barber-Surgeons' Company, to poorer apothecaries, and to midwives'.[71] Learned physicians, on the other hand, possessed a social and cultural cachet; disproportionately represented in the entourages of popes, kings, and the higher nobles, they assiduously cultivated and were cultivated by the wealthy urban families that could afford their substantial fees. The stratification by class was not absolute, however. The social elites called on surgeons, barbers, midwives, and empirical specialists when they required their particular services, and the middle orders and the poor had access to university-educated physicians in parts of Europe other than England, where medical institutions were more developed and physicians thicker on the ground.

In general, the period after about 1250 produced specialized institutions and strategies devoted not only to overseeing the licensing and practice of doctors but also to monitoring the health of the population as a whole and to providing medical care to a broader clientele than could otherwise afford it. The central and northern Italian city-states were the earliest and most active in this respect, but a number of their initiatives – notably the state-salaried doctor, the hospital for the sick poor, and the public health board – eventually spread to other parts of Europe. The motives behind these developments were complicated. They combined obvious social and economic interests with a public and private commitment to Christian charity, a growing sense of the state's responsibilities towards its citizens, and a new perception (rooted largely in the recurring epidemics of plague after 1348) of the poor as carriers of contagion and disease. These forces produced a variety of experiments and institutions designed to mediate between doctor and patient and to defray the costs of health care in a way that benefited all parties involved.

Not all of these practices and institutions served the indigent. In Italy, for example, and possibly elsewhere in Europe – research on the practice of pharmacy in this period is practically non-existent – the apothecary's shop emerged as the main centre of community medical practice.[72] From at least the mid-fourteenth century, apothecaries employed doctors, most of them university-trained physicians, to see patients in their shops,

---

[71] Pelling and Webster, 'Medical Practitioners', p. 182.
[72] Richard Palmer, 'Pharmacy in the Republic of Venice in the Sixteenth Century', in A. Wear, R. K. French and I. M. Lonie (eds.), *The Medical Renaissance of the Sixteenth Century* (Cambridge, 1985), p. 105.

offsetting part or all of their fees to individual clients – a cheaper and more convenient alternative to the house call. In addition, especially toward the end of the fifteenth century, religious confraternities and other fraternal organizations began to hire doctors to provide free medical treatment to their members, along with other social services such as burial or illness benefits. Other institutions, including monasteries and convents, also salaried doctors to attend their members and employees.[73]

In addition to these private arrangements, various public authorities subsidized the medical care of their citizens. From the early thirteenth century on, Italian communes began to employ doctors not only to treat soldiers, prisoners, and condemned criminals, but also to attend their other inhabitants, especially the poor; this practice later spread northward to France, Switzerland, and Germany, where the emperor Sigismund in 1436 required all towns to hire a town physician.[74] Like most medical institutions in this period, the office of municipal doctor assumed many forms according to local resources and needs. Although some cities hired surgeons, barbers, or empirics, many town doctors were physicians trained at the university, and some were rising stars in their profession, later going on to serve at princely courts.

The most important institution evolved in this period to broaden access to medical care was the hospital for the sick poor. During the early Middle Ages, as we have already seen, hospitals were small – rarely accommodating more than fifteen or twenty people – and they usually functioned as general hospices for the needy, including pilgrims and travellers as well as the homeless, the sick, and the infirm. During the high and later Middle Ages, however, pious Christians founded many new hospitals, most in the renascent cities. Some of these began to specialize in the treatment of the sick, developing an impressive set of medical strategies and practices.[75]

In his *History of the West*, written about 1225, Jacques de Vitry described these new foundations:

Both male and female communities, having renounced the world, live under a rule in leproseries or hospitals for the poor – of which there are untold numbers

---

[73] Park, *Doctors and Medicine*, pp. 99–100, 106–10.
[74] Nutton, 'Continuity or Rediscovery?', pp. 26–34; Park, *Doctors and Medicine*, pp. 87–94; Jacquart, *Milieu médical*, pp. 131–7.
[75] See in general the chapters by Michel Mollat in Jean Imbert (ed.), *Histoire des hôpitaux en France* (Toulouse, 1982), chs. 2–3 (bibliography on pp. 529–31); Kealey, *Medieval Medicine*, chs. 4–5; Jesko von Steynitz, *Mittelalterliche Hospitäler der Orden und städte als Einrichtung der sozialen Sicherung* (Berlin, 1970); Thompson and Goldin, *The Hospital*.

in the West – humbly devoted to serving the sick and the poor...Men and women live and eat separately, in modesty and chastity. Day and night, they observe the canonical offices, insofar as their commitment to hospitality and their ministry to the poor permits.[76]

Some of these communities were independent, while others belonged to one of the various hospital orders founded in this period, including the Knights of St John (later known as the Hospitallers) and the orders of the Holy Spirit and of St Anthony, which was established to care for victims of ergotism (St Anthony's fire).[77] In the early fourteenth century, a few of the new foundations began to reject the incurables that had made up the bulk of their clients, in order to specialize in the care of the acutely ill, joined in some institutions by young children and pregnant women. (The initial impetus seems to have come from Islamic and Byzantine models, transmitted through the rule of the Knights of St John.)[78] These institutions varied enormously from region to region and from town to town, but some, particularly in Italy, developed impressive medical organizations.

Most of the larger medical hospitals for the sick employed at least one xdoctor – and in many cases both a physician and a surgeon – as well as auxiliary personnel such as midwives, barbers, and apothecaries.[79] By the late fifteenth century, some were separating patients with different illnesses, often providing special rooms for the mentally ill and those requiring intensive care, and isolating those with contagious skin diseases. In the most advanced hospitals, such as Santa Maria Nuova in Florence, doctors saw each patient daily and prescribed individual treatment and medication, all provided free of charge. These doctors often came from the highest ranks of the profession, attracted both by the range of medical experience offered by the hospitals and by the opportunity to gain merit by aiding the poor. In 1434, for example, the city consuls of Lyon took this situation for granted, censuring several hospitals where the sick were 'treated by ignorant hospital brothers, superstitious monks,

[76] Jacques de Vitry, *The Historia occidentalis of Jacques de Vitry*, ed. J. F. Hinnebusch (Fribourg, 1972), ch. 39; see A.-M. Bonenfant-Feynman, 'Les organisations hospitalières vues par Jacques de Vitry (1225)', *Annales de la Société Belge d'Histoire des Hôpitaux*, 18 (1980), 17–45.

[77] Timothy S. Miller, 'The Knights of Saint John and the Hospitals of the Italian West', *Speculum*, 53 (1978), 709–33; Adalbert Mischlewski, *Grundzüge der Geschichte des Antoniterordens bis zum Ausgang des 15. Jahrhunderts* (Cologne, 1976); Chaumartin, *Mal des ardents*.

[78] Miller, 'The Knights of Saint John', pp. 719–23. See also Michael W. Dols, 'The Origins of the Islamic Hospital: Myth and Reality', *Bulletin of the History of Medicine*, 61 (1987), 367–90.

[79] Jacquart, *Milieu médical*, pp. 127–31; Mollat in Imbert, *Histoire des hôpitaux*, ch. 3; K. Park, 'The Renaissance Hospital', *FMR*, no. 8 (Jan./Feb. 1985), pp. 132–3; K. Park, 'Healing the poor: Hospitals and Medicine in Renaissance Florence', in Jonathan Barry and Colin Jones (eds.), *Medicine and Charity* (London, 1991).

empirics, or self-proclaimed sorcerors,' and 'languished and died for lack of real doctors.'[80]

It is difficult to reconstruct daily life inside the hospitals and to estimate mortality rates. But surviving records indicate that the late medieval hospital was not necessarily a way-station to the cemetery. Death rates in the hospitals that took in young children or accepted chronically ill and infirm patients were high, as one would expect. In some late fifteenth-century and sixteenth-century institutions for the acutely ill, however, discharge rates approached 90 per cent.[81] In addition to mild herbal medication, the best hospitals provided their patients good and abundant food, warmth, and rest in clean beds – the preoccupation with hygiene was considerable – as well as round-the-clock nursing and simple surgery, and their patients responded, as the acutely ill frequently do, by getting well.

Although medieval hospitals originated as charitable institutions, intended to alleviate the suffering of the sick and the poor, they gradually acquired another set of functions having to do with public health, as municipal authorities began to incorporate them into a broader programme of public hygiene focused on the prevention of epidemic disease. Epidemics were the bane of the late medieval city; dysentery, smallpox, influenza, typhus, and plague spread rapidly in the dirty and crowded urban quarters, exacting a heavy periodic toll in lives and suffering. In the thirteenth century, many city governments began to take systematic measures to deal with this threat to public order and public health. Drawing on contemporary medical theory, which blamed the spread of most epidemic diseases on fetid and corrupted air, they passed laws governing the disposal of wastes, the cleaning of streets and sewers, and the practice of trades such as butchery, tanning, and dying that polluted the water and produced foul smells.[82]

Public measures against leprosy, thought to spread through human contact, had a somewhat different thrust.[83] Although the separation of

[80] Nicole Gonthier, 'Les hôpitaux et les pauvres à la fin du Moyen Age; l'exemple de Lyon', Le Moyen Age, 84 (1978), 304. On Santa Maria Nuova, K. Park and John Henderson '"The First Hospital among Christians": the Ospedale di Santa Maria Nuova in Early Sixteenth-Century Florence', Medical History, 35 (1991).

[81] Park, 'The Renaissance Hospital', p. 133, drawing on records from two Florentine hospitals.

[82] Lynn Thorndike, 'Sanitation, Baths and Street-Cleaning in the Middle Ages', Speculum, 3 (1928), 192–203; Arlette Higounet-Nadal, 'Hygiène, salubrité, pollutions au Moyen Age: l'exemple de Périgueux', Annales de Démographie Historique (1975), pp. 81–86; Carmichael, Plague and the Poor, pp. 96–8; and in general George Rosen, A History of Public Health (New York, 1958), ch. 3.

[83] On leprosy in general, Richards, Medieval Leper; Saul Nathaniel Brody, The Disease of the Soul: Leprosy in Medieval Literature (Ithaca, NY, 1974); and Albert Bourgeois, Lépreux et maladreries

the leper seems to have sprung initially from ritual rather than medical concerns, the thirteenth century and early fourteenth century increasingly interpreted leprosy as contagious, and cities began to revise their statutes to prevent physical contact between the sick and the well. Although the isolation of lepers was never as universal or absolute as is often portrayed, it became more common after 1300 for cities to require citizens to denounce suspected lepers, to appoint juries of doctors or other lepers to examine them, and to expel victims or intern them in hospitals or small communities outside the city walls.[84]

It was the appearance of plague in 1348, however, and its periodic return throughout the later fourteenth and fifteenth centuries, that crystallized the concern with public health. The mortality rates in the first epidemics were appalling – up to half of the population of some cities died in 1348 – and they inspired new and more stringent strategies against epidemic disease. At first, city governments merely resurrected traditional measures, reiterating prohibitions against dirt and odors and appointing temporary committees of officials to enforce them. Increasingly, however, they resorted to novel means. In Italy, where the organization of public health, like that of medical practice, was most developed, these temporary committees evolved into permanent magistracies, charged with overseeing moral as well as physical hygiene.[85] Some cities compiled 'books of the dead', comprehensive mortality records, in order to identify epidemics and follow their course. Above all, since they were convinced very early that plague was contagious, they began to elaborate new techniques for isolating the sick. The initial measures were defensive, requiring relatives to destroy the clothing and effects of the dead, controlling burials and visits to the sick, and imposing restrictions on travel and trade with infected areas. By the fifteenth century, however, Italian cities were experimenting with more active and selective measures, placing ships and travellers under regular quarantine for observation and establishing special isolation hospitals for victims of plague. Some built new hospitals for the purpose, while others converted older hospitals, including leprosaria, left conveniently empty

---

du Pas-de-Calais, Xe–XVIIIe siècles (Arras, 1972). On leper hospitals in particular: Imbert, *Les hôpitaux en droit canonique*, pp. 149–95; Mollat in Imbert (ed.), *Histoire des hôpitaux*, pp. 36–47; Kealey *Medieval Medicus*, pp. 101–4. Danielle Jacquart and Claude Thomasset, *Sexuality and Medicine in the Middle Ages* (Princeton, NJ, 1988), pp. 183–8.

[84] Regulations in Léon Le Grand, *Statuts d'Hôtels-Dieu et de léproseries: recueil de textes du XIIe au XIVe siècle* (Paris, 1901), pp. 181–252. See also Luke Demaitre, 'The Descriptions and Diagnosis of Leprosy by Fourteenth-Century Physicians', *Bulletin of the History of Medicine*, 59 (1985), 327–44.

[85] Carlo M. Cipolla, *Public Health and the Medical Profession in the Renaissance* (Cambridge, 1976), ch. 1; Carmichael, *Plague and the Poor*, ch. 5, with many references.

by the rapid retreat of leprosy in recent years. It took much longer for similar measures to appear in northern Europe, where the municipal reactions to plague tended to reflect the earlier hygienic approach.[86]

Michel Foucault has argued that as leprosy declined over the course of the fifteenth century, a casualty of better living conditions and shifting disease patterns, another group began to move into the physical and moral space previously occupied by lepers. These new 'ritual exiles' were the insane. Originally venerated for their special vision and allowed to wander from town to town, the mentally ill were increasingly shut up and shut in.[87] Foucault describes the general shift in attitudes evocatively, but his explanations for it are less convincing. Insanity had never been primarily a moral category. Unlike leprosy, it had long been integrated into the medical order and treated as a physical state with moral ramifications rather than the reverse. Even in the early Middle Ages, doctors and lay writers alike drew a clear distinction between the insane (furiosi) and the possessed (demoniaci); by the thirteenth century, even borderline moral and spiritual conditions such as acedia, or sloth, were solidly embedded in medical discussions.[88] Doctors identified most mental disorders as diseases of the brain and their treatments included standard medical procedures, such as medication to restore humoral imbalance, purgation, phlebotomy, and occasional trephination.

Unlike leprosy again, insanity was not considered contagious. It is for this reason that we find the insane not only in general medieval hospices, where lepers were never admitted, but also, beginning in the later Middle Ages, in the new specialized hospitals for the sick.[89] The violent or disruptive were often separated from other patients, as were, for

[86] Sylvette Guilbert, 'A Châlons-sur-Marne au XVe siècle; un conseil municipal face aux épidémies', Annales: Economies, sociétés, civilisations, 23 (1968), pp. 1289–96.

[87] Michel Foucault, Madness and Civilization: A History of Insanity in the Age of Reason, trans. Richard Howard (New York, 1965), ch. 1.

[88] Stanley W. Jackson, 'Acedia the Sin and its Relationship to Sorrow and Melancholia in Medieval Times', Bulletin of the History of Medicine, 55 (1981), 172–85; and in general Judith Neaman, Suggestion of the Devil: the Origins of Madness (Garden City, NY, 1975), ch. 1; Stanley W. Jackson, 'Unusual Mental States in Medieval Europe, I: Medical Syndromes of Mental Disorder', Journal of the History of Medicine, 27 (1972), pp. 262–97; see also H. C. Erik Midelfort's critique of Foucault, 'Madness and Civilization in Early Modern Europe: A Reappraisal of Michel Foucault', in Barbara C. Malament (ed.), After the Reformation: Essays in Honor of J. H. Hexter (Philadelphia, 1980), pp. 247–65.

[89] See in general George Rosen, 'The Mentally Ill and the Community in Western and Central Europe during the Late Middle Ages and the Renaissance', Journal of the History of Medicine, 19 (1964), 377–88; idem, Madness in Society: Chapters in the Historical Sociology of Mental Illness (London, 1968), ch. 4; Dieter Jetter, Grundzüge der Geschichte des Irrenhauses (Darmstadt, 1981); Patricia Allderidge, 'Hospitals, Madhouses and Asylums: Cycles in the Care of the Insane', British Journal of Psychiatry, 134 (1979), 312–24; Rotha Maria Clay, The Medieval Hospitals of England (London, 1909), ch. 3.

example, those with head wounds or communicable skin conditions, but this was a practical measure rather than a serious attempt at moral or physical isolation. Like other hospital patients and unlike the inmates of leprosaria, the mentally ill were treated by hospital doctors, and they were generally expected to recover: the statute of Holy Trinity hospital, for example, in late fourteenth-century Salisbury, allowed them to stay 'until they come to their sense'.[90] If neither their families nor local hospitals could accommodate them, they were interned in cages – in late medieval Nuremberg it was possible to rent one from the city magistrates – and in jails.

In other words, the general problem posed by insanity was one of public order and social welfare rather than public health. This problem concerned not insanity *per se*, but one particular group of insane, the chronically ill poor. Being poor, they lacked families with the space and the resources to care for them at home. Being chronically ill – the usual term was 'incurable' – they were excluded from many hospitals for the sick, which increasingly admitted only the acutely ill. Beginning in the fifteenth century we see a general and growing preoccupation on the part of city authorities and charitable associations with chronic illness among the poor. The reasons for this were complicated, involving both a new fear of the homeless and rootless as threats to public health and social order, and a genuine concern for their plight. In some areas, such as northern Italy, the principal catalyst seems to have been the arrival of syphilis in the 1490s, which focused lay attention on chronic disease just as the plague had done for acute illness.[91] Moved by these considerations, individuals and municipalities began to found large and specialized hospitals for the incurably ill. Some were general institutions, while others admitted only particular groups: the blind, syphilitics, epileptics, the insane. Thus the early fifteenth century saw the creation of the first new hospitals for the mentally ill, in Valencia and Seville. During the same period a few pre-existing general hospitals such as St Mary's Bethlehem, in England, also began to make a speciality of the insane, while a different type of institution, centred on home care, grew up

[90] Quoted in Clay, *Medieval Hospitals*, pp. 33–4.
[91] We lack a general study of this subject, although see (for syphilis) Cassiano da Langasco, *Gli spedali degli incurabili* (Genoa, 1938). On the fifteenth- and sixteenth-century shift in attitudes toward poverty: Bronislaw Grmek, 'Renfermement des pauvres en Italie (xiv–xviie siècle): Remarques préliminaires', in *Melanges en l'honneur de Fernand Braudel*, 2 vols. (Toulouse, 1973), i, esp. pp. 209–10; Natalie Zemon Davis, 'Poor Relief, Humanism, and Heresy – The Case of Lyon', in her *Society and Culture in Early Modern France* (Stanford, 1965), pp. 17–64; and Brian Pullan, *Rich and Poor in Renaissance Venice: The Social Institutions of a Catholic State* (Cambridge, MA, 1971), part ii.

around the healing shrine of St Dympna in Gheel.[92] After 1500, some empty leprosaria were also given over to this new purpose, although others went to house other groups. In its earliest phases, therefore, Foucault's 'great confinement' was a response to a genuine social need – the lack of alternatives for indigents who were chronically ill – and its punitive aspects were rooted less in changing attitudes toward mental illness than in changing attitudes toward the poor.

It is scarcely surprising to find medieval administrators and medical practitioners grappling with many problems, like chronic illness among the poor, that we still find intractable today. It is more striking to discover the extent to which our solutions echo their own. This represents no coincidence, for our medical order is historically continuous with theirs. The towns and cities of the later Middle Ages invented many of the strategies and institutions that still structure western medical practice: professional organizations and licensing procedures, public health boards and agencies, university education in medicine, and institutions such as hospitals that mediate between the doctor and his or her patients. This fact does not minimize the differences between our society and theirs, between their medicine and our own. But it encourages us to understand our own order as the product of a long historical evolution, full of contingent elements, and it lends new interest to the workings of medicine in the medieval world.

[92] Grace Goldin, 'A Painting in Gheel', *Journal of the History of Medicine*, 26 (1971), 400–12; Jetter, *Geschichte des Irrenhauses*, pp. 79–80, 179–85; Giulio J. Dominguez, 'The Hospital of Innocents: Humane Treatment of the Mentally Ill in Spain, 1409–1512', *Bulletin of the Menninger Clinic*, 31 (1937), 285–97.

The patient in England, c. 1660–c. 1800

ROY PORTER

If the development of medicine is to be seen to have any progressive unity which relates its past to its present and future, the focus of that study must lie with the evolution of the medical profession, the development of clinical techniques, the rise of scientific medicine and the institutions within which it is pursued and practised. All of this – the stuff of regular medical history – presupposes, silently, the existence of the very *raison d'être* of medicine, the sick person. The history of the sick cannot be written in the same sequential way in which one tells the chronicle of medicine and doctors, of Falloppio being the teacher of Fabricius, who in his turn was the teacher of William Harvey, who discovered the circulation of the blood, and 'founded' modern scientific medicine. But that does not mean that it cannot, or should not, be written at all. Nor does it imply that medical patients are in some sense 'subhistorical', timeless objects merely waiting to be treated by doctors who are part of progress.[1]

For the sick too have had their own medical culture, one with profound links to the wider consciousness of their times – religious, political, moral, aesthetic. Moreover, in important ways, the sick have not just been 'patients' but 'agents' as well, both looking after their own health, and playing active roles in managing their dealings with medical professionals and the institutions of regular medicine. The interplay between laity and 'faculty' in negotiating medical transactions has varied enormously down the ages, being responsive to a range of different factors (e.g. how much esoteric scientific expertise the professional doctors have possessed, beyond the control of sick people, or how far the

[1] For a development of these arguments, and full bibliography see Roy Porter, 'The Patient's View: Doing Medical History from Below', *Theory and Society*, 14 (1985), 175–98.

state has been prepared to back the medical professions' claims to a monopoly of practice). The history of patient–doctor relations is neither unilinear nor simple. For instance, we might be tempted to suppose that the rise of state and scientific medicine during the present century would have tipped the balance in favour of giving more power to the profession. This may be so. But even today within orthodox medicine, the scope for the manipulation of medical relations by the sick person remains enormous, and the rising demand for alternative and fringe therapies demonstrates the continued capacity of popular medical choice to reassert itself.

This chapter does not try to map out a millennia-long account of changes in lay medicine, or in patient–doctor dynamics as viewed from the sick person's point of view. Instead it takes a slice of time – the period roughly from the Restoration (1660) to the Regency (1811) in England, and probes the structure of the lay role in the healing of the sick. It will be divided up into three sections. The first part will offer a very elementary account of the range of medicine and healing available to sick people in England over that period, stressing continuities with the past and exploring the rough distribution of lay medicine and professional medicine. The second part will focus upon the nuances of the practice of self-medication amongst sick people, exploring how self-medication ('from below') was not a tradition utterly distinct from professional medicine ('from above'), but rather one which fell – probably increasingly over time – within the gravitational pull of the traditions of learned physic (people's medicine and professional medicine thus constitute a dialectical relationship, not 'separate spheres'). The third part will briefly explore the consciousness of sick people themselves. This can fruitfully be done for many categories of the sick. What being ill meant within a religious world-view, for example is particularly revealing. Here I briefly attempt to examine what it felt like to be insane (or to be labelled and treated as mad).

The map of medicine

When people fell sick in 1660 or 1700, what did they do? The affluent might have access to three kinds of regular practitioner. At the top was the physician, whose job was to diagnose, and provide attendance and advice. Members of a liberal profession, founded upon a university education, physicians were expected to have a gentlemanly bearing to match that of their wealthy patients. Top physicians crowded into the capital, where Fellows and Licentiates of the Royal College of Physicians enjoyed a monopoly. Outside London, physicians practised in corporate towns and cathedral cities. Out in the sticks, the presence of university educated physicians was haphazard.[2]

Lower in status than the physician was the surgeon. His was a craft not a science, involving the 'hand' not the 'head'; and it was a skill taught by apprenticeship. His job (sometimes hers: there were a few female surgeons) was to treat external complaints (boils, wounds, etc.), to set bones and perform simple operations. As arts of the knife, surgery and barbering had long been yoked together, the Barber Surgeons Company of London dating from 1540 (they did not split up till 1745).[3]

Parallel to the surgeon was the apothecary, the physician's underlining. The physician prescribed; the apothecary dispensed. In practice, however, particularly in the countryside, the apothecary increasingly acted the physician's part. Indeed the surgeon and the apothecary also overlapped. In small towns, for example, there would be just one single practitioner who would turn his hand to all branches of healing. By the eighteenth century the name 'surgeon–apothecary' was the commonest title given to the country or small-town practitioner. In all but name, he was becoming the general practitioner.[4]

We do not know how many regularly trained practitioners were at work in Stuart England. Numbers steadily rose, however, during the eighteenth century. The first 'medical register', published in 1779 and 1783, lists about 3,000 (there must have been more).[5] Even if regulars were in short supply, however, there was never any shortage of other people experienced in caring for the sick. Such 'irregulars' came in many guises. Some practised full-time, others occasionally; some for money, others out of charity; some were licensed, most were tolerated, a few were prosecuted. Amongst certified practitioners were authorized midwives (all female). These required a bishop's license to testify to the woman's good character.

Another type of medical practitioner who might have the legal

[2] See Charles Webster (ed.), *Health, Medicine and Mortality in the Sixteenth Century* (Cambridge, 1979); H. J. Cook, *The Decline of the Old Medical Regime in Stuart London* (Ithaca and London, 1986).
[3] Z. Cope, *The Royal College of Surgeons of England. A History* (London, 1959).
[4] J. G. L. Burnby, *A Study of the English Apothecary from 1660 to 1760, Medical History*, Suppl. 3, (London, 1983); I. S. L. Loudon, 'The Nature of Provincial Medical Practice in Eighteenth Century England', *Medical History*, 29 (1985), 1–32; *idem*, 'The Origin and Growth of the Dispensary Movement', *Bulletin of the History of Medicine*, 55 (1981), 323–42; G. Holmes, *Augustan England: Professions, State and Society 1680–1730* (London, 1982).
[5] Joan Lane, 'The Medical Practitioners of Provincial England in 1783', *Medical History*, 28 (1984), 353–71.

protection of a licence was – odd though it may seem – the quack or mountebank. Often coming from France or Italy, charlatans could purchase royal privileges to practise, just as 'empirics' could patent their nostrums and proprietary medicines.[6]

Thousands of people made a living, or topped up their incomes, from medicine at this time. Grocers and pedlars sold drugs. Blacksmiths and farriers drew teeth and set bones. Itinerants toured the country, selling bottles of brightly coloured 'wonder cures'. Some were probably simply rogues. Other travelling doctors possessed genuine skills in treating eye, teeth, or ear complaints, thus performing a useful service in the days before business was brisk enough to support permanent medical specialists in every town.

Far more people, however, practised healing without any view to reward, but rather out of neighbourliness, paternalism, good house-keeping, religion or simple self-help. Every village had its 'nurses' and 'wise women', well-versed in herbal lore. The gentry and clergy prided themselves upon treating their tenantry as a matter of piety, duty, and sheer necessity. Their wives would play 'lady bountiful'.

Sometimes this lay medicine was attacked by regular practitioners. But almost all was perfectly legal (only irregulars who brazenly trespassed upon the privileges of the London College and Companies found themselves before the courts). And it filled a gap. Thus, although professional doctors were fewer in Stuart times than later centuries, the presence of an abundance of popular healers meant that few who needed medical attention would have gone without. And that includes even the very poor. Physicians and quacks alike often made a point of treating poor patients gratis, out of charity.

Moreover, parish paternalism frequently involved no small outlay of ratepayers' money on the sick or infirm, out of a mixture of genuine community feeling and enlightened self-interest. Sometimes the amounts laid out on individuals appear surprisingly generous. It was not unknown to pay to send a sick person to a spa or up to London for treatment, doubtless in the hope that such outlays would prove a long-term economy. In the days before friendly societies, charity and Poor Law relief combined to offer at least some medical attention to the lower orders.

As other chapters in this volume demonstrate, the period under discussion was one of extremely high morbidity and mortality. Sickness

---

[6] See W. F. Bynum and R. Porter, *Medical Fringe and Medical Orthodoxy* (London, 1986).

and death were all around.[7] Few young adults would not have had several brothers and sisters already in their graves. In such a society, illness was typically not seen as a random accident striking from outside, but as a deeply significant life event, integral to the sufferer's whole being – spiritual, moral, physical. This was partly because of contemporary assumptions about what caused illness. Both the explanations of the doctors, and the outlooks of lay 'common sense', regarded health as a measure of the proper workings of the individual constitution, and sickness as a sign of its malfunctioning. To maintain good health, one needed to ensure proper diet, exercise, evacuations, adequate sleep, a healthy environment and one had to regulate one's passions. More particularly, the different qualities vital for life had to be kept in a good balance. The body must not be allowed to become too hot or cold, too wet or dry (fevers or colds would result).

Thus sickness was seen largely as something personal and internal, rather than, as nowadays, primarily the result of 'invasion' by 'germs'. Careful attention to 'regimen', or life style, would, it was hoped, prevent disease (literally 'dis-ease'). This preventative view made good sense at a time when curative medicine was little advanced. One way in which people in traditional society coped with the fact that doctors weren't miracle workers was to view their health as ultimately their own personal responsibility.

That still left the question of why people fell sick in the first place. There were several plausible explanations. For one thing, far too many people lived in unhealthy environments or pursued unhealthy occupations. Since the Greeks, it had been well known that cramped, slummy areas of towns were hotbeds of epidemics, or that people who lived in marshy areas got pestilential fever.

Second, it was widely believed that disease might be the result of *maleficium*, or spells cast by witches, or of satanic or demonic possession. Of course belief in the real powers of witchcraft and in demonism very gradually declined during the seventeenth century, and attributing disease and death to evil spirits became confined to the lower classes, as did the use of magic to ward them off. Survivals of medical magic still persisted into the nineteenth century amongst the common people (e.g. passing a child with whooping cough under a donkey).[8]

Third, and extremely importantly, the fallen condition of mankind was blamed for the ubiquity of sickness, suffering and death. Through

[7] C. Gittings, *Death, Burial and the Individual in Early Modern England* (London, 1984).
[8] K. V. Thomas, *Religion and the Decline of Magic* (London, 1971).

original sin, Adam and Eve had brought death and disease into the world. The Bible warned that women would bring forth children in pain, as a consequence of the sins of the flesh. Disease could be a perpetual *memento mori*, and death itself a release from this vale of tears.[9]

Such views could make general sense of disease and death. In themselves they did not solve the question: why did it happen to me? For this, more particular moral theories (disease as punishment) and providentialist explanations were developed. For above all, disease was seen in the seventeenth century (though decreasingly so thereafter) as the finger of Providence. God used illness for a multitude of higher purposes. It could be an affliction against the ungodly, as with the plagues of Egypt. It could be a trial, or even a mark of divine favour.[10] Few people thought that medicine and the Divine Will were likely to be seriously at odds, though some Scottish Calvinists resisted the introduction of smallpox inoculation in the eighteenth century, on the grounds that if God wanted people to die of smallpox, it was not for man to prevent it.

Overall, the medical culture of pre-industrial England focused heavily upon the individual, and God's purposes for him, when it came to explaining sickness. As we shall see in the next section, this had important consequences for what people did in the teeth of actually falling sick.

Self-medication and lay healing

'Porter has been very ill in the workhouse', recorded the Somerset parson, William Holland, in 1802: 'I went into him, he was in a fit. I gave them some gin to put into his mouth.' Apparently the treatment worked. 'I called afterwards and he told me he was much better and that the gin relieved him much from the wind. He is very violent at times, but seemed very rational and tractable.' That was not the end of Parson Holland's parochial medical ministrations at the parish poorhouse. A week later – on a day he missed family breakfast because 'I cut myself shaving and it bleeds so plentifully that I know not how to stop it' – he

[9] *Ibid.*; see also, W. Sheils (ed.), *The Church and Healing* (Oxford, 1982).

[10] A. Wear, 'Puritan Perceptions of Illness in Seventeenth Century England', in R. Porter (ed.), *Patients and Practitioners. Lay Perceptions of Medicine in Pre-industrial England* (Cambridge, 1985), pp. 55–99; Lucinda Beier, 'In Sickness and in Health: A Seventeenth Century Family's Experience', in *ibid.*, pp. 101–28; Jonathan Barry, 'Piety and the Patient: Medicine and Religion in Eighteenth Century Bristol', in *ibid.*, pp. 145–75; Johanna Geyer-Kordesch, 'Cultural Habits of Illness: The Enlightened and the Pious in Eighteenth Century Germany', in *ibid.*, pp. 177–204.

returned there and 'gave to Porter today a glass of gin as he apprehended a fit coming on'.[11]

Spiritual physic as plied by Holland forms but one strand in the rich texture of lay medicine within the community, which has been practised time out of mind. It has taken many forms. At the most elementary level, there has been self-dosing, in the sense of one individual setting out his own rules of health, establishing a regimen – diet, exercise etc. – diagnosing his own complaints, making and applying his own medicines, and even carrying out his own auto-surgery (self-bleeding was not uncommon: early in the nineteenth century, the self-medication fanatic, Charles Waterton, claimed to have bled himself no fewer than 110 times.[12]

In reality, however, self-healing has been enmeshed in wider social networks. 'Medicine without doctors'[13] has rarely been medicine without family or community obligations and expectations: the clergy have healed their flocks, Lady Bountifuls their servants, and fathers their children. 'Agues are much about', wrote Parson George Woodward in the mid eighteenth century, 'and my wife being a professed Sangrado for that distemper, has multitude of patients, that come to her three or four miles round, and great success she has with her powders'.[14] Before the eighteenth century, doctors were rarely present at childbirth.[15] But that doesn't mean to say it was a private event; rather, giving birth was a protracted public ritual, involving the mother's female friends and family. Likewise, the knowledge and skills possessed by lay people who practised healing were only very exceptionally seen as unique, personal gifts or callings; typically they were regarded as applications of a body of lore that was in essence public, handed down orally, sometimes preserved in family manuscript recipe books, or culled out of printed volumes. In the 'world we have lost', self-medication was part and parcel of a comprehensive lay medical culture, which in turn was rooted in the community and its wisdom.

[11] Jack Ayres (ed.), *Paupers and Pig Killers. The Diary of William Holland a Somerset Parson 1799–1818* (Gloucester, 1984), p. 69. Holland confessed that 'gin is bad physick'.
[12] R. Aldington, *The Strange Life of Charles Waterton 1782–1865* (London, 1948).
[13] G. Risse, R. L. Numbers and J. Walzer Leavitt (eds.), *Medicine Without Doctors* (New York, 1977); A. C. Fellman and M. Fellman, *Making Sense of Self. Medical Advice Literature in Late Nineteenth-Century America* (Philadelphia, 1981); J. C. Whorton, *Crusaders for Fitness. The History of American Health Reformers* (Princeton, NJ, 1982).
[14] D. Gibson (ed.), *A Parson in the Vale of White Horse* (Gloucester, 1982), p. 129. Sangrado was a Spanish fictional doctor, notorious for bloodletting.
[15] A. Wilson, 'Participant or Patient? Seventeenth Century Childbirth from the Mother's Point of View', in Porter, *Patients and Practitioners*, pp. 129–44.

Most people in early modern England medicated themselves and largely did without professional doctors not through choice – not because they had opted for an 'alternative medicine' – but through necessity. The routine services of professionally trained doctors were too expensive for most people to afford, except in case of direst emergency. Even then, in a mainly rural society, practitioners commonly lived too many hours' ride away to make summoning their services convenient or practicable. The dissenting minister, Richard Baxter, noted in the late seventeenth century that he 'had been forced by the Peoples Necessity to practise Physick...no Physician being near',[16] and Hugh Smythson's *Compleat Family Physician* justified its publication a century later on the grounds that 'in the remoter provinces of the kingdom of Great Britain (and indeed, in every part of it, except the metropolis and its environs), medical assistance is placed at such a distance from the major part of the inhabitants, and the expence of obtaining it is so considerable', that self-medication, guided by a trusty *vade mecum*, was the only preservative of health.[17]

Doubtless, over the centuries many lay people were deeply suspicious of doctors (back in 1464, Margaret Paston had warned her husband, 'For Goddys sake be war what medesyns ye take of any fysissyans of London');[18] and some took the view, advanced from the Puritan radicals through to John Wesley,[19] that the medical trade was a recent conspiracy, designed to cheat the laity out of both their health and their money. Healing had been corrupted from paternalism to professionalism. Nevertheless, before the nineteenth century, there were few true precursors of Christian Scientists and those rebellious dissenting autodidact Victorian medical sectaries who insisted that the only doctor was Dr Nature. Even Wesley told sufferers in his *Primitive Physick*: 'In uncommon or complicated cases...I again advise every man without delay to apply to a Physician that fears God.'[20]

The sick in Stuart and Georgian England habitually treated themselves (for them primary care was self-care), but they did so for reasons of practicality or the purse not of principle. Living in mid-seventeenth-century rural Essex, the vicar, Ralph Josselin, and his family were frequently ill, but they almost never consulted professional doctors. This

[16] Quoted in R. Hunter and Ida Macalpine, *Three Hundred Years of Psychiatry 1535–1860* (London, 1963), p. 240.   [17] H. Smythson, *Compleat Family Physician* (London, 1781), pp. v-vi.

[18] Quoted in M. Chamberlain, *Old Wives Tales: Their History, Remedies and Spells* (London, 1981), 68.

[19] John Wesley, *Primitive Physick* (London, 1747); see also, G. S. Rousseau, 'John Wesley's *Primitive Physic* (1747)', *Harvard Library Bulletin*, 16 (1968), 242–56.   [20] *Ibid*.

was probably for reasons of expense and distance. It certainly wasn't because Josselin repudiated physick for prayer or was dismissive of the ideas and medicines of regular practitioners. Josselin read orthodox enough medical books; his frequent comments in his diary upon the causes and cures of sickness chime with regular medicine, and the pills and potions he made up, or obtained from local gentry such as Lady Honeywell, would have found no quarrel amongst the faculty.[21] Josselin's metropolitan contemporary, Samuel Pepys, was continually preoccupied with illness – his own, his wife's, his household's, the city's; despite being friendly with numerous practitioners, he rarely drew upon their professional services, preferring to protect his health and rectify sickness by regimen and self-dosing. But once again this was not because Pepys was involved in any ideological championing of self-help against what Ivan Illich would call an iatrogenic disabling profession. It was simply because, as Pepys saw it, the person best placed to understand his own complaints and safeguard his own health was generally himself.[22]

The practice of taking care of one's own health was heartily endorsed, at some level at least, by the faculty itself. After all, traditional, learned Hippocratic medicine set great store by the individual's duty to regulate his own life style, via the so-called six 'non-naturals' (diet, evacuations, exercise, air, sleep, and the passions), stressing the therapeutic importance of temperance, and condemning undue faith in specifics or automatic recourse to medicaments as quackish.[23] Text-books and case-notes reveal just how commonly learned Humanist physicians recommended relatively 'non-medical' remedies to their patients: riding, a change of air or diet, a trip to the waters, a holiday. Within that framework, which required the patient to be active not merely passive, self-treatment could complement rather than countermand the recommendations of orthodox physic. Thus it was natural for Benjamin Furly, recovering from illness in the late seventeenth century, to write: 'I am so far advanced that both my Doctors have quit me (for I had no less than 2) and left me to the Kitchen, and my Nurse.'[24]

---

[21] A. Macfarlane (ed.), *The Diary of Ralph Josselin, 1616–1683* (London, 1976); Beier, 'In Sickness and in Health'; *idem*, 'Sufferers and Healers; Health Choices in Seventeenth Century England', (University of Lancaster Ph.D Thesis, 1984).

[22] See Porter, 'Patient's View'; *idem*, 'Introduction' in Porter (ed.), *Patients and Practitioners*, pp. 1–22; Barry, 'Piety and the Patient'; see I. Illich, *Limits to Medicine* (Harmondsworth, 1976).

[23] L. J. Rather, 'The Six Things Non-Natural: a Note on the Non-Naturals', *Clio Medica*, 3 (1968), 337–47; P. Niebyl, 'The Non-Naturals', *Bulletin of the History of Medicine*, 13 (1971), 486–92.

[24] E. S. de Beer (ed.), *The Correspondence of John Locke*, in progress (1950–), vol. IV (Oxford, 1976), p. 188 (Benjamin Furly to Locke, 23 January 1691; no. 1354).

All the indications are that the presence of regular medicine increased markedly, indeed, quite disproportionately, from the late seventeenth century onwards. Of course, as the research above all of Charles Webster and Margaret Pelling has demonstrated,[25] it would be wrong to regard the Stuart market towns or countryside entirely as a medical desert, with just the occasional oasis of practitioners in big cities. Even so, it is clear that it was during the eighteenth century that England became quite well populated with surgeon–apothecaries, the prototype of general practitioners or family doctors (there were some four thousand by the 1780s). In contrast to their predecessors, these everyday practitioners were better educated and qualified (a significant percentage had studied at Leyden, Edinburgh, or taken courses or walked the wards in London hospitals), and, as Loudon has demonstrated, they became more highly esteemed and better rewarded.[26]

In London, and in a few other prestigious cities – above all, Bath – top physicians concentrated, drawing custom, fees and acclaim on a scale hitherto unknown (what predecessors could match a Mead, Sloane, Lettsom, Heberden or Baillie?). By 1800, voluntary hospitals and dispensaries crowned England's major cities and population centres, providing care for the labouring poor; and a growing proportion of parishes had contracted with a surgeon–apothecary to provide medical services for paupers.[27] Quantification is not yet possible, but it is indisputable that professional medicine became readily more available to a growing segment of the population, and being treated by the doctor became a way of life. A century after Josselin, Parson Woodforde routinely summoned the local doctor. Though he used kitchen physic too, he was grateful to have regular practitioners on call, writing, when his servant Betty fell sick,[28]

[25] Webster, *Health, Medicine and Mortality*; M. Pelling, 'Barbers and Barber-Surgeons: an Occupational Group in an English Provincial Town, 1550–1640', *The Society for the Social History of Medicine Bulletin*, 28 (1981), 14–16; *idem*, 'Medical Practice in the Early Modern Period: Trade or Profession?', *The Society for the Social History of Medicine Society Bulletin*, 32 (1983), 27–30.

[26] Loudon, 'Provincial Medical Practice'; *idem*, 'The Doctor's Cash-Book: The Economy of General Practice in the 1830s', *Medical History*, 27 (1983), 249–68; J. Lane, 'Medical Practitioners'; *idem*, 'The Provincial Practitioner and His Services to the Poor 1750–1800', *The Society for the Social History of Medicine Bulletin*, 28 (1981), 10–14; Holmes, *Augustan England*; Burnby, *English Apothecary*.

[27] J. Woodward, *To Do the Sick no Harm. A Study of the British Voluntary Hospital System* (London, 1974); E. G. Thomas, 'The Old Poor Law and Medicine', *Medical History*, 24 (1980), 1–19; Lane, 'Medical Practitioners'; Loudon, 'Provincial Medical Practice'.

[28] John Beresford (ed.), *The Diary of a Country Parson*, 5 vols. (Oxford, 1981), IV, p. 85. For Woodforde see N. C. Hultin, 'Medicine and Magic in the Eighteenth Century. The Diaries of James Woodforde', *Journal of the History of Medicine and Allied Sciences*, 30 (1975), 349–66.

Am well pleased however that I sent her to the Doctor which I should have done before had I known that she was worse than usual, which by meer chance I heard this morning by Nancy. I thought, as she did not complain to me, that she was brave and better by drinking Wine daily.

Put in crude terms England was becoming more 'medicalized'.

This 'medicalization' undoubtedly made inroads upon certain traditional areas of popular or lay healing. It is reasonable to suppose, for example, that the extension of official (Poor Law) or charitable medical provision was an important factor in the decline of magical medicine and the marginalization of wise women and cunning men.[29] Both amongst the more affluent classes and in new lying-in hospitals for the poor, new male accoucheurs replaced traditional midwives and the community rituals of giving birth.[30] The age-old treatment of the mad at home or within the parish began to give way to the public or private lunatic asylum, often presided over by a regular medical man, and increasingly involving techniques – moral management – granting the practitioner a heroic role.[31] Did such 'medicalization' also erode routine self-medication, or lay health culture at large?

The answer is clearly no. We have access to what literate lay people thought and did about health and sickness in the Georgian century through a multitude of sources – letters, diaries, journals, commonplace books, periodical publications and so forth[32] – and their collective testimony makes it plain that all ranks of society continued to take a presiding interest over their own health. A veritable mailbag of lay remedies was sent to George III in 1788 when he went mad.[33] Court cases likewise bring self-medication to light, as the trial at Huntingdon in 1736 of a soldier:[34]

who pretended [i.e., claimed] to cure a Boy of the Ague; and thinking to frighten it away, by firing his Piece over the Boy's Head, levell'd it too low, and shot his Brains out.

[29] Thomas, *Religion and the Decline of Magic*; Chamberlain, *Old Wives Tales*; R. Porter, 'Medicine and the Decline of Magic', *Strawberry Fayre* (Autumn 1986), 88–94.

[30] W. F. Bynum and R. Porter (eds.), *William Hunter and the Eighteenth Century Medical World* (Cambridge, 1985); M. C. Versluysen, 'Midwives, Medical Men and "Poor Women Labouring of Child"; Lying-in Hospitals in the Eighteenth Century', in H. Roberts (ed.), *Women, Health and Reproduction* (London, 1981), pp. 18–49.

[31] R. Porter, *Mind Forg'd Manacles* (London, 1987).

[32] Joan Lane, '"The Doctor Scolds me": The Diaries and Correspondence of Patients in Eighteenth Century England', in Porter (ed.), *Patients and Practitioners*, pp. 205–48.

[33] I. Macalpine and R. Hunter, *George III and the Mad Business* (London, 1969). George himself said his physician was the Queen.

[34] J. Grange, 'Cambridgeshire Country Cures', *Life Magazine* (May 1985), p. 29.

Letters passing between friends and family reveal endless inquiries after and information about health, and judgements upon various doctors. Moreover, they are crammed with detailed recommendations about particular cures and recipes, and advice about how to preserve or restore one's health. And people kept on treating themselves. The Cambridge don and poet, Thomas Gray, recorded how Ridlington, a Fellow of Trinity Hall, dying of dropsy, 'prescribed himself boiled chicken entire and five quarts of small beer', and recovered.[35] Some self-doctors mixed physical and spiritual remedies. 'Took Caster Oil – read Tristram Shandy', wrote John Baker in his mid-eighteenth-century diary[36] (sensible self-medication, as Sterne had composed his novel 'against the spleen', arguing that true Shandeism was good for the health).[37]

'I am sorry that you have been plagu'd with yt cursed Distemper, the Piles', commiserated David Garrick to his friend John Moody, in a letter of 1771:[38]

live abstemiously for a little time, & take Every Night a large tea spoonfull of flower of Brimstone (night & morning) mix'd up with honey or treacle, & you will be ye better for it – You should make up a Gallipot of it & take it by way of Sweetmeat thank ye Stars for ye Piles – if you had not them, you would have gout, or Stone or both & ye Devil and – While I had ye Piles, I had Nothing Else, now I am quit of them, I have Every other disorder –

Garrick was no enemy to the faculty – he used top London doctors as well as quacks such as the uroscopist, Myersbach[39] – but it was clearly the most natural thing in the world for him to offer physical advice to a comrade, without any suggestion that for his own good Moody ought to hurry along to his physician.[40]

Many other types of evidence confirm how active, how resilient, lay habits of self-medication remained throughout the Georgian century. Every well-stocked gentry house had its calf-bound ledger of family

---

[35] Quoted in R. Porter, *English Society in the Eighteenth Century* (Harmondsworth, 1982), p. 34.

[36] Philip. C. Yorke (ed.), *The Diary of John Baker, Barrister of the Middle Temple, Solicitor-General to the Leeward Isles* (London, 1931), p. 133.

[37] For Sterne, see R. Porter, 'Against the Spleen' in V. G. Myer (ed.), *Laurence Sterne: Riddles and Mysteries* (London and New York, 1984), pp. 84–99.

[38] D. Lyhee and G. Kahre (ed.), *The Letters of David Garrick*, 3 vols. (London, 1963), II, 743 (Garrick to John Moody, 6 June 1771, no. 635).

[39] Roy Porter, '"I Think Ye Both Quacks": The Controversy between Dr Theodor Myersbach and Dr John Coakley Lettsom', in W. F. Bynum and Roy Porter (eds.), *Medical Fringe and Medical Orthodoxy, 1750–1850* (London, 1986), pp. 56–78.

[40] Porter, 'Medicine and the Decline of Magic'.

remedies kept on the kitchen dresser, full of cures for diseases alongside recipes for plum pudding and syllabub, soap and polish. Similarly, when a gentleman such as John Byng, Viscount Torrington, went on his horseback travels around the country, he made sure he packed his own medicines, including proprietary preparations such as Dr James's Powders ('shou'd a fever overtake me, I will hope that by taking some of his doses and being well wrap'd up in blankets, I shall chase away sickness, without consulting the medical country blockheads, who kill, or cure, by chance').[41]

Another traveller who forearmed against falling sick was John Wesley. For the years covered by his journal show that his invariable response to illness was to medicate himself. It always worked. His face became swollen; he cured it with nettles. He had lumbago; it went when he applied garlic to his feet. He was believed to be dying of a consumption. 'A thought came into my mind to make an experiment. So I ordered some brimstone to be powdered, mixed with the white of an egg, and spread on brown paper, which I applied to my side. The pain ceased in five minutes, the fever in half an hour; and from this hour I began to recover strength.' When fellow methodists fell sick, Wesley played doctor to them, and was all for giving them electrical treatment: 'I prepared and gave them physic myself, having for six or seven and twenty years made physic the diversion of my leisure hours.' But for himself, the true panacea was riding: 'I must be on horse-back for life, if I would be healthy.'[42]

What is quite conspicuously absent during the eighteenth century is any sign that lay people began to entrust or resign the care of their bodies solely to medical professionals. The precise relations of authority, of duty and obligation, between patients and doctors were complex, open to negotiation, and often fraught (that is perhaps why it was an age notable for major new formulations of medical ethics, culminating in Thomas Percival's *Medical Ethics* of 1803). Medical authority was often uneasily received ('the doctor scolds me' complained John Stedman) and many sick people were clearly prepared to call in the doctor only as a last resort. As the Quaker William Stout put it:[43]

---

[41] C. Bruyn Andrews, *The Torrington Diaries*, 4 vols. (London, 1970; New York, 1970), I, 8.

[42] R. A. Knox, *Enthusiasm* (London, 1950), p. 425. See also Rousseau, 'Wesley's *Primitive Physick*'.

[43] J. D. Marshall (ed.), *The Autobiography of William Stout* (New York, 1976), p. 178. For Stedman, see Lane, 'Diaries and Correspondence'. See J. Pickstone, 'Establishment and Dissent in the Nineteenth Century. Exploration of Some Correspondence Between Religious and Medical

In the 2nd month this year, I was seized with great paine in my bowels and violent purging and other distempers. Which much weakened me, and was advised to doctors, which I had not hitherto done for thirty years last past; but always let nature and time worke a cure, as it has hitherto done, and now did, with patience and resignation.

Indeed, Stout's first substantial contact with the medical profession in thirty years came when he was run over by the local surgeon's horse. From the doctor's point of view, this seemed like cussedness. Edward Jenner – a country practitioner as well as the pioneer of smallpox vaccination – griped that the sick 'seldom ask my advice until things come to extremes; they go to so-and-so, who has "a desperate good receipt"'.[44]

On the other hand, the lasting failure of medicine to conquer the great killer and chronic diseases only confirmed the retreat into either self-medication or into a kind of philosophical stoicism. As Elizabeth Montagu was to remark:[45]

I have swallowed the weight of an Apothecary in medicine, and what I am better for it, except more patient and less credulous I know not. I have learnt to bear my infirmities and not to trust to the skill of Physicians for curing them. I endeavour to drink deeply of Philosophy, and to be wise when I cannot be merry, easy when I cannot be glad, content with what cannot be mended, and patient where there can be no redress. The mighty can do no more, and the wise seldome do as much.

It would, however, be a mistake to focus too much on friction between patients and their practitioners in this period. It was bound to arise in an exchange relationship when the demand-side was so desperate (we are talking about people wanting life not tea-services) and the supply so self-confessedly inadequate. For surely the truly important fact is that the expanding empire of regular medicine did not actually swallow up, or silence, lay medical culture. Nor did it even create a serious rift between lay people and professionals of the kinds that arguably came about between (say) the legal profession and its clients, or notably between the Anglican clergy and their alienated, apathetic or antagonistic parishioners. The extension of regular medicine did not curtail self-

Belief Systems in Early Industrial England', in W. Sheils (ed.), *Church and Healing*, pp.. 165–90. For confirmation of the resilience of lay medical culture see E. Shorter, *Bedside Manners* (Harmondsworth, 1986).

[44] P. L. L. Saunders, *Edward Jenner: the Cheltenham Years 1795–1823* (Hanover and London, 1982), p. 49.

[45] Emily Climenson (ed.), *Elizabeth Montagu, The Queen of the Blue Stockings. Her Correspondence from 1720–1761*, 2 vols. (London, 1906), I, 36.

medication, but rather coopted it. Aiming to control it, a collusive relationship set in which ultimately succeeded only in giving lay medicine a new lease of life.

Some indication of the hydra-like quality of medical self-help is given by the Jeremiads issued throughout the eighteenth century by medical men lamenting how consumer self-choice was raging out of control. 'Lady and Gentlemen doctors', deplored Dr James McKittrick Adair, were the bane of the national health. Puffed up with a few ideas derived from 'dispensatories and practical compilations', and from their peers, such people of fashion were in danger – so great was the power of their patronage – of subverting independent medical judgement and of poisoning their servants and retainers.

Worst of all, in some doctors' eyes, lady and gentlemen doctors were reducing physic to fashion. Time was when the fashionable disease was the vapours. Then the new-fangled medical language of the nerves caught on:[46]

Upwards of thirty years ago [Adair noted] a treatise on nervous diseases was published by my quondam learned and ingenious preceptor Dr Whytt, professor of physic, at Edinburgh. Before the publication of this book, people of fashion had not the least idea that they had nerves; but a fashionable apothecary of my acquaintance, having cast his eye over the book, and having been often puzzled by the enquiries of his patients concerning the nature and causes of their complaints, derived from thence a hint, by which he readily cut the gordian knot – 'Madam, you are nervous!' The solution was quite satisfactory, the term became fashionable, and spleen, vapours, and hyp [i.e., fashionable hypochondria] were forgotten.

Nowadays, Adair contended, nerves were decidedly *demodé*, and it was essential to be bilious. Not only was fashion dictating the choice of sickness, but in an affluent society full of bored people with time weighing heavily upon their hands, being ill was now the thing of fashion.[47]

What Adair particularly deplored was that patients had apparently made up their minds willy-nilly to have fashionable conditions, and were dictating terms to their physicians:[48]

instead of my patients giving me a detail of their symptoms, by which I might judge of the nature of the disease, the answer generally was, 'Doctor, I am bilious'; and, on enquiry, I found that they had generally been in the habit of taking medicines to carry off the supposed offensive bile.

[46] J. McKittrick Adair, *Essays on Fashionable Diseases* (London, 1790), p. 60.
[47] *Ibid.*, p. 7.   [48] *Ibid.*, p. 7.

If the lay medical voice, with its desire to call the medical tune, imposed terms of service which many doctors deplored, they were – as Adair's own anecdote demonstrates – little more than the profession's own chickens come home to roost. For (as critics and satirists never tired of pointing out) never before had the medical profession so saturated the market with writings, from sixpenny pamphlets to weighty tomes, directed specifically at a health-conscious lay readership. The genre of medical advice literature had a long history of course. As Paul Slack has shown, works such as Thomas Moulton's *Mirror or Glass of Health* (written, said Moulton, so that 'every man, woman and child could be their own physician in time of need') were almost as old as the printed book itself.[49] But Virginia Smith has convincingly documented how the literature of self-care and self-cures both grew substantially in scale and also developed improved techniques for influencing its target audience during the Georgian age.[50] Literally hundreds of books came on the market aiming to make *Every Man his Own Physician*, or claiming to be *The Family Physician* (1807), or *The Poor Man's Medicine Chest* (1791), offering *Physick for Families* (1674), or *Domestic Medicine* (1769), many of them going through multiple editions. Mirroring such books, journals such as the *Gentleman's Magazine* acted as exchanges – from laymen to laymen, from doctors to laymen – of medical information: diagnostic, therapeutic, pharmaceutical.[51] Though some of the most popular books of regimen – e.g. John Wesley's *Primitive Physick* – were the work of laymen, a large, and, indeed, Smith has found, increasing proportion, were penned by orthodox doctors, most influentially of all William Buchan's *Domestic Medicine*, which first appeared in 1769 and continued in print through to 1846; Buchan was said in the early nineteenth century to sit alongside the Bible in every Scottish household.

Not infrequently, such works were linked to the sale of ready-stocked medicine chests. Today's bathroom cabinet, with its scatter of aspirins, cough mixtures and antiseptic creams, looks positively spartan compared to the medicine chests – one for gentlemen, one for ladies, one for horses – containing well over a hundred different preparations which Richard Reece was advertising in his *The Domestic Medical Guide* at the beginning of the nineteenth century. Reece's chests included laudanum, calomel,

[49] P. Slack, 'Mirrors of Health and Treasures of Poor Men: the Uses of the Vernacular Medical Literature of Tudor England', in Webster, *Health, Medicine and Mortality*, pp. 237–73.

[50] V. Smith, 'Prescribing the Rules of Health: Self-Help and Advice in Late Eighteenth Century England', in Porter (ed.), *Patients and Practitioners*, pp. 249–82.

[51] R. Porter, 'Lay Medical Knowledge in the Eighteenth Century: the Case of the *Gentleman's Magazine*', *Medical History*, 29 (1985), 138–68.

antimony, guiacum and extract of lead. William Buchan for his part –
though deploring excessive reliance upon druggings – recommended
that every well-equipped home should have supplies of:[52]

Adhesive Plaster, Agaric of Oak, Ash coloured Ground liverwort, Burgundy
pitch, Cinnamon water, Crabs claw prepared, Cream of Tartar, Elixir of vitriol,
Flowers of sulphur, Gentian root, Glauber's salts, Gum ammoniac, Gum arabic,
Gum asafoetida, Gum Camphor, Ipecacuanha, Jalap, Jesuit's Bark, Liquid
laudanum, Liquorice root, Magnesia alba, Manna, Nitre or Salt peter, Oil of
almonds, Olive oil, Pennyroyal water, Peppermint water, Rhubarb, Sal
ammoniac, Sal prunell, Seneka root, Senna, Snake root, Spirits of hartshorn,
Spirits of wine, Sweet spirits of nitrate, Sweet spirits of vitriol, Syrup of lemons,
Syrup of oranges, Syrup of poppies, Tamarind, Turner's cerate, Vinegar of
squills, Wax plaster, White ointment, Wild Valerian root, and Yellow
basilicum ointment.

Doctors doubtless had mixed motives for writing home-care books,
reward and reputation being amongst them. But one should not
underestimate how far a sector at least of the regular medical profession
positively advocated enlightened self-care and educated auto-medication.
In the light of 'the progress of knowledge', the right to health was as
important, as natural, as all the other rights of man, proclaimed
Buchan.[53] Whether doctors liked it or not, sick people would medicate
themselves. Kept ignorant, Buchan warned, they would do this badly,
falling victim to cunning women, quacks and nostrum-mongers.
Discussing syphilis, he wrote:[54]

While men are kept in the dark, and told that they are not to use their own
understanding, in matters that concern their health, they will be the dupes of
designing knaves; and a disease, the most tractable in its nature, and almost the
only one for which we possess a specific remedy, will be suffered to commit its
ravages on the human race and to embitter the most delicious draught that
Heaven has bestowed for the solace of human life.

Enlightened people, educated by best faculty advice, would treasure
their health effectively, and could be instructed to recognize when
summoning of professional aid was vital.[55] In any case, stressed Buchan,
the optimal therapeutics for most complaints rarely required recondite
medication – the province, assuredly, only of the physician and the
apothecary – but typically demanded strategies well within the control

[52] Quoted in Chamberlain, *Old Wives Tales*, p. 184.
[53] W. Buchan, *Observations Concerning the Prevention and Cure of the Venereal Disease* (London,
1796), p. xxvi. Buchan is quoting this phrase from Benjamin Rush.   [54] *Ibid.*, p. 5.
[55] C. Lawrence, 'William Buchan: Medicine Laid Open', *Medical History*, 19 (1975), 20–35.

of the patient: bed-rest, simple diet, attention to the non-naturals, hygiene, cleanliness and, not least, trust in the healing powers of Nature. This applied even to venereal disease: 'in nineteen out of twenty cases, where this disease occurs, the patient may be his own physician'.[56]

There is thus every reason to believe that the expansion of professional medicine in the eighteenth century stimulated rather than suppressed lay medication. For one thing, the flood of self-care literature clearly fostered people's involvement in, and care for, their health. This is not to contend, in a crass, psychologically reductionist way, that it turned people into morbid hypochondriacs, still less that it was conspiratorially aiming to do just that (though there is a grain of truth here, to which I shall return). But much circumstantial evidence suggests that the Georgians were quite exceptionally preoccupied with personal health management (possibly because in their relatively secularizing culture, the well-being of the body was increasingly replacing the attention formerly devoted to the cleansing of the soul). And contemporaries undoubtedly linked this concern with the influence exerted by do-it-yourself medical works. Oliver Goldsmith, himself a medical doctor – indeed, a man whose self-dosing habits with Dr James's Powders apparently hastened his own death – put it all in a nutshell in *She Stoops to Conquer*. To prove her undying maternal concern for her son, Mrs Hardcastle insists how she's nursed and doctored him:[57]

MRS HARDCASTLE: Did I not prescribe for you every day, and weep while the receipt was operating?
TONY LUMPKIN: Ecod; you had reason to weep, for you have been dosing me ever since I was born. I have gone through every receipt in the Family Physician ten times over; and you have thoughts of coursing me through Quincy next spring.

Adair deplored the flood of books such as *Domestic Medicine* and its ilk, because they turned patients into medical prisoners.

Two dimensions of the rising supply-side of physic need further mention. On the one hand, the medicine which patients read in books or heard from their practitioners was, to a large degree, a *rational* medicine, which set great store by offering causal accounts of maladies, grounded in a wider economy of life and physiology (commonly the theory of the humours, latterly the model of the body as a plumbing system or as a set of nervous electrical circuits). Rational physic was

---

[56] Buchan, *Observations*, p. 9.
[57] Oliver Goldsmith, *She Stoops to Conquer*, Act II. John Quincy authored a best-selling medical dictionary.

graphic, coherent, and capable of being intellectually internalized by the sufferer, in such a way as to make sense of himself.[58] Andrew Wear has moreover contended this could be as true for quack as for the most orthodox Galenic physic.[59] In the interpretation of Nicholas Jewson, this sharing of medical consciousness – an inevitable consequence of the doctor's dependence upon the patient's own verbal 'history' – engendered a rough parity in the doctor–patient relationship, indeed an element of client control, in sharp contrast to the relative authoritarianism of later scientific and hospital medicine.[60] There is a truth here. Indeed, some Georgian patients were notoriously unbiddable. Dr Johnson writes to Mrs Thrale:[61]

I have begun to take valerian; the two last nights I took half an ounce each night; a very loathsome quantity. Dr Lawrence talked of a decoction, but I say, all or nothing.

In return, such attitudes begot a moral-tale literature in which doctors depicted the sticky ends disobedient patients came to. But patient power consequent upon access to rational medicine also had ambiguous consequences. For it made the sick person party to medical rationalizations, a consumer of potentially unlimited medical stories, one who could generate for himself endless diagnostic tales. Bernard Mandeville perceptively if cynically noted the implications in his *Treatise of the Hysterick and Hypochondriack Diseases*, a book professedly written 'by way of Information to Patients rather than to teach other Practitioners'. As soon as his character, Misomedon, began to exercise his 'Prerogative of a Man of Letters' – he was an Oxford-educated scholar gentleman – to delve into medicine's mysteries, to hear from his physicians the precise anatomy of his ailments, as soon as he fell 'in love with the Reasoning Physician', he was a lost man.[62] His fancy took over, he conceived of

---

[58] Lester King, *The Medical World of the Eighteenth Century* (Chicago, 1958); Cook, *Decline of the Old Medical Regime*.

[59] A. Wear, 'Medical Practice in Late Seventeenth and Early Eighteenth Century England: Continuity and Union', in Roger French and Andrew Wear, *The Medical Revolution of the Seventeenth Century* (Cambridge, 1989), pp. 294–320.

[60] N. Jewson, 'The Disappearance of the Sick Man from Medical Cosmology 1770–1870', *Sociology*, 10 (1976), 225–44; *idem*, 'Medical Knowledge and the Patronage System in Eighteenth Century England', *Sociology*, 8 (1974), 369–85.

[61] R. W. Chapman (ed.) *Letters of Samuel Johnson*, 3 vols. (Oxford, 1984), II, p. 268 (Johnson to Mrs Thrale, 14 Nov. 1788, no. 591); see also J. Mulhallen and D. J. M. Wright, 'Samuel Johnson: Amateur Physician', *Journal of the Royal Society of Medicine*, 76 (1983), 217–22.

[62] B. Mandeville, *A Treatise of the Hysterick and Hypocondriack Diseases*, 2nd edn (London, 1730; reprinted Hildesheim, 1981), pp. iv, 8 (Misomedon also 'digested' a course of medical reading). See also J. Marlow, *Letters to a Sick Friend* (London, 1682).

appalling new pathological sequelae and deduced their necessary causes, he multiplied his symptoms and his physicians. Between them, Mandeville said, such patients and such doctors will reason 'a trifling Distemper into a Consumption'.[63] And not least, by endless self-druggings, morbid self-medicators produced new rounds of side-effects, whose symptoms added another twist to the spiral. John Wesley made the same point. Physic held no dangers so long as it remained empirical, a matter of 'Are you sick? Drink the juice of this herb and your sickness will be at an end.'[64] Once party to all the palaver about causation, rationalizations and theory, however, the sick person was done for.

This leads to a second and parallel point: self-druggings. One of the key reasons enlightened physicians such as William Buchan advanced for educating the public in proper medical self-care was precisely the hope of stemming the tide of what they saw as drug abuse. The Georgian pharmacopoeia was not necessarily very effective, but it contained strong stuff, including opium (often prescribed in heroic doses), antimonial preparations, mercury for syphilis, and other mineral and metal remedies.[65] The 'pudding time' of the apothecary in the eighteenth century undoubtedly lay in his capacity to sell the public more, and ever more costly drugs.[66] Hard on his heels came the new trade of druggist.[67] If the apothecary's training and clinical attention went some way to minimize the dangers of excessive consumption of potentially lethal medicaments, no such safeguards surrounded the druggist's trade.

Moreover, and no less important, the logic of capitalist profit turned the old face-to-face empiric or mountebank into a new-style mass wholesaler of nostrums, proprietary or patent medicines. Dr James's Powders, Anderson's Scots Pills, Turlington's Pills, Bateman's Pectoral Drops, Daffy's Elixir, Stoughton's Great Cordial Elixir (advertised as ('approved by about twenty Eminent physicians of the College'), Godfrey's Cordial, Fryar's Balsam, Joshua Ward's Pill and Drop, Velno's Vegetable Syrup, Samuel Solomon's Balm of Gilead – all these and many more came to be advertised nationwide in the press, and were available at hundreds of retail outlets. Sales of many nostrums rose to phenomenal heights. Dr Robert James claimed to have sold 1,812,000 doses of his powders in twenty years, and Isaac Swainson boasted of

[63] Mandeville, *Treatise*, p. 6.   [64] Wesley, *Primitive Physick*, p. 12.
[65] V. Berridge and G. Edwards, *Opium and the People* (London, 1981).
[66] Burnby, *English Apothecary*.
[67] Irvine Loudon, '"The Vile Race of Quacks with which this Country is infested"', in Bynum and Porter (eds.), *Medical Fringe*, pp. 106–28.

vending 20,000 bottles of Velno's Vegetable Syrup a year, of which he bragged 'two thirds are ordered directly or indirectly by the faculty'.[68]

In the seventeenth century, Ralph Josselin had medicated himself chiefly with simple herbal remedies, culled from the meadows. The eighteenth-century self-medicator, by contrast, had unparalleled access – utterly unrestricted by law – to fairly cheap but potent – often lethal – medical brews, many of them, highly laced with opium and alcohol, addictive. As is evident from the correspondence of people such as Horace Walpole, taking proprietary medicines became almost a daily habit (Walpole called James's Powders a 'panacea' and puffed them to all his friends). Dr Adair complained of the habit which had grown up – encouraged in part by the cult of self-medication literature and exacerbated by the ready availability of medicaments, of habitual daily self-purging (the long term effects often were dire).[69]

In his satirical fiction, Bernard Mandeville depicted Misomedon's wife, Polytheca, utterly hooked on medicinal drugs which had wrecked her health (the blame, for Mandeville, lay at the door of unscrupulous apothecaries). When, in Mandeville's tale, the good physician prescribed to her exercise but no drugs she was outraged.[70] In this area of drug addiction such fictions have been frequently mirrored by reality. Medically prescribed opiates undoubtedly set Samuel Taylor Coleridge upon the road to chronic morphine addiction.[71] And the fate of Percy Shelley may be comparable.[72]

It is highly probable that while at either Eton or Oxford, Shelley contracted – or thought he contracted – a venereal infection, probably syphilis. Over the years, he consulted scores of doctors about his (supposed) condition, undergoing a whole range of orthodox therapies to treat what he took to be the long-term sequelae of his infection (these may largely have been the side effects of his heroic and chronic medication). But, under the ghastly stimulus of his own crash-course reading in the medical literature – Fracastoro on syphilis was one of his favourites – and a spell of walking the wards at St Barts Hospital, Shelley seems also to have subjected himself to self-cures, including aqua fortis

[68] Roy Porter, 'Before the Fringe', in Roger Cooter (ed.), *Studies in the History of Alternative Medicine* (London, 1988). For Swainson see Isaac Swainson, *Directions for the Use of Velno's Vegetable Syrup* (London, 1790). More broadly see Porter, '"I Think Ye Both Quacks"', in Bynum and Porter (eds.), *Medical Fringe*. [69] Adair, *Fashionable Diseases*, 7.

[70] Mandeville, *Treatise*.

[71] M. Lefebure, *Samuel Taylor Coleridge: A Bondage of Opium* (London, 1974).

[72] The following discussion depends upon N. Crook and D. Guiton, *Shelley's Venomed Melody* (Cambridge, 1986).

and arsenical preparations, mercurials and laudanum. His famous espousal of vegetarianism may also largely have been a self-medicating strategy, designed to purge his constitution of venereal taint. In Shelley's case, medical self-education and self-drugging reached positively terrifying proportions. After reading about elephantiasis in Sir William Jones's *Asiatic Researchers*, and coming across about two extraordinary cases of leprosy in London hospitals, Shelley convinced himself over a period of some months that he too was a victim of leprosy (traditionally seen as one possible consequence of venereal disease).[73]

Shelley, a poet wild with imagination, was, we may dismissively note, after all, a hypochondriac. But more requires to be said. For one thing, it was during the course of the eighteenth century that the very conception of hypochrondia steadily changed its meaning.[74] Up to the late seventeenth century, hypochondriasis was classed essentially as a regular organic disease of the lower abdomen. By the early nineteenth century, it had turned into the psychiatric condition of being morbidly anxious about health. Would it be totally fanciful to suggest that this sea-change was due, in part at least, to the very economy of medical self-help obtaining in the Georgian age, in which individual self-care remained a duty, sufferers were exposed as never before to a Gothick horror literature of medical cautions, and the sick had unexampled access to an arsenal of drugs which certainly – as in Shelley's case – would create real pain and malaise where there was none before?

Physicians, of course, ridiculed and deplored the hypochondriac, and his cousin, the Mr Woodhouse-like valetudinarian, seeing them all as egoistic attention cravers; those, mocked Adair, 'who are sick by way of amusement and melancholy to keep up their spirits'.[75] But more perceptive souls rightly recognized that as well as being the doctors' bane, the hypochondriac was also their victim. To patients long encouraged by trains of physicians and apothecaries to swallow medicines

[73] Some ended up worse than Shelley. Take this patient in James Mason Cox's lunatic asylum:
CASE III
Mr –, aged 25, of fair complexion, though his hair and eyes were dark, of exemplary morals, and most amiable manners: fond of anatomy, and had dissected some few animals; very desultory in his studies, but had read several medical authors with much attention, and was in the constant habit of quacking himself. Though no apparent alteration took place in his countenance, yet he constantly complained of his health, to which all his attention was confined, till at length he was rendered absolutely incapable. After the repeated and anxious inquiries of his friends, it was discovered that he believed himself affected with syphilis, connected, not by any unfortunate connection, but from sitting on the same seat after an infected person. Deaf to all reasoning and every attempt to prove the extreme improbability of the disease being propagated in such a way, his case was referred to some medical man of his proposing of whom he had read or heard; and he being previously instructed, pronounced it venereal, sent a prescription, which very soon dissipated the absurd idea, and restored him to himself, his friends, and family.
See J. M. Cox, *Practical Observations on Insanity* (London, 1806), pp. 52–3.
[74] Porter, *Mind Forg'd Manacles*.   [75] Adair, *Fashionable Diseases*, p. 95.

by the gallon, to be told by a sagacious physician to leave off and let Dr Nature do her work could be traumatic in the extreme. Hypochondriasis, Dr Robert James pointed out, was a peculiarly tough nut to crack, precisely because – as with psychoanalysis nowadays – the patient, while ostensibly seeking to be cured, nevertheless wanted his relationship with the doctor to be interminable:[76]

No disease is more troublesome, either to the Patient or Physician, than hypochondriac Disorders; and it often happens, that, thro' the Fault of both, the Cure is either unneccessarily protracted, or totally frustrated; for the Patients are so delighted, not only with a Variety of Medicines, but also of Physicians.

Interestingly, Dr Peter Shaw argued in the mid eighteenth century that the only cure for the disease of hypochondriasis was for the patient to wean himself off his doctor dependence: you must become 'your own physician'.[77] As Sir John Hill put it, 'the patient must do a great deal for himself'.[78] In other words, doctor's orders were: patient, heal thyself, or a renewed vindication of medical self-help.[79]

The thrust of this section has been to argue that it would be a mistake to regard amateur self-medicare before the nineteenth century as radically opposed to regular professional medicine. Ideologies of medical self-help, stipulating the root-and-branch rejection of professional knowledge or care (the medical equivalent of radical Protestantism),

[76] Quoted in A. M. Ingram, *Boswell's Creative Gloom* (London, 1982), p. 104.

[77] Quoted in Hunter and Macalpine, *Three Hundred Years of Psychiatry*, p. 312.

[78] J. Hill, *Hypochondriasis* (London, 1756), Cf. p. 24:

Though the physician can do something toward the cure, much more depends upon the patient; and here his constancy of mind will be employed most happily. No one is better qualified to judge on a fair hearing what course is the most fit; and having made that choice, he must with patience wait his good effects. Diseases that come on slowly must have time for curing; an attention to the first appearances of the disorder will be always happiest; because when least established it is easiest overthrown: but when that happy period has been neglected, he must wait the effects of such a course as will dilute and melt the obstructing matter gradually; for till that be done it is not only vain, but sometimes dangerous to attempt its expulsion from the body.

But prior to the course of any medicine, and as an essential to any good hope from it, the patient must prescribe himself a proper course of life, and a well chosen diet: let us assist him in his choice; and speak of this first, as it comes first in order.

[79] A more sober parallel would be Samuel Johnson, wrestling with his own melancholy. When Johnson asked of his friend Dr Brocklesby:

> Canst thou not minister to a mind diseased;
> Pluck from the memory a rooted sorrow;
> And with some sweet oblivious antidote
> Cleanse the stuffed bosom of that perilous stuff
> Which weighs upon the breast?

Brocklesby also knew his Shakespeare, replying:

> Therein the patient must minister to himself

quoted in Porter, '"The Hunger of Imagination": Approaching Samuel Johnson's Melancholy', in W. F. Bynum, Roy Porter and Michael Shepherd (eds.), *The Anatomy of Madness*, 2 vols. (London, 1985), I, pp. 63–88.

were largely outgrowths of the nineteenth century in America and England.[80] Because personal and professional healing were essentially complementary rather than in competition,[81] the massive extension of orthodox and commercial medicine, developing from the eighteenth century and accelerating into the nineteenth, actually augmented lay medical culture and self-medication. That necessarily happened, one might say, because without acutely health- and medicine-conscious consumers, the blossoming of the doctors within the commercial market place could never have been sustained. The extension of medicalization did not spell the impoverishment or expropriation of lay medical culture.[82] Rather, in a way that Foucault has helped us to understand,[83] it stimulated the proliferation of a repertoire of new discourses and practices about sickness. Only within a flourishing lay medical culture could a love letter open, as Lady Caroline Lamb poured out her affections to Lord Hartington:[84]

My most sanative elixir of Julep, my most precious cordial confection, my most dilutable sal polychrist and marsh mallows paste, truly comfortable spirit of hartshorn tincture of rhubarb and purgative senna tea! It is impossible, my most exquisite medecine chest, for me to describe the delightful effect the potion you sent me this morning had upon me Prescribe such powders to all the EPHEMERA [sic] who die for love of your Lordship's tricoloured eyes, and remember, cousin my heart and heart of my cousin, that your all faithful gallipot was only waiting for a line to dose you with letters every day, and how dost do, my dear Roderick due?

Experiences of illness

I have been discussing sick people's experiences of illness in general. I wish to close by examining personal experiences of one particular illness at this time: mental illness.

We possess a rough-and-ready picture of the main features of the treatment of the insane in this period. It is discussed in some detail in my chapter later in this book, 'Madness and its institutions', but it will be

---

[80] Whorton, *Crusaders for Fitness*.

[81] M. E. Rundell, *The New Family Receipt Book* (London, 1814), p. 262, stressed, at the opening of ch. 26, 'Health':

The following Chapter will be found to contain some receipts, which perhaps may appear to infringe on the medical profession. It should however be understood, that only such popular articles are here introduced, as may, in ordinary cases, afford help or mitigation, until medical aid can be obtained; and also in such cases as require instantaneous assistance.

[82] *Pace* Illich, *Limits to Medicine*.

[83] The parallel is with his argument about the proliferation of discourse about sex. M. Foucault, *A History of Sexuality*, vol. I, *Introduction* (London, 1979).

[84] Earl of Besborough (ed.), *Lady Besborough and Her Family Circle* (London, 1940), p. 206.

helpful, as context for examining the views of the mad themselves, to sketch in the broadest picture here. In 1660, people regarded as mad were generally kept at home, or under some sort of parochial care. Few received much medical attention. They were widely assumed to be incurable. Most probably suffered neglect, and casual cruelty was common.[85]

Over the next century and a half, it gradually became more common – perhaps, by 1800, normal – to lock mad people away in madhouses or asylums. Alongside Bethlem Hospital, England's one traditional public asylum, public asylums were founded in many big cities. But more importantly, private asylums were set up too (the 'trade in lunacy'). Many of these were abysmal and exploitative; a few gave high-quality care. The trend towards confinement, however, accompanied a major transformation in attitudes towards insanity: a new belief that it was a condition which could not merely be contained and secured, but cured. Isolation and attention in the asylum ('far from the madding crowd') would, it was hoped prove therapeutic. The eighteenth century closed on a note of optimism towards the mad, coming from doctors and society alike. They were (it was claimed) being treated more humanely; their reason would be restored.[86]

That was the official view, the view of reformers and doctors. Did mad people themselves share this optimism? What were their views about being diagnosed as mad and receiving the treatment which they did? Here we run into grave problems of evidence and interpretation. It is difficult enough to get under the skin of ordinary sick people in the past, and to try to grasp what their pain felt like, and how precisely they reacted to terrifying illnesses and the prospects of death. It is doubly difficult – yet particularly fascinating – to try to probe what it felt like to be (or to be thought to be) mad. For one thing, there is an inevitable ambiguity of consciousness (if such people were mad, can we actually believe, take at face value, or indeed make any sense of, anything they recorded?). For another, the number of accounts which we actually possess, penned by people treated as insane, is pitiably small. In the period in question, we have fewer than a dozen extended, connected testimonies written by people treated as insane, often locked up in madhouses, describing their experiences. Typically, they were written after the event, and they are clearly socially unrepresentative (for one

[85] M. MacDonald, *Mystical Bedlam: Madness, Anxiety and Healing in Seventeenth Century England* (Cambridge 1981); Porter, *Mind Forg'd Manacles*, ch. 1.

[86] W. L. Parry-Jones, *The Trade in Lunacy, A Study of Private Madhouses in England in the Eighteenth and Nineteenth Centuries* (London, 1971); A. Scull, *Museums of Madness* (London, 1979).

thing, almost all were the work of men, though we know that a substantial minority of people in asylums were women);[87] so the problems of interpretation are quite acute.

Even so, mad people's writings actually form themselves into certain patterns. One division is quite fundamental. Some 'mad people' (i.e. those regarded and treated by society and doctors as mad) themselves accepted the reality of their own insanity. Typically, such people wrote after their own recovery, to prove to themselves and to the world that they were rational again. Other 'mad people' wrote to deny that they were or ever had been insane, and to vindicate their own rationality against those whom they believed to be their malicious persecutors (it is of course a matter for our historical judgement as to whether we see these often wild self-vindications as proof of the original diagnosis, or at least as evidence that, locked away in madhouses, such people became disturbed and unbalanced).

Crucially, all those who wrote *apologiae* for themselves, confessing their former madness but claiming to be sane once more, did so from within a religious framework. In the seventeenth century, George Trosse (who became a Presbyterian minister), in the eighteenth century, William Cowper, the poet, and in the nineteenth century, John Perceval (later campaigner on behalf of lunatics), all argued that their own insanity had come upon them either through literal persecution and possession by the Devil and his minions, or through despair of salvation or of the justice of God.[88] The condition of being mad, and possessing what Perceval called a 'head of fire', was that of wrestling with evil spirits. These sufferers recognized that they had spoken in strange voices, as a result of being turned into ventriloquist's dummies by forces from Beyond. They had recovered, either when God had overcome Satan in the 'psychomachy' – the struggle for possession of the soul – taking place in them, or, put another way, when they themselves had seen the light of true religion. William Cowper explained how, placed in an asylum, he became well after reading in the Bible that Christ had died for his sins:[89]

But the happy period which was to shake off my fetters and afford me a clear opening of the free mercy of God in Christ Jesus was now arrived. I flung

[87] D. A. Peterson, 'The Literature of Madness, Autobiographical Writings by Mad People and Mental Patients in England and America from 1436–1975' (University of Stanford Ph.D. Thesis, 1977); idem, *A Mad People's History of Madness* (Pittsburgh, 1982); Porter, *Mind Forg'd Manacles*, ch. 5.

[88] See, W. Cowper, *Memoir of the Early Life of William Cowper Esq.*, 2nd edn (London, 1816); J. T. Perceval, *A Narrative of the Treatment Received by a Gentleman During a State of Derangement* (London, 1851); G. Trosse, *The Life of Mr George Trosse…* (Exeter, 1714).

[89] Cowper, *Memoir*, p. 44.

myself in a chair near the window, and seeing a Bible there, ventured once more to apply to it for comfort and instruction. The first verse I saw, was the 25th of the 3rd of Romans: 'Whom God sent forth to be a propitiation through faith in his blood, to declare his righteousness for the remission of sins that are past, through the forebearance of God.'

Immediately I received strength to believe and the full beams of the Sun of righteousness shone upon me. I saw the sufficiency of the atonement he had made, my pardon sealed in his blood, and justification.

In the increasingly secular society of the eighteenth century, doctors frequently argued that evangelical religion posed a dangerous threat to people's sanity. Fundamentalism with its threats of hell-fire, bred religious melancholy, which often led to derangement or suicide. There is some truth in the charge. On the other hand, autobiographical testaments such as these show that people who became disturbed within the framework of a religious consciousness, also frequently possessed the spiritual resources, strength and support to recover their sanity, and to make sense of an episode of madness within a wider meaning of life. Trosse, for example, regarded his recovery from insanity rather like the spiritual conversions recorded by John Bunyan and other sinners saved from the brink; Trosse abandoned his former evil ways and became a Presbyterian minister.

Very different are the writings of those 'mad people' (such as Alexander Cruden, Samuel Bruckshaw, and William Belcher in the eighteenth century) who wrote to deny, root and branch, that they ever had been mad. Their writings provide no explicit recognition of inner struggle and spiritual torment (we as historians can read between the lines of course).[90] Rather they depict the battle (as they see it) of a persecuted individual against malicious and tormenting doctors and captors, and create an image of the lunatic asylum as a kind of 'English Bastille', an institution not for treating the mad but simply for shutting them away and punishing them. It was widely claimed in Georgian England that private madhouses were abused as places to sequestrate difficult family members. Certainly, the testimony of autobiographical accounts such as Alexander Cruden's gives support to such allegations. It is no accident that Cruden titled one of his books *The London Citizen Exceedingly Injured, or A British Inquisition Display'd. In an Account of the Unparalleled Case of a Citizen of London, Bookseller to the late Queen, who was in a most Unjust and Arbitrary manner sent on the 23rd March last by one Robert Wightman, a mere Stranger, to a Private Madhouse* (1739). In rather

[90] See A. Cruden, *The London Citizen Exceedingly Injured* (London, 1739); S. Bruckshaw, *The Case, Petition and Address of Samuel Bruckshaw* ... (London, 1774); compare Porter, *Mind Forg'd Manacles* ch. 5.

similar vein, John Perceval, held in two of the most liberal asylums in England in the 1830s, made comparable protests against the arbitrariness (and hence counter-productiveness) of his treatment. Unlike the sufferers from somatic illnesses dealt with earlier in this chapter, he complained that he was totally under medical dominance:[91]

Men acted as though my body, and soul, were fairly given up to their control, to work their mischief and folly upon. My silence, I suppose, gave consent. I mean that I was never told such things we are going to do; we think it advisable to administer such and such medicine... I was fastened down in bed; a meagre diet forced down my throat... my will, my wishes, my repugnancies, my habits, my delicacy, my inclinations, my necessities, were not consulted, I may say thought of. I did not find the respect paid usually to a child.

These linkages between the hospital and the prison, the doctor and the jailer, are lurid, and perhaps evidence of the unbalanced minds of such autobiographers. But they remind us in a graphic way that medicine is not a hermetically sealed world of purely therapeutic relations, but one in which wider questions of social relations, power, and authority, matter as much as in the outside world. Focusing attention upon the position of the patient helps remind us of those relations.

[91] Perceval, *Narrative*, p. 179.

Making sense of health and the environment in early modern England

ANDREW WEAR

Meanings of health and illness

Most of the chapters in this volume concentrate on medicine, its theories, organization, relations with the state and its general place in society. It is clear from them that 'medicine' has to be taken in a very wide sense, and its history is not just that of a limited, elite group of practitioners but encompasses many other groups in society (for instance the patients of the previous chapter). What is also obvious is that the ways in which health and illness were made sense of extend well beyond any single account of the theories of medical practitioners. In early modern England (1550–1750) some aspects of life which today are strongly 'medicalized' (under the control of doctors and medicine) were then less influenced by medicine, especially that of the elite or 'learned' medicine of the university-trained physicians. Childbirth and death were two such important events. Conversely, we might expect that the environment, the context in which all the stages of life took place, would not be related very closely to health in this period. After all, it was in the nineteenth century that the hygienic and sanitary revolutions took place, and it might seem that only in recent years has the environment been valued in its own right. However, in early modern England there were clear ways of making sense of the relationship between health and the environment. In this chapter I will first briefly sketch out an argument for putting the medical theories of this period into a social, economic and religious framework, and so lessening the sense that they are autonomous and separate from society. This will make it easier to understand how

Note: The editions of sixteenth- and seventeenth-century works that I have used are often later than the first edition.

childbirth and health, whose histories I also briefly discuss, were often placed into non-medical settings. The major part of the chapter deals with perceptions of health and the environment; less has been written on this and the topic deserves more extensive treatment. The emphasis will be on the ways in which meaning was given to significant aspects of health and illness.

Medical theories

Medical theories underwent radical change at this time. At the beginning of the period (1550) learned medicine, that is the medicine taught in the universities and practised by the Fellows of the London College of Physicians, was based on the classical authority of Galen and described the body in humoral, qualitative terms. At the end of the period (1750) Galenic medicine was in decline and had been replaced by chemical and mechanical explanations of the body. During the Civil War and Interregnum Paracelsian medicine, with its stress on chemical explanations of disease and chemical remedies, and with its radical opposition to Galenic learned medicine, became popular with the sectarian reformers of medicine. They felt that it provided the appropriate aetiological and therapeutic body of knowledge (its roots being popular rather than traditional and learned) for a new type of Christian, charitable medicine that would be available to all, especially the poor.[1] Politics and medicine were clearly connected. However, the most radical change in medical theory was produced by 'the scientific revolution' of the seventeenth century when a new natural philosophy (later called physics) and chemistry replaced the Aristotelian world of the four causes, four qualities and four elements (the four humours of the body being the analogues to the elements that made up the world).[2] This 'new science' was based on the idea that the world and the body were alike made from particles of matter of different sizes, shapes and motions. Although the theoretical shift appears to be very radical, for medicine this was less so. In the last three decades of the seventeenth century and during most of

[1] See Charles Webster, *The Great Instauration: Science, Medicine, and Reform 1626–1660* (London, 1975); for a revisionary view see Peter Elmer 'Medicine, Religion and the Puritan Revolution', in Roger French and Andrew Wear (eds.), *The Medical Revolution of the Seventeenth Century* (Cambridge, 1989), pp. 10–45.

[2] Put simply the four causes were the material, formal, efficient and final cause. A statue, for instance, was made of material (marble), it was given form (the formal cause) by a sculptor (the efficient cause) who had a purpose in mind (the final cause). The four qualities were hot, cold, dry, moist; in combination they produced the elements, water (moist and cold), earth (dry and cold), air (moist and hot), fire (hot and dry). The humours were phlegm (moist and cold) blood (moist and hot), yellow bile (hot and dry), black bile (dry and cold).

the eighteenth century there was a proliferation of new theories – iatrochemical, iatromechanical, iatromathematical – but they did not improve life expectancy nor did they produce better cures than the old Galenic ones. Indeed, a case can be made that most of medicine remained unchanged.[3] For instance, many therapeutic procedures such as the use of bleeding, cupping, purging, the emphasis on diet and regimen (which was especially present in learned medicine) retained their popularity throughout the period; the one major change being that chemical remedies came increasingly to the fore. Moreover, the existence of a large number of empirics at the end of the seventeenth century who used a variety of theories, often mixing Galenic with newer chemical and mechanical ones, indicates that medical theories often were employed more as a means of gaining patients (the appeal of traditional scholarly learning, the attraction of the latest most fashionable philosophy) than for any desire to identify any 'truth'.[4] The changing theories of medical practitioners are most appropriately placed within the changing commercial structure of the medical market place as described in the previous chapter. If political and commercial considerations influenced the type of medical knowledge that practitioners chose, then this is an indication that medical theories of whatever type did not enjoy an autonomous existence as 'objective' knowledge independent of society, and that claims for their universal acceptance would fail.

There is, in fact, much more to the meaning of health and illness than the story of how learned medical theories changed. In the early modern period, professional medicine with its strong claims to authority and monopoly in medical matters had not come into existence, the types of knowledge that could be used to make sense of health and illness went beyond medicine to include magic, witchcraft and religion as well as lay or folk medical knowledge. The decline in magic throughout the seventeenth century, which has been traced by Keith Thomas in his magisterial *Religion and the Decline of Magic*, and the secularization that occurred after the Restoration of Charles II in 1660 meant that magical and religious explanations of illness became less widespread. For instance, the Anglican establishment of the Restoration attacked the 'enthusiasm'

[3] See Andrew Wear, 'Medical Practice in the late Seventeenth and early Eighteenth-Century England: Continuity and Union', in R. French and A. Wear (eds.), *Medical Revolution*, pp. 294–320. One new effective remedy was Chinchona bark (later 'quinine') which was used for fevers (it worked against malaria); this was a plant and not a chemical remedy.

[4] On empirics see Roy Porter, 'The Language of Quackery in England 1660–1880', in P. Burke and R. Porter (eds.), *The Social History of Language* (Cambridge, 1986), pp. 73–103; Roy Porter, *Health For Sale. Quackery in England 1660–1850* (Manchester, 1989).

of the religious sects that flourished during the Civil War and in the Interregnum. Therefore recourse to God to explain physical illness as providential or madness as possession became suspect.[5] Such explanations were still used amongst non-conformist groups such as Quakers through the eighteenth century, but overall significant changes did occur in the non-medical meanings given to health and illness.

Birth and death

Two aspects of the life cycle, birth and death, which today are strongly medicalized, at the start of the period were very much in lay and religious hands, but as we come to the end of the seventeenth century the medicalization of birth increased and later it did for death as well. Adrian Wilson has shown[6] that in the early seventeenth century birth was an all female ceremony orchestrated by the midwife who was accompanied by the pregnant woman's friends and neighbours, the gossips. Men were excluded from the house during the birth. Only when there was a complication during labour was a male practitioner brought in and then normally only to extract or dismember the dead foetus.[7] At the end of the seventeenth century and the beginning of the eighteenth men became increasingly involved in delivery. Men midwives such as William Giffard claimed that their knowledge of anatomy enabled them to 'touch', and explore, the womb and to reposition the foetus to ensure that it would be born alive.[8] Additionally, in the early eighteenth century the public became aware of the use of the forceps (they had been

[5] See the conclusion of Michael MacDonald's, *Mystical Bedlam* (Cambridge, 1981) where he argues that the period from the Restoration to the end of the eighteenth century was a 'disaster for the insane.' Also Michael MacDonald, 'Religion, Social Change and Psychological Healing in England 1600–1800', in W. J. Shiels (ed.), *The Church and Healing* (Oxford, 1982), pp. 101–25; David Harley, 'Mental Illness, Magical Medicine and the Devil in Northern England, 1650–1700', in French and Wear (eds.), *Medical Revolution*.

[6] Adrian Wilson, 'Participant or Patient? Seventeenth Century Childbirth from the Mother's Point of View', in R. Porter (ed.), *Patients and Practitioners: Lay Perceptions of Medicine in Pre-Industrial Society* (Cambridge, 1985), pp. 129–44; but see also his 'The Ceremony of Childbirth and its Interpretation', in Valerie Fildes (ed.), *Women as Mothers in Pre-Industrial England* (London, 1990), pp. 68–107, where he rejects his former interpretation of childbirth as a rite of passage, he now sees it as an example of the 'world turned upside down' and as reinforcing the cohesion of women's culture.

[7] See the essays by Adrian Wilson, 'William Hunter and the Varieties of Man-Midwifery' and by Edward Shorter, 'The Management of Normal Deliveries and the Generation of William Hunter', in W. F. Bynum and Roy Porter (eds.), *William Hunter and the Eighteenth-Century Medical World* (Cambridge, 1985), pp. 343–69 and 371–83 respectively.

[8] See William Giffard, *Cases in Midwifery* (London, 1734). Giffard constantly contrasted his knowledge of anatomy and technique with the lack of it in the midwives whose mistakes, he claimed, he was constantly being brought in to correct.

a secret of the Chamberlen family throughout the previous century). Although forceps were not employed by all men midwives, female midwives were particularly discouraged from using them and this further downgraded their status. By the middle of the eighteenth century, men increasingly took charge of normal deliveries (though female midwives still delivered the majority of women) as well as being brought in as a matter of course for complicated deliveries. Historians are not agreed on the reasons why the childbirth scene changed from a female social ceremony (together with female expertise) to a male technical operation. Some feminist historians have seen the changeover as a deliberate male takeover of a female activity, as an attempt to have male control of all of medicine, an attempt which makes the female midwife subservient to the male practitioner and which begins the process whereby men assert the right, through claims of education and technological expertise, to control and manipulate women's bodies.[9] Other interpretations have pointed out that women themselves began increasingly to prefer male midwives and that fashion was important in getting male midwives accepted. In commercial eighteenth-century England a 'trickle-down' effect occurred whereby the elite levels of society influenced those lower down, and geographically as London led, the provinces followed.[10] The acceptance of male midwives is seen to fit this process. Additionally, the rational and scientific ethos of the eighteenth-century Enlightenment, in which the ideas of the natural were changing and the body was seen increasingly as a machine, may have allowed the presence of the men midwives to become more acceptable, since they claimed a superior knowledge and technical skill which was not possessed by women midwives. This is a point that appears to have been accepted by women. (Or, perhaps, as some women writers at the time implied, women preferred men to women.)[11]

None of the interpretations is completely satisfactory, all of them have been placed into larger interpretations with limited concrete evidence of

[9] See B. Ehrenreich and D. English, *Witches, Midwives and Nurses* (New York, 1973) and their, *Complaints and Disorders: the Sexual Politics of Sickness* (New York, 1974); Jean Donnison, *Midwives and Medical Men. A History of Interprofessional Rivalries and Women's Rights* (London, 1979).

[10] See, for instance Adrian Wilson, footnotes 6 and 7 above; Roy Porter, 'A Touch of Danger: the Man-midwife as Sexual Predator', in G. S, Rousseau and R. Porter (eds.), *Sexual Underworlds of the Enlightenment* (Manchester, 1988), pp. 206–32; Dorothy and Roy Porter, *Patient's Progress. Doctors and Doctoring in Eighteenth-Century England* (London, 1989), pp. 172–7; for the view that the man midwife represented a positive gain in health terms see E. Shorter, *A History of Women's Bodies* (London, 1983).

[11] See Sarah Stone, *A Complete Practice of Midwifery* (London, 1738), pp. xi–xii, on the 'finish'd assurance' of 'young Gentlemen-Professors'.

why women altered their choice over who delivered them. Nevertheless, it is clear that the meaning of childbirth changed.

Death also was a largely non-medical ceremony in the sixteenth and in the first half of the seventeenth century.[12] There were differences at the deathbed between Protestant and Catholic countries. For instance, the Catholic anointing with holy oil, the giving of the sacraments and the deathbed confession were viewed as Papist superstitions by many Protestants who believed the age of miracles was past.[13] But both religions insisted that a priest or minister should be in charge at the deathbed, the medical practitioner having departed when it was clear that no more could be done medically.

The process of dying was part of social life. Family and friends were present together with the minister to give the dying person encouragement at the moment when the temptations of the devil were at their greatest, and when the powers of good and evil fought for the soul of the dying. To help the dying meet the challenge books explaining the art of dying (*Ars Moriendi*) had been published from the Middle Ages onwards. Additionally, the dying had to give outward signs that they had died well. They were in a sense actors, who by showing calmness, rationality, fortitude, faith, forgiving their enemies and welcoming death and the chance of making the transition to heaven died 'a good death'. These actions gave the onlookers hope and expectation that the dying person had gone to heaven.[14] The public and religious nature of the

[12] On the history of death see Phillipe Ariès, *The Hour of our Death* (London, 1983); Michel Vovelle, *La mort et l'occident de 1300 à nos jours* (Paris, 1983); David E. Stannard, *The Puritan Way of Death* (New York, 1977); Gordon E. Geddes, *Welcome Joy, Death in Puritan New England*, Studies in American History and Culture; no. 28 (Ann Arbor, 1981); John McManners, *Death and the Enlightenment* (Oxford, 1981).

[13] William Perkins, the puritan theologian, condemned the anointing with holy oil as 'this greasy sacrament of the Papists' writing that 'anointing of the body was a ceremony used by the Apostles and others, when they put in practise this miraculous gift of healing which gift is now ceased', William Perkins, *A Golden Chaine* (London, 1612), p. 501. For a discussion of puritan attitudes in England to death see Andrew Wear, 'Puritan Perceptions of Illness in Seventeenth Century England', in Porter (ed.), *Patients and Practitioners*, pp. 55–99, especially pp. 64–70.

[14] John Donne in his 'Sermon of Commemoration of the Lady Danvers, Late Wife of Sir John Danvers, 1627' expressed the conventional actions expected of the dying: 'And in that forme of Common Prayer, which is ordain'd by that Church...she joyn'd with that company, which was about her death-bed, in answering to every part thereof, which the Congregation is directed to answer to, with a cleere understanding, with a constant memory, with a distinct voyce, not two houres before she died...Wee lost the earthly Paradise by death then; but wee get not Heaven, but by death, now. This shee expected till it came, and embrac't when it came. How may we thinke, shee was joy'd to see that face that Angels delight to looke upon, the face of her Saviour, that did not abhor the face of his fearfullest Messenger, Death? Shee shew'd no fears of his face, in any change of her owne; but died without any change of conternance or posture; without any struggling, any disorder; but her Death-bed was as quiet as her Grave.' John Hayward (ed.), *John Donne, Complete Poetry and Selected Prose* (London, 1929), pp. 574–5. For a discussion of the death-

deathbed was far different from today's medicalized death, which in western countries often takes place in medical institutions such as hospitals. The emphasis on the welcome transition from this world to the other world and its rational performance also militated against trying to concentrate on extending the last moments of life or on deadening the agonies of death.

The religious stress upon dying appears to have lessened in the second half of the seventeenth century. The Anglican Jeremy Taylor wrote that the struggle between good and evil did not occur in a special way at death but throughout life.[15] As Enlightenment ideals came to emphasize this present life, the existence of an after world was sometimes doubted. Thus, at least for parts of elite society, the religious meaning of death was lessened. John McManners has emphasized in his *Death and the Enlightenment* that most classes of society in France, the focus of his study, still saw death in religious terms. England, with its larger middle class was likely to have had a more extensive secularization of death, even though the process was not as thoroughgoing as some of the French *philosophes* would have hoped. In the latter half of the eighteenth century some doctors remained at the deathbed and 'managed' death, using opiates to deaden pain.[16] But in doing so they reduced both the independence of the dying and their role in the process of dying. If religious imperatives determined the ideal death in the sixteenth century, by the end of the eighteenth century the medicalized death was beginning to take shape. Again, this alteration reflects and confirms the decline of religion and the process of secularization which encouraged a medicalization of life and death.

The recent interest in the history of birth and death owes much to the present day concerns in western society with the way medicine controls the process of giving birth and of dying. Another modern-day concern is with the way our environment shapes our health. This topic was also of interest for the early modern period, though in this case, the forces of religion and of secularization were less evident. Despite attempts at sanitation and street cleaning, despite the ordinances controlling food markets, stinks and overcrowding, England at this time was often preceived as crowded, dirty, smelly and unhygienic. Probably many

---

bed and the behaviour expected of the dying 'actor' see A. Wear, 'Puritan Perceptions of Illness in Seventeenth Century England', and 'Interfaces: Perceptions of Health and Illness in Early Modern England', in Roy Porter and Andrew Wear (eds.), *Problems and Methods in the History of Medicine* (London, 1987), pp. 230–55.

[15] Jeremy Taylor, *Holy Living and Dying* (London, 1650, 1651).

[16] Dorothy and Roy Porter, *Patient's Progress*, pp. 144–52.

people were used to this but we rarely hear from them.[17] Many others, however, thought that this environment posed a danger to health and pictured a healthier alternative. I will first discuss how the environment and people were related at a general level, and then I shall consider how the environment was seen to affect health.

Health and the environment

England was perceived by the English, or at least by English eulogists as the best possible environment for English people. William Harrison in *The Description of England* (1577) and William Camden in his *Britannia* (Latin first edition, 1586) both agreed, at a time of intense national feeling, that the country was situated in the most temperate climate in the world, being neither too hot nor too cold.[18] As Camden put it 'Britaine is seated as well for aire as soile, in a right fruitful and most milde place.'[19] Harrison also argued that the English were taller, stronger, whiter and more courageous than those nearer the equator who were more feeble, delicate, fearful and blacker.[20] The way in which the connection was made between a country and its people was not an objective account, but often involved large doses of propaganda and patriotism.

From the point of view of health, the opinion was often expressed that the country in which one was born was the best and most healthy to live in, a view in keeping with the contemporary growth of the nation-state. A person's constitution or humoral balance was influenced by the constitution of the country of their birth. There was, therefore, an intimate correspondence between the two. William Vaughan, the Welsh writer and unsuccessful colonist of Newfoundland, asked in his *Directions for Health* 'What is the best Ayre?'. He replied:

[17] The physician Henry Brooke was one person who was satisfied with the environment. In ΥΓΙΕΝΗ, *Or A Conservatory of Health* (London, 1650), pp. 67–8 he wrote that many men not of the strongest constitution lived long and without sickness, 'amidst noysom and unpleasant Smells, as Oyl-men, Sope-boylers, Tallow-Chandlers' and those who dealt with 'Dung, cleaning of Common-shores and Jaxes' came to no harm 'because of the familiarity that by long use is begotton between such Smells and their Natures'. Brooke also robustly decried the too sensitive sensibilities of those who made themselves ill with the fear of imaginary dangers: 'However 'tis best for them that are any thing Healthful not be over -solicitous in the choice of Aire...for they do thereby very much deject Nature, and opinionate themselves into Sickness. Such Imaginations keep the mind in continuall doubts and perplexities, and make us sickly, out of a fear of being sick.
[18] William Harrison, *The Descripton of England*, ed. George Edelen (Ithaca, NY, 1968), pp. 428–9; William Camden, *Britannia, or a Chorographical Description of...England, Scotland and Ireland* (London, 1637), p. 2. [19] Camden, *Britannia*, p. 2.
[20] Harrison, *Description of England*, pp. 445–6.

That which is a mans usuall soyle, and Countries ayre is best. This by the Philosophers is approved in this principle: 'Every mans naturall place preserveth him which is placed in it'. And by the Poet confirmed: 'Sweet is the smell of Countries soyle.'[21]

The enterprise of colonizing America forced people to articulate their ideas of how to judge whether a place was healthy or not, and the evidence from the North American colonies provides a good insight into how the environment and health were related. The many letters, pamphlets and books which gave optimistic accounts of Newfoundland, New England and Virginia written at the end of the sixteenth and the first half of the seventeenth centuries in the course of trying to attract prospective colonists and setting their minds at rest about the unknown frequently referred to the idea that a person's country of birth was most healthy for them. In the *Planter's Plea* (1630), a tract encouraging the development of the New England settlement, the writer extolled the air of the colony. Air, 'the very food of life' as Richard Whitbourne the promoter of Newfoundland had put it,[22] was probably the most important of all the characteristics that were considered when judging the healthiness of a place. *The Planter's Plea* stated:

No country yields a more propitious ayre for our temper [constitution], than New-England, as experience hath made manifest, by all relations: manie of our people that have found themselves alway weake and sickly at home, have become strong and healthy there perhaps by the dryness of the ayre and constant temper of it which seldome varies suddenly from cold to heate as it doth with us: so that Rhumes are very rare among our English there.[23]

The relationship between bodily constitution and the land was thus even better in New England than back home in Old England.

The connection between people and their country of birth was used in other contexts. When English writers such as Nicholas Culpeper in the mid seventeenth century argued for cheap medicines which could be collected locally from fields and used by the poor, or like William Harrison extolled home-grown remedies simply on a nationalistic dislike of anything foreign,[24] they drew upon this view of how people were related to their country of birth. Additionally, Culpeper referred to

---

[21] William Vaughan, *Directions for Health*, 5th edn (London, 1617), p. 4.

[22] Richard Whitbourne, *A Discourse and Discovery of New-Found-Land* (London, 1622), in Gillian T. Cell (ed.), *Newfoundland Discovered*, Hakluyt Society (London, 1982), p. 165.

[23] *The Planter's Plea*, in Peter Force (ed.), *Tracts and Other Papers Relating Principally to the Origin, Settlement and Progress of the Colonies of North America*, 4 vols. (New York, 1836–47; reprinted New York, 1947), II, tract 3. p. 13. [24] Harrison, *Description of England*, pp. 266–8.

God's providence and wisdom in the creation in having provided not only food, but also appropriate remedies to cure the diseases of one's native country. This was a common sentiment amongst writers who were concerned with charity. In his *School of Physick* (1659) Culpeper wrote:

As the Earth is called the Mother of all things, not because it bringeth them forth onely, but yieldeth them perpetual nourishment, so is the Country of all people so then named, the Parent of all parents. Then by Nature's laws, all things being abundantly ministered unto us for the preservation of Health at home in our own Fields, Pastures, Rivers etc, how can the Wisdom of God, and his Goodness stand with the absence of Medicines and Remedies necessary for the Recovery of Health, the need being as urgent of the one as the other...it followeth necessarily that the Medicine should be as ready for the sick, as meat and drink for the hungry and thirsty: which except it be applied by the Native Country, cannot else be performed.[25]

Culpeper added that animals are given 'knowledge of Medicines to help themselves, if haply disease [occur] among them; neither out of India nor Arabia, but from their very haunt', and much more is given to us, 'the Lords of all Creatures'.[26]

Ideas about health and illness often reflect the different intentions of specific social groups. Most learned physicians, educated in the universities and charging high fees, would have been hearty prescribers of expensive foreign drugs. However, outside of London and one or two large towns, such physicians were few on the ground, and, in any case, were too expensive for most people.[27] As Roy Porter has pointed out in the previous chapter, the medical market place was composed of family members, neighbours, ministers and their wives, together with the wives of country gentry who might all give advice and treatment for free and practitioners such as wise women, uroscopists, astrologers, empirics and apothecaries who normally charged low fees. The ethos of much of medical practice was that it was demotic and open to all. Because of this ethos, the self-sufficiency appeal of native herbs for native diseases had added force, especially in the context of charity for the poor. The biographical sketch of Culpeper produced soon after his death stated:

[25] Nicholas Culpeper, *School of Physick* (London, 1659), p. 7.

[26] *Ibid.*, p. 8. Culpeper was drawing upon, sometimes word for word, Timothie Bright's *A Treatise Wherein is Declar'd the Sufficiencie of English Medicine* (London, 1580).

[27] See Margaret Pelling and Charles Webster 'Medical Practitioners', in Charles Webster (ed.), *Health, Medicine and Mortality in the Sixteenth Century* (Cambridge, 1979), pp. 164–235 who show that although medical graduates were few, the number of medical practitioners of all sorts was high. Also Doreen G. Nagy, *Popular Medicine in Seventeenth Century Medicine* (Bowling Green, Ohio, 1988).

To the poor he prescribed cheap but wholesome Medicines; not removing, as many in our times do, the Consumption out of their bodies into their purses; not sending them to the East Indies for Drugs, when they may fetch better of their own Gardens.[28]

The countryside and the city

The link between people and their environment (their native land) that has been discussed so far, treated both the country and its people as undifferentiated. What was different was other peoples, other countries and their climates, and foreign illnesses and remedies. Not only was the doctrine used for patriotic propaganda purposes (implying a sense of belonging and of excluding), and for expressing a political view about medicine, but it also had a moralizing aspect where categories such as natural and unnatural came into play. For instance, Thomas Tryon, a fervent exponent of vegetarianism in the later seventeenth century, deplored the use of exotic drugs as a sign of the degeneration of society from its pure natural state.[29]

The environment, however, was not always seen as an undifferentiated whole, to be patriotically idealized if it was one's own country or to be suspiciously sniffed at if foreign. When people came to look at England in detail they saw many different types of environment.

The major distinction between town and countryside, which was current amongst writers on health and the environment as well as in literary culture, forms the backbone of the rest of the chapter. The countryside was perceived to be much healthier than towns or cities. This view is confirmed by modern historical demography. The population of London, which had grown from 120,000 in 1550 to 490,000 by 1700, would have declined over this period if it had not been for the continued influx of people from the countryside that made up for the drain on the city's population caused by its high mortality.[30] This was realized by John Graunt whose *Natural and Political Observations…upon the Bills of Mortality* (1662) was the first study of population demography. It was based on a quantitative analysis of the weekly bills of mortality compiled by London parish clerks which gave numbers and causes of death. The book's numerate approach was very much in

[28] In Culpeper, *School of Physick*, sig. C4.
[29] Thomas Tryon, *The Way to Health, Long Life and Happiness* (London, 1697), pp. 382–8.
[30] See R. Finlay, *Population and Metropolis: the Demography of London 1580–1650* (Cambridge, 1981) and Roger Finlay and Beatrice Shearer 'Population Growth and Suburban Expansion', in A. L. Beier and Roger Finlay (eds.), *The Making of the Metropolis. London 1500–1700* (London, 1986), pp. 37–60.

keeping with the 'new science' of the Royal Society, and it also marks the start of the endeavour of relating deaths and types of death to environmental causes in a quantitative way. Nevertheless, Graunt's ideas of the environmental factors causing illness and death were traditional.

On the population of London Graunt noted that between 1603 and 1644 burials (363,935) exceeded christenings (330,747) and he concluded:

> From this single Observation it will follow, that London should have decreased in its People; the contrary whereof we see by its daily increases of Buildings upon new Foundations, and by turning of great Palacious Houses into small Tenements. It is therefore certain, that London is supplied with People from out of the Country, whereby not only to supply the overplus differences of Burials above mentioned, but likewise to increase its Inhabitants according to the said increase of housing.[31]

Graunt discussed the reasons for this imbalance between London and the countryside. He wrote that the number of breeders (women of childbearing age) was fewer in London than in the countryside.[32] But he also believed that London itself was less healthy than the country, though those who were 'seasoned' (whose bodies had adapted over time to the environment of London) could live long:

> As for unhealthiness, it may well be supposed, that although seasoned Bodies may, and do live near as long in *London*, as elsewhere, yet new-comers and Children do not: for the *Smoaks*, *Stinks* and close *Air*, are less healthful than that of the Country; otherwise why do sickly Persons remove into the Country-Air? And why are there more old men in Countries than in London, per rata?[33]

Graunt indicted both the pressure of people and the air they breathed:

> I considered, whether a City, as it becomes more populous, doth not, for that very cause, become more unhealthful: and inclined to believe, that London now is more unhealthful than heretofore; partly for that it is more populous, but chiefly because I have heard, that sixty years ago few Sea Coals were burnt in London, which are now universally used. For I have heard that Newcastle is more unhealthful than other places, and that many People cannot at all endure the smoak of London, not only for its unpleasantness but for the suffocation which it causes.[34]

Thomas Short, one of Graunt's eighteenth-century successors, whose demographic studies ranged across England, also believed that high population densities caused ill health. A sense of the suffocating closeness of towns helped to explain the figures from the parish registers:

---

[31] John Graunt, *Natural and Political Observations...upon the Bills of Mortality* (London, 1676), pp. 57–8. [32] Graunt, *Observations*, p. 62. [33] *Ibid.*, p. 63.
[34] *Ibid.*, p. 94–5.

The closer Towns and Villages stand, the more pent-up the Houses, the lower and closer the Rooms, the narrower the Streets, the smaller the Windows, the more numerous the Inhabitants, the unhealthier the Place. This is evident from several Towns in our Tables.[35]

Graunt did not believe that London's air produced barrenness in the same way as it produced a greater degree of death and disease than was found in the countryside (though he did blame London for its greater adulteries and fornications which 'do certainly hinder Breeding').[36] But, like many early modern writers, he made the connection between the body and the mind, and wrote that city life could produce psychological barriers to natural activities:

The minds of men in *London* are more thoughtful of business than in the country, where their work is corporal Labour and Exercises; All of which promote Breeding, whereas Anxieties of the mind hinder it.[37]

The countryside was the norm, from which urban living was an unnatural departure that incurred additional health risks. The health advice books, of which a very large number were printed in this period,[38] structured the relationship between health and the environment by means of the traditional 'six non-naturals' (air, food and drink, sleep and waking, retention and evacuation, exercise and rest, and the passions). These books were aimed at sedentary readers such as merchants, clerics and the studious, and they extolled the virtues of country air, food and exercise. (What the illiterate, who comprised the majority of the population thought about health remains largely a blank: the history of how people perceived health and the environment in this period is based on evidence from the literate.) Works such as Thomas Cogan's *Haven of Health* (1584) and the English translation of Leonard Lessius' *Hygiasticon* (1634) emphasized that country people took a lot of exercise and were generally longer lived. As Cogan, a physician and a Fellow of Oriel College, Oxford, put it:

Husbandman and Craftsmen for the most part doe live longer, and in better health than Gentlemen and learned men, and such as live in bodily rest.[39]

The country gentleman could live in the countryside, benefit from

[35] Thomas Short, *New Observations on City, Town and Country Bills of Mortality*, London 1750, ed. Richard Wall (London, 1973), p. 65.   [36] Graunt, *Observations*, pp. 63–4.
[37] *Ibid.*, p. 64.
[38] See Paul Slack 'Mirrors of Health and Treasures of Poor Men: the Uses of the Vernacular Medical Literature of Tudor England', in Charles Webster (ed.), *Health, Medicine and Mortality in the Sixteenth Century* (Cambridge, 1979), pp. 237–73.
[39] Thomas Cogan, *The Haven of Health* (London, 1636).

country air, yet suffer the same ills as his town counterpart. As well as country air, it was the way of life associated with the country, hard labour, a meagre diet and a lack of luxury which produced health. The well-to-do part of society, those 'increasing the wealth of the kingdom' (just under half the population in Gregory King's calculation for 1688),[40] was being advised that the poorer part of the population, if it lived in the countryside, was healthier than they were.

William Bullein in the *Government of Health* (1558) wrote in dialogue form:

JOHN. I have found verie much disquietnes in my body, when my servants and labouring familie have found ease and yet we are partakers of one aire.
HUMPHREY. The cause why thy labouring servants in the field at plough, pastures, or woode, have such good health, is exercise labour, and the disquietness commeth partly of idleness and lack of travail [work], which moderately used, is a thing most sovereign in nature.[41]

What John's labouring servants thought about their master's way of life compared to their own we do not know; the illiterate remain silent, but the equation of health with the poorest sections of society can be interpreted as an implied justification for doing nothing about their condition of life, and fits that strand of sixteenth and seventeenth-century English social policy which held that there was no necessity to ameliorate the lot of the poor.[42]

The distinction between the healthy countryside and unhealthy towns and cities was made throughout the early modern period, and many people felt that they could express opinions with some authority about health and the environment. Much of the knowledge was traditional, based on long experience or on authorities such as Galen. Sometimes it was founded on personal observation and experience, which through the sixteenth and seventeenth century was being given increasingly high status in subjects like astronomy, medicine and natural philosophy and was taken to be a guarantee of truth. This view was also current in society at large. It was used by American settlers when they tried to convince their readers back in England of the truth of the claims about

[40] Cited by Peter Laslett, *The World We Have Lost – Further Explored* (London, 1983), pp. 32–3, Laslett cautions against the accuracy of King's figures, p. 298 note 4. Keith Wrightson, *English Society 1580–1680* (London, 1982), p. 148, finds King's results of value: 'in [his] opinion at least half of his countrymen in 1688 were scarcely able to simply provide an adequate maintenance for their families. The poor had emerged as a massive and permanent element in English society.'
[41] William Bullein, *Government of Health* (London, 1591), p. 31v.
[42] See Paul Slack, *Poverty and Policy in Tudor and Stuart England* (London, 1988) for a discussion of the underlying attitudes of government to the poor and their relief.

the health and riches to be found in the new lands. One writer asserted that the temperate nature of the New England climate was 'made manifest by experience, the most infallible proof of all assertions'.[43] A leading puritan, Francis Higginson, writing back to England to prospective immigrants took care to stress not only that as a preacher he could not lie, but that he reported nothing unless he had:

seen it with my own eyes and partly heard and inquired from the mouths of very honest and religious person(s), who by living in the country a good space of time had had experience and knowledge of the state thereof and whose testimonies I do believe as myself.[44]

Anyone could be an authority about health and the environment, because anyone could draw upon personal experience and upon traditional knowledge. This mirrors the way in which anyone could set up as an authority in the medical market place of the time.

Despite the possibility of individual differences of opinion there was a consensus as to the topography of health and illness that held, on the whole, for most of the early modern period. What constituted healthy places, airs and waters was generally agreed upon, and everyone believed that healthy places meant healthy bodies. In 1576 William Lombarde had commented in his *A Perambulation of Kent* that Romney Marsh was sparsely populated because 'most men be yet still of Porcius Cato his minde, who held them starke madde, that would dwell in an unwholsome Aire.'[45] (Modern historical demographers also agree that low-lying marsh ground produced a higher death rate.)[46] Tobias Venner, the Bath physician, in his book on regiment, *Via Recta ad Vitam Longam* (1628), wrote at length on the relationship between health and low-lying places:

Therefore he that desireth to live a long and healthy life, must dwell in an eminent and champion country, or at least, in a place that is free from muddy and waterish impurities: for it is impossible, that a man should live long and healthily in a place, where the spirits are with impure ayre daily affected.[47]

Marshy air produced nearly all 'the diseases of the braine and sinews, as

[43] G. Mount (pseudonymous), *An Historicall Discoverie and Relation of the English Plantations of New England* (London, 1627), sig. D2v.
[44] Everett Emerson (ed.), *Letters From New England. The Massachusetts Bay Colony, 1629–1638* (Amherst, 1976), p. 30.
[45] William Lambarde, *A Perambulation of Kent* (London, 1576), p. 159.
[46] Mary Dobson, '"Marsh Fever": A Geography of Malaria in England', *Journal of Historical Geography* 6 (1980), 359–89, and idem, 'The Last Hiccup of the Old Demographic Regime: Population Stagnation and Decline in Late Seventeenth and Early Eighteenth-Century England', *Continuity and Change*, 4 (1989), 395–428.
[47] Tobias Venner, *Via Recta ad Vitam Longam* (London, 1628), p. 8.

Crampes, Palsies etc. with paines in the joynts; and to speake all in a word, a general torpidity both of minde and body'.[48] Venner elaborated on how the mind was affected, 'those living in eminent and champion Countrys' were 'witty, nimble, magnanimous and *alta petentes*'. However he warned:

the contrary is seene in low and marish places: for there, the Inhabitants, by reason of the evilnesse of the Ayre, have grosse and earthy spirits, whereof it is, that they are for the most part men, *humun tantum sapientes*, dull, sluggish, sordid, sensual, plainly irreligious, or perhaps some of them, which is little worse, religious in shewe, external honest men, deceitfull, malicious, disdainfull.

From this stance of environmental determinism Venner advised, in conclusion that 'all such as are ingenious, generous, and desirous of perfection, both in minde and body, that they endeavour by all means, to live in a pure and healthy Ayre'.[49]

In the second half of the seventeenth century a more distinctly 'scientific' style of reporting on the climate, health and natural history of a place began to emerge. The new Baconian and Royal Society ideology of exactness and exhaustiveness in observation can be discerned in reports such as John Clayton's letters to the Royal Society 'of several observables in Virginia' (1688), John Ray's *Observations ...made on a journey through part of the Low Countries, Germany, Italy and France* (1673), Hans Sloane's *A Voyage to the Islands of Madera, Barbadoes, Nieves, St Christopher's and Jamaica, with the Natural History of the last* (2 vols. 1707, 1725), William Hillary's *An Account of the Principal Variations of the Weather, and the concomitant Epidemic Disease, as they appeared at Rippon and the circumjacent Parts of Yorkshire from the Year 1726 to the End of 1734* (1740), and Thomas Short's *New Observations on City, Town and Country Bills of Mortality* (1750).

Nevertheless, despite the new style of writing, little had essentially changed from the early seventeenth century. Thomas Short no longer agreed that England had the healthiest climate in the world,[50] but he did concur that the countryside was the healthiest place in which to live. He wrote that he had begun with the country registers:

as a rural life was the first State of Man and as it is still the healthiest, and affords the truest and most innocent Pleasures: For there (except in great, rich, or opulent Men's Houses) still remains such Vestiges of Virtue, Sobriety,

---

[48] *Ibid.*, p. 3.   [49] *Ibid.*, p. 9.   [50] Short, *New Observations*, pp. 1–2.

Regularity, Plainness, and simplicity of Diet as bears some small Image or Resemblance of the primeval State.[51]

Short used information from parish registers of births, marriages and deaths to draw epidemiological conclusions which were not much different from those of a hundred or more years before that had been based upon common experience and tradition. Short concluded from his data that:

Dry, open Situations meanly elevated, neither like Beacons on the Tops of lofty Mountains, nor like Reeds in the marshy Vallies, are above all others (*caeteris paribus*) the healthiest; for such Habitations have a free, pure, open Air...[52]

The unhealthiest places were:

Low Habitations, especially on stiff Clay, rotten Earth, or near a Level with the sea, great Rivers, Marshes, Lakes or putrid standing Waters. These are worst of all; for their Air is always moist, gross, and loaded with Exhalations often putrid.[53]

There was also a stream of advice on creating the best environment. This could involve, for instance, the siting of a house. Garvase Markham, in his *The English Husbandman* (1635) which was addressed to a newly prosperous group in English society, advised:

let not your house be too neere great Rivers or Brookes, they may smile in Summer, but they will be angrie in Winter, and it is better to have them wash your Grounds than wet your house, Besides they oft vomit forth ill ayres, and are in their owne natures Aguish and unwholesome.[54]

Robert Burton wrote in the *Anatomy of Melancholy* (1621) that:

A clear air cheers up the spirits, exhilarates the mind; a thick, black misty, tempestuous, contracts, overthrows. Great heed is therefore to be taken at what times we walk, how we place our windows, lights and houses, how we let in or exclude this ambient air.[55]

How far anyone acted on such advice is unclear. When the mortality in Jamestown, Virginia, became too great, plans were made to move the settlement to high ground away from its marshy air which was blamed for the deaths. Such action at this time was rare. Romney Marsh, despite its reputation, was not deserted. Lambarde noted that it was 'famous throughout the Realme, as well for the fertilitie and quantitie of the

---

[51] *Ibid.*, p. 1.   [52] *Ibid.*, p. 13.   [53] *Ibid.*, p. 19.
[54] Gervase Markham, *The English Husbandman* (London, 1635), p. 22.
[55] Robert Burton, *The Anatomy of Melancholy*, ed. Floyd Dell and Paul Jordan-Smith (New York, 1938), p. 435.

soile...' and that 'it offered Wealth without healthe'.[56] If a place was economically attractive then its reputation for ill health was ignored. This was certainly the case with the most populous place in England, London.

As we have seen, too many people in one place could, it was believed, be a cause of disease and death (an idea which also finds approval today). The authorities were aware of the dangers of overcrowding. A royal proclamation of 1580 tried to limit new buildings in London and to prevent more than one family living in a house (like others of its kind it was unsuccessful). The proclamation argued that disease, especially plague, could spread in crowded conditions:

Where there are such great multitudes of people brought to inhabit in small houses, whereof a great part are seen very poor, and they heaped up together, and in a sort smothered with many families of children and servants in one house or small tenement, it must needs follow (if any plague or popular sickness should by God's permission enter amongst those multitudes) that the same would ... spread itself and invade the whole city and confines, as great mortality should ensue to the same.[57]

Despite the fear of plague, despite the acknowledged higher risk of disease and death, people still flocked to London from the healthy countryside and the city grew inexorably. As today, knowledge about

[56] Lambarde, *A Perambulation of Kent*, p. 158. William Strachy's account of the healthiness of Jamestown in 1610, the need to settle on a hill and the analogy with England illustrates some of the points of the chapter so far: 'True it is, I may not excuse this our Fort, or James Towne, as yet seated in some what an unwholesome and sickly ayre, by reason it is in a marish ground, low, flat to the River, and hath no fresh water Springs serving the Towne, but what wee drew from a Well sixe or seven fathom deepe, fed by the brackish River owzing into it, from whence I verily beleeve, the chiefe causes have proceeded of many diseases and sicknesses which have happened to our people, who are indeede strangely afflicted with Fluxes and Agues; and every particular season (by the relation of the old inhabitants) hath his particular infirmity too, all which (if it had bin our fortunes, to have seated upon some hill, accommodated with fresh Springs and cleere ayre, as doe the Natives of the Country) we might have, I believe, well escaped: and some experience we have to perswade our selves that it may be so, for of foure hundred and odde men, which were seated at the Fals, the last yeere when the Fleete came in with fresh and yong able spirits, under the government of Captain Francis West, and of one hundred to the Seawards (on the South side of our River) in the Country of the Nansumundes, under the charge of Captaine John Martin, there did not so much as one man miscarry, and but very few or none fall sicke, whereas at James Towne, the same time, and the same moneths, one hundred sickened, & halfe the number died: howbeit, as we condemne not Kent in England, for a small Towne called Plumsted, continually assaulting the dwellers there (especially new commers) with Agues and Fevers; no more let us lay scandall, and imputation upon the Country of Virginia, because the little Quarter wherein we are set down (unadvisedly so chosed) appears to be unwholesome, and subject to many ill ayres, which accompany the like marish places.' William Strachy 'A true Reportorie of the Wreck and Redemption of Sir Thomas Gates, Knight; upon and from the ilands of the Bermudas: his comming to Virginia and the Estate of that colonie then ... July 15. 1610', in 'Samuel Purchas, *Hakluytus Postumus or Purchas His Pilgrimes*, 20 vols. (1625; reprinted Glasgow, 1905), XIX, pp. 58–9.

[57] Cited in Lawrence Manley, *London in the Age of Shakespeare* (London, 1986), pp. 184–5.

health risks does not easily change people's behaviour when faced with the economic opportunity or the social magnet of the city.

Understanding knowledge about the environment

Medical theories came and went in the early modern period – Galenic humouralism, alchemy, iatrochemistry, chemistry, iatromechanism. The changes are easy to discern. Tobias Venner rationalized in a traditional Galenic manner that marshy air was bad 'for impure, grosse and intemperate ayre doth corrupt the spirits and humours'.[58] Over a hundred years later Thomas Short was urging parents living in towns or cities to place their children in the countryside, if they could. He justified his argument by using the mechanical and chemical language of his time which had replaced that of the humours. The town's or city's

Atmosphere is loaded, and has its Spring lessened by sulphurous, and other Steams, so as it cannot duly inflate and distend the Lungs, nor compress the sanguinous Vessels, cool the Blood, nor communicate fresh Fewel to it, for the City Air is full of perspired Matter, discharged from both dead and living animal bodies, and other noxious Matter; Matter as well from diseased as healthy Bodies, and many insensibly convey the Seeds of several Distempers with the unhealthy State of those Juices they exhaled from.[59]

By and large both humoral and mechanical writers agreed on the facts of the case – city air was bad – but they explained why this was so in different ways.

There were, however, other ways of understanding the relationships between health and the environment apart from the learned theories of medicine, chemistry and natural philosophy. How did early modern society judge whether an environment (or food and drink) was bad? People used their senses: smell, for instance, was very important.[60] Not only could smell indicate that something was healthy or unhealthy, but smells were employed in an active manner to maintain health and to keep out disease. In times of plague bunches of sweet-smelling flowers or herbs were carried to counter the foul-smelling vapour or miasma (infectious air) coming from places like cesspits that was believed to cause plague. Thomas Muffet, in his *Health's Improvement* (1655) published fifty-one years after his death, advised that plague air was to be corrected with 'good fires, and burning of Lignum Aloes, Ebony, Cinamon bark, Sassaphras and Juniper. Burn also the piths of Oranges, Citrons and

---

[58] Venner, *Via Recta*, p. 8.   [59] Short, *New Observations*, p. 63.
[60] For a slightly later period see Alain Corbin, *The Foul and the Fragrant* (Leamington Spa, 1986).

Lemons, and Myrrh and Rosen; and the poorer sort may perfume their chambers with Baies, Rosemary, and Broom itself.'[61]

More generally, Robert Burton extolled the virtues of 'artificial air' as a way 'to correct nature by art', this was 'to be made hot and moist, and to be seasoned with sweet perfumes, pleasant and lightsome as may be; to have Roses, Violets, and sweet smelling flowers ever in their windows, Posies in their hand'.[62] John Evelyn in his *Fumifugium* (1661) outlined a grandiose scheme to counteract London's foul air which he believed came from the burning of sea coal and from the stench of church yards, charnel houses, chandlers and butchers.[63] A mass of sweet-smelling trees, bushes and plants would be planted to surround and vivify London.[64] Evelyn argued that London's air 'carries away multitudes by languishing and deep Consumptions, as the Bills of Mortality do weekly inform us', and that 'almost half of them who perish in London, dye of phthisical and pulmonic distempers; That the inhabitants are never free from Coughs and importunate Rheumatisms, spitting of Impostumated and corrupt matter, for remedy whereof, there is none so infallible, as that in time, the Patient change his Aer, and remove into the Country'.[65]

Behind such a scheme seems to lie the smells and images of the paradisical garden and of exotic worlds. The Dedication to Charles II of the *Fumifugium* was perhaps hyperbolic and other worldly even for its own time, but this was still an age of strange new worlds. Evelyn explained that he wrote:

'to render not only Your Majesties Palace, but the whole City likewise of the sweetest and most delicious Habitations in the World; and this with little or no expense; but by improving those Plantations which Your Majesty so laudably affects in the moyst, depressed and Marshy grounds about the Town...upon every gentle emmission through the Aer, should so perfume the adjacent places with their breath, as if by a certain charm, or innocent Magick, they were transferred to that part of Arabia, which is therefore styl'd the Happy, because it is amongst the Gums and precious spices.[66]

[61] Thomas Muffet, *Health's Improvement* (London, 1655), p. 25. Muffet added, p. 26: 'But here a great question ariseth, whether sweet smels correct the pestilent aire, or rather be as a guide to bring it the sooner into our hearts? To determin which question I call all the dwellers in Bucklers Berry in London to give their sentence: which only street (by reason that it is wholly replenished with Physick Drugs, and Spicery and was daily perfumed in the time of the plague with pounding of Spices, melting of gums, and making perfumes for others) escaped that great plague brought from Newhaven, whereof, there died so many, that scarce any house was left unvisited.'
[62] Burton, *Anatomy of Melancholy*, p. 436.
[63] John Evelyn, *Fumifugium or the Inconvenience of the Aer and Smoak of London Dissipated* (London, 1661), pp. 56, 21. [64] *Ibid.*, pp. 24–5. [65] *Ibid.*, 12–13.
[66] *Ibid.*, sig. A3r.

This language of sweet sensation should not be dismissed merely as the effusions of a keen gardener (Evelyn was the gentleman-gardener of Sayes Court where he had retreated to during the Interregnum, and was to write treatises on forest and fruit trees). The enterprise of bringing the country into the city is still with us in the shape of public parks and gardens and in the ethos of the suburban garden. Moreover, Evelyn rightly used as evidence of a longing for the countryside and its health the common practice of the ill and convalescent of travelling into the countryside for a change of air and to escape the diseases of the city.

Behind the idea of *rus in urbe* lay, I think, the Garden of Eden,[67] the paradisical garden where the smells of the plants were the most fragrant. and where there was neither death nor disease. In a sense, paradise was the absolute measure against which all other environments were measured. The power of Christianity in this period made the Garden of Eden a potent symbol, but paradise had also the functional role of representing perfection in a society which lacked today's instruments and scales that give us our measure of objective degrees of impurity (as for chemicals or bacteria in water).

The ideal perfection of paradise was not attainable on earth by human art. As John Parkinson put it in the title page of his botanical work the *Paradisi in Sole Paradisus Terrestris* (1629), 'who wishes to compare art with nature and our parks with Eden, without wisdom measures the stride of the elephant by the stride of the mite and the flight of the eagle by that of the midge'. Nevertheless, Thomas Short noted that the 'rural life' still bore 'some small image or Resemblance of the Primeval State'. Perfection did not now exist, but we could still glimpse in the countryside what it had been like. There were different opinions on whether the pale images of paradise to be found on earth were creations of nature or of man. Virgin America was often likened to paradise, and the noble savage, the Indian, enjoyed the good health appropriate to such a place.[68]

On the other hand, nature could be seen as hostile with demi-paradise having to be worked for. The cartographer, John Norden, in his

---

[67] For a much wider cultural context to the perception of the environment, gardens, paradise and the treatment of animals see Keith Thomas, *Man and the Natural World. Changing Attitudes in England 1500–1800* (Harmondsworth, 1984), which is the standard work on the subject. Also Raymond Williams, *The Country and the City* (London, 1985).

[68] See H. C. Porter, *The Inconstant Savage, England and the North American Indian 1500–1660* (London, 1979); C. Clacken, *Traces on the Rhodian Shore* (Berkeley, 1976). Peter Hulme, *Colonial Encounters. Europe and the Native Caribbean 1492–1797* (London, 1986).

Surveiors Dialogue (1610) discussed the different types of agricultural land in England. He felt that if left to nature even:

the fairest pastures, and greenest meadows, would become in short time, over-grown with bushes, woods, weeds and things unprofitable, as they were before they were rid and cleansed of the same by the industry of man, who was inioyened that use and travaile to manure the earth, which for his disobedience should bring forth these things.[69]

After the Fall there could be no natural paradise, though it could be hoped and worked for. In the *Dialogue* the 'Surveyor' speaks of 'Tandeane' in Somerset as 'the paradise of England' which is a product of its natural fruitfulness but also of its people doing 'their best by art and industry' and 'they take extraordinarie paines in soyling, plowing and dressing their lands'.[70]

Paradise might be perceived for a while in the *terra nova* of America with its noble savages and its gardens of Eden until epidemics, famine and the need to shape the land, and to take the Indian's lands changed the perception of both land and Indians to hostile and unpleasant entities. Paradise could also be found in a vestigial form in the countryside whether in its natural state or as something to be worked for, never reached perhaps but distantly approached by art and industry. In a sense the Fall ensured that the environment, like man and woman, would always be tainted and unhealthy to some degree.

Paradise and the Fall is a useful way of showing how the perception of the countryside as healthy had its counterpart in the revealed truth of religion. The story of the Fall also gave a Biblical origin for the need for curative medicine to counteract newly arrived death and disease. The means to ameliorate the consequences of the Fall were given by God to man but they likewise could not restore the original situation. Tobias Whitaker, a Norwich and London physician, wrote in 1638 in a work extolling the health-giving virtues of wine:

for had Adam never sinned, yet must his body have been preserved and maintained by diet, which is part of physick. But after his fall so violated his equall temper [constitution] that as then he became subject to mortalitie and naturall decay. Then came in the necessity of medicine and ever since for this necessitie sake, hath the Almighty commanded an honour to be given to the Phisician for he heath created him an Angell of mercy.[71]

The environment was not merely a place where people lived, whether

[69] John Norden, *The Surveiors Dialogue* (London, 1610), p. 184.
[70] *Ibid.*, pp. 191–2.
[71] Tobias Whitaker, *The Tree of Humane Life or The Bloud of the Grape* (London, 1638) sig. A 3r.

in cities, on mountains or in swampy land. From it came food and drink. Just as a healthy environment provided healthy people, so too a healthy environment was thought to produce healthy plants and animals and pure water, and hence health-giving food and drink. Mrs Ann (possibly Aphra) Behn's poem in support of Thomas Tryon's call for vegetarianism pointed to the example of Adam and the long-lived Patriarchs who did not eat meat, but it also evoked the golden-age environment of 'Christal Streams' and 'plenteous Wood' which provided 'harmless drink and wholsom food'.

> In that blest golden Age, when Man was young,
> When the whole Race was vigorous and strong.
> When Nature did her wonderous dictates give,
> And taught the Noble Savage how to live.
> When Christal Streams and every plenteous Wood
> Afforded harmless drink and wholsom food;
> ...E'er that ingratitude in Man was found
> And ev'ry Age produced a feebler Race,
> Sickly their days and those declin'd apace,...
> Give us long life and lasting Vertue too:
> Such were the mighty Patriarchs of old
> Who in God in all his glory did behold,
> Inspir'd like you [Tryon], they Heavens
>   Instructions show'd
> And were as Gods amidst the wondring Croud;
> Not he that love th' Almighty Wand cou'd give
> Diviner Dictates, how to eat and live
> And so essential was this cleanly Food,
> For Man's eternal health eternal, eternal good,
> That God did for his first – lov'd Race provide
> What thou, by God's example, best prescribed...[72]

The allusion to paradise gave a benchmark for judging the health of the environment and its products, but it was of little use in the practical daily business of deciding which products one should select to eat and drink. Ideas of cleanliness and dirt, of the natural and unnatural, of light and darkness, of movement and sluggishness underlay many of the descriptions of healthy and unhealthy food and drink. These are to be found in the health advice books of the time and judging from the large numbers written there was a market for them amongst the literate section of the population.[73] The link between medicine and food is still a strong one today (diet and heart disease, cancer etc.); in the early

[72] In Thomas Tryon, *The Way to Health*, sig. A 4r.   [73] See note 38 above.

modern period advice on how to judge not only the healthiness but also the goodness or freshness of water, fish and meat was prominent. Effective official inspection of food and analysis of water was developed in the nineteenth and twentieth centuries. Consumers in the early modern period had to judge for themselves. Moreover, medicine was closely connected to cooking. A Hippocratic view had been that internal medicine was a specialized form of dietetics and that preparing food was analogous to preparing medicines.[74] Sixteenth- and seventeenth-century manuscript collections of medical prescriptions or recipes often included recipes for food, and as Thomas Cogan put it 'the learned Physition … is, or ought to be a perfect cooke in many points'.[75]

Animals were judged to be healthy (hence to be healthy food) in the same way as humans. As the husbandman working in the fields was thought to be healthier and longer lived than the city merchant or student so animals and fish coming from the wild were equated with health and cleanliness. Thomas Venner wrote that eating fish produced 'much grosse, slimie superflous flegme' which in turn could cause gout, bladder stone, leprosy, scurvy and other skin diseases. He advised great care in the choice of fish 'as that it be not of a clammie, slimie, neither of a very grosse and hard substance … neither of ill smell and unpleasant savour'. Venner considered what conditions produced the healthiest fish:

Wherefore of sea-fish, that is best which swimmeth in a pure sea, and is tossed and hoysed with winds and surges: for by reason of continuall agitation, it becometh of a purer, and lesse slimie substance, and consequently of easier concoction [digestion], and of a purer iuyce.[76]

Similarly fresh-water fish was best:

Which is bred in pure, stonie or gravelly rivers, running swiftly. For that which is taken in muddie waters in standing pooles, in fennes, mores and ditches, by reason of the impuritie of the place, and water, is unwholesome …[77]

The concepts (and language) can be found in a number of writers. Sir Thomas Elyot in the sixteenth century had written in his best-selling *Castell of Health* (1534):

The best fish after the opinion of Galen is that which swymmeth in a pure sea and is tossed and lift up with wynds and surges. The more calme that the water

---

[74] A point made in the Hippocratic treatise *On Ancient Medicine*.
[75] Cogan, *Haven of Health*, p. 112.
[76] Venner, *Via Recta*, p. 69; see also Cogan, *Haven of Health*, p. 161.
[77] Venner, *Via Recta*, p. 70.

is, the worse the fish. They which are in muddy waters, do make much fleume and ordure, taken in fennes and dyckes be worst.[78]

Just as fish could be polluted, so could water. The best water was that which came from rain water or from fountains or springs, and flowed swiftly. William Vaughan indicated that good water was known 'By the clearnesse of it. That water is best which is light, transparent, agreeable to the sight, Christalline, and which runneth from an higher to a lower ground'. (He also added that 'some use to try [test] water by putting a clean Napkin in it and if any spots appeare upon the same they suspect the goodnesse of the water'.)[79] Bad water was found in standing pools, marshy ground; river water could also be of poor quality, if, as Venner wrote, 'it be polluted by the mixture of other things, as it commeth to passe in Rivers, that run thorow marish places, or neere unto populous Townes and Cities: for then, by reason of all manner of filth running, or cast into them, they become very corrupt and unwholesome'.[80] Venner added that it was up to the inhabitants of towns to find and to select wholesome river water which 'runneth with a full streame upon gravell, Pebble-stones, Rockes, or pure earth: for that water, by reason of the purity of the place, motion, and radiant splendor of the Sun is thinner, sweeter and therefore more pure and wholesome'.[81]

There are some common factors underlying these types of explanation. There was a holistic approach to the environment and its products. Not only did the environment affect living things and its own substances such as water, but the explanations used to make sense of the environment and plants and animals were often the same. As we have seen above, motion was a common key to the healthiness of fish and of water. Cogan expressed this in explicit terms:

For the flowing water doth not lightly corrupt, but that which standeth still: Even so bodies exercised, are for the most part more healthfull, and such as bee idle more subject to sicknesse.[82]

[78] Sir Thomas Elyot, *The Castell of Health* (London, 1580), p. 32v
[79] Vaughan, *Directions for Health*, pp. 25–6. Burton, *Anatomy of Melancholy*, p. 397, described the sensory qualities of good water: 'Pure, thin, light water by all means use, of good smell and taste, like to the air in sight, such as is soon hot, soon cold...'
[80] Venner, *Via Recta*, p. 10.   [81] *Ibid.*, p. 11.
[82] Cogan, *Haven of Health*, p. 2. Lack of exercise was often thought to lead to disease. Sir Richard Hawkins gave as one of the causes of scurvy 'the want of exercise also either in persons or elements, as in calmes. And were it not for the moving of the Sea by the force of windes, tydes and current, it would corrupt all the world'. He advised 'to keepe the company occupied in some bodily exercise of worke, of agilitie, of pastimes, of dancing, of use of Armes; these helpe much to banish this imfirmitie'. 'The Observations of Sir Richard Hawkins, knight, in this Voyage into the South Sea, An. Dom. 1593', in Purchas, *Hakluytus Postumus* XVII, pp. 76–7.

More general and unifying types of explanation were also used. The earth itself could be seen anthropomorphically, to be cared for in the same way as people. John Norden described the land in terms of hot, dry, cold and moist, the four qualities that made up both the world and the body,[83] and he advised the farmer to give the best care to his land:

For land is like the body, if it bee not nourished with noutriture and comforted and adorned with the most expedient commodities, it will pine away, and become forlorne, as is the minde that hath, no rest nor recreation waxe the lumpish and heavy.[84]

Farmers also treated the illnesses and hurts of their animals in ways that mirrored the medical practice that was applied to humans. Henry Best, a farmer from Elmswell in Yorkshire, wrote about the health of sheep in his manuscript Farming Book (1641). One entry has:

It is usuall with sheepe, and especially with hogges and lambs, to fall blind by reason of an humour that falleth out of the head into the eyes, whereby groweth (as it weare) a scumme over the stine [the cornea] of the eye. Many Shepheards will undertake to cure this by bloodinge them in the wykes of the eyes with a penne-knife, but the only way is to take ground-Ivy-leaves and to chewe them in your mouth, and to take the leafe with your finger after yow have sucked the Juice from it. This Juice you are to spurte into the eye morninge and eveninge, or if you will, thrice a day.[85]

A humoral explanation, use of bleeding, and disagreement about remedies was typical of medical practice for people. The use of the same types of theories and practices for animals as for people must have helped to produce a sense of interrelatedness. A sense which, for the link between humans and the environment, was formally expressed in the quasi-philosophical belief that the microcosm (the body of man) was a miniature version of the macrocosm (the greater world of the universe), and that events in the latter affected the former.[86]

Moreover the unity between the environment, living organisms like plants and animals and humans was expressed in the food cycle. Animals

---

[83] Norden, *Surveiors Dialogue*, p. 196.   [84] *Ibid.*, p. 76.

[85] David Woodward (ed.), *The Farming and Memorandum Books of Henry Best of Elsmwell 1642*, British Academy Records of Social and Economic History, New Series VIII, 1982. In the sixteenth century William Turner argued that medicinal baths should be made in Bath for animals in addition to those for humans. William Turner, *The Rare Treasor of the English Bathes*, in Thomas Vicary, *The Englishmen's Treasure* (London, 1586). p. 108.

[86] A small illustration of this is in Henry Whitmore, *Febris Anomala Or, The New Disease that Now Rageth Throughout England* (London, 1659) at p. 126 where the author notes that the new disease begun 'to visibly abade and slacken; which if I mistake not was about the latter end of November, when the cold weather begun to break forth, which on a sudden growing sharp made in the microcosm, the body of man a change as well as in the macrocosm'.

were what they ate, and we in turn were what we ate of them. As Cogan put it: 'Such as the food is, such is the blood: and such as the blood, such is the flesh.' [87] He went on to argue that our health depends on what we eat. This also applied to animals:

Yet the goodnesse of the pasture helpeth much to the goodnesse of the milke: for ill pastures made ill milke, and good pastures made good milke: for such as the food is such is the bloud and such as the bloud is, such is the milke.[88]

Given the view that there was a close union between all the parts of the organic and inorganic worlds it is not surprising that specific ideas such as the healthiness of motion were applied to a wide range of objects and creatures. At the level of these specific ideas there was a perceived dichotomy between town and country, short life and long life, the unhealthy and the healthy, the stultifying and the fresh, the stagnant and the moving, dark and light, crowded and uncrowded, the tame and the wild, ('unhealthy places in the countryside' could be substituted for town or city in the first pair of opposites). These were not merely opposing pairs of ideas, but towns, for instance, could be associated with one part of each pair, with tameness, bad stagnant air or water, darkness and smoke, overcrowding, bad health etc. That such contrasts really were current is clear from the example of the pig.

Swine's flesh was looked on with some suspicion, but it was believed to be healthy if the pig had been allowed to roam in the wild and to eat natural foodstuffs. Cogan wrote:

Also better [to eat] of a wilde swine than of a tame, because as Galen saith, the flesh of swine fed at home is more full of superflous moysture for want of motion, beside they live in a more grosse ayre than those that live wild. But our use in England is for the most part to breed our swine at home, except it be for the time of mast falling, for then they feed abroad in the woods, which kinde of feeding in my judgement is most wholesome: wherefore brawne, which is of a bore long fed in a stie can in no wise be wholesome meat, although it be young. For beside that it is hard of digestion (as common experience proveth) it must needs breed ill iuce in the body, considering the want of motion and grosse feeding thereof for which course we use commonly to drinke strong wine with brawne to help digestion.[89]

Thomas Fuller in his *History of the Worthies of England* (1662) praised 'Hampshire Hoggs' as producing the best bacon because:

Here the swine feed in the Forrest on plenty of Acorns (mens meat in the Golden, Hog's food in this Iron Age); which going out lean, return home fat,

---

[87] Cogan, *Haven of Health*, Epistle Dedicatory.   [88] *Ibid.*, p. 176.   [89] *Ibid.*, p. 133.

without either care or cost of their owners. Nothing but fulness stinteth their feeding on the mast falling from the Trees, where also they lodge at liberty (not pent up, as in other places to stacks of Pease), which some assign the reason of the fineness of their flesh.[90]

Thomas Muffet agreed that the pig was especially nourishing 'if he feed abroad upon sweet grass, good mast and roots; for that which is penn'd up and fed at home with taps droppings, kitchin offal, soure grains and all manner of drosse cannot be wholsom'.[91] And Thomas Tryon at the end of the century held a similar view: 'That Bacon and Pork, which is fed with Corn and Acorns and have their liberty to run, is much sweeter and wholsomer, easier of digestion and breeds better blood than that which is shut up in the Hogg-sties, such Bacon for want of motion becomes more of a gross phlegmatic Nature'.[92]

The idea that fresh air, fresh food and freedom to move were good for pigs (and for men and women) remained the same despite changes in theoretical perspectives, and these ideas can also be found today amongst the 'green' or environmental movements as well as amongst many other groups. A characteristic of such 'natural' ideas is that they were generalized enough to be applicable to many different types of situation. Thomas Muffet, for instance, wrote about the fattening of fowl and he united the view that lack of exercise produced unhealthy food with another basic concept (already referred to) that there is a close connection between the qualities (psychological as well as physical) of the bodies that we eat and our own:

But here a question may be moved, Whether this penning up of birds, and want of exercise, and depriving them of light, and cramming them so often with strange meat, makes not their flesh as unwholesome to us as well as fat? To which I answer that to cramb Capons, or any bird and to deprive them of all light, is ill for them and us too: for though their body be puffed up, yet their flesh is not natural and wholesom; witness their small discoloured and rotten livers; whereas Hens and Capons feeding themselves in an open and clean place with good corn have large, ruddy and firm livers...[do not feed them] in a coope or close roome, for then the aire and themselves will smell of their own dung, but in a cleane house spacious enough for their little exercise; not in a dark place, or stitching up their eyes, for that will cause them to be timerous, or ever sleepy; both which are enemies to their bodies, and consequently ours.[93]

[90] Thomas Fuller, *The History of the Worthies of England*, 2 vols. (London, 1811), I, p. 400.
[91] Thomas Muffet, *Health's Improvement* (London, 1655), p. 68.
[92] Tryon, *The Way to Health*, p. 67.
[93] Muffet, *Health's Improvement*, pp. 43–4. Thomas, *Man and the Natural World*, p. 189 cites this in part when discussing the perceived cruelty of poultry farming.

Despite the great changes that have taken place in medical ideas, many views about the healthiness of the environment and its products have remained largely unchanged. In a sense, they express the aspirations of certain parts of society: condemnation of present-day developments and a yearning for a natural world whose attributes – clean, light, spacious allowing motion, uncrowded etc. – are still viewed today, unquestioningly, as good and positive characteristics. Perhaps an anthropologist would use such attributes, and the pairs of opposites listed earlier, as evidence from which to construct a picture of the type of society that created them. A historian of medicine, after cautious caveats about the limited currency of such ideas, can note that early modern England possessed a well-articulated body of knowledge about the health of the environment. At a time when cities and towns were growing in size and in unhealthiness a set of values was present which acted as a counter weight, which some of the literate classes, at least, could refer to even if they did not always act on them. (Though as Philip Curtin has shown in his study of mortality in the tropics, the mortality of European armies declined when some of these ideas such as siting camps on hill stations, good ventilation, clear water were put into practice in the nineteenth century.)[94]

I would like to thank Lindsay Granshaw, Roy Porter and Phillip Wilson for their helpful comments on this chapter.

[94] Philip Curtin, *Death by Migration. Europe's Encounter with the Tropical World in the Nineteenth Century* (Cambridge, 1989).

Medicine in the age of Enlightenment

GUENTER B. RISSE

Introduction

Historical scholarship usually assigns the term Enlightenment to a period which began with the Glorious Revolution of 1688 in England and ended either with the 1776 Declaration of Independence by the United States, or the French Revolution of 1789. As a European reform movement, the new era witnessed a shift in values and social policy that profoundly shaped subsequent human history. Among the most prominent beliefs operative during the Enlightenment was faith in the progress and perfectibility of society with the help of science and technology. On the methodological front, the power of reason – variously interpreted as mathematical–deductive or sensualist–inductive – characterized the debates concerning human understanding.

A rejection of previous theological hierarchies and social constraints was initiated by Enlightenment thinkers under the banner of a desirable 'natural' evolution of the innate intellectual and moral tendencies of man. Finally, the condition of liberty as a right for the attainment of happiness and fulfilment was coupled with the principle of utility – greater benefits for the greatest number. Both constituted the fundamental pillars for the envisioned reconstruction of human institutions.[1]

---

[1] For brief overviews, consult C. Brinton's article, 'Enlightenment', in Paul Edwards (ed.), *The Encyclopedia of Philosophy*, 8 vols. (New York, 1967), II, pp. 519–25; and H. O. Pappe, 'Enlightenment', in Philip P. Wiener (ed.), *Dictionary of the History of Ideas*, 4 vols. (New York, 1973), II, pp. 89–100. For further details, see Paul Hazard, *European Thought in the Eighteenth Century*, trans. J. Lewis May (New York, 1963); and Ernst Cassirer, *The Philosophy of the Enlightenment*, trans. F. C. A. Koelln and J. P. Pettegrove (Boston, 1955); and Peter Hulme and Ludmilla Jordanova

In health-related fields, the Enlightenment established a much more optimistic outlook concerning the role and benefits of medicine. In their quest towards progress, most contemporary thinkers believed that health was a natural state of the body which could be maintained and protected. In turn, they were confident that, eventually all diseases could be eradicated. Such a positive view of health and medicine permeated a large number of professional and lay writings of the period which described in great detail the conditions needed for the prevention and cure of sickness.[2]

Programme and theories

In their works a number of prominent Enlightenment thinkers outlined the conditions under which well-being could be preserved. This programme of health conservation was initially designed for the upper and middle classes of society based on the classical model of the so-called 'non-natural' elements.[3] These comprised environmental factors such as air, food and drink, functions including motion and rest, and natural bodily sleep and wakefulness, evacuation and retention of nutritive elements, and finally psychological influences such as the passions of the soul. Together, the 'non-naturals' were seen as the factors primarily responsible for human health and they were subject to appropriate

(eds.), *The Enlightenment and Its Shadows* (London, 1990); and Roy Porter and Midulas Teich, *The Enlightenment in National Context* (Cambridge, 1981). Broad linkages between science and the Enlightenment are explained in I. B. Cohen, 'Scientific Revolution and Creativity in the Enlightenment', *Eighteenth-Century Life*, 7 (1982), 41–54; and the first four chapters of Colin A. Russell, *Science and Social Change, 1700–1900* (London, 1983); see also Thomas L. Hankins, *Science and the Enlightenment* (Cambridge, 1985).

[2] For a general overview of the role of medicine see Peter Gay, 'Enlightenment: Medicine and Cure', in *The Enlightenment*, 2 vols. (New York, 1966–9), II, pp. 12–23. Background information on biology is available from a recent article by Francesca Rigotti, 'Biology and Society in the Age of Enlightenment', *Journal of the History of Ideas*, 47 (1986), 215–33. A brief view of eighteenth-century medicine is available in L. S. King, 'The Debt of Modern Medicine to the Eighteenth Century', *Journal of the American Medical Association*, 190 (1964), 829–32; and W. F. Bynum, 'Health, Disease and Medical Care', in G. S. Rousseau and R. Porter (eds.), *The Ferment of Knowledge* (Cambridge, 1980), pp. 211–53. A more extensive background treatment of the subject can be found in Lester S. King, *The Road to Medical Enlightenment, 1650–1695* (London, 1970); and by the same author, *The Philosophy of Medicine; The Early Eighteenth Century* (Cambridge, MA, 1978). See also the various contributions in *The Medical Enlightenment of the Eighteenth Century*, ed. A. Cunningham and R. French (Cambridge, 1990); and James C. Riley, *The Eighteenth-Century Campaign to Avoid Disease* (Basingstoke, England, 1987).

[3] L. J. Rather, 'The Six Things "Non-Natural": A Note on the Origins and Fate of a Doctrine and a Phrase', *Clio Medica*, 3 (1968), 337–47. More details are contained in P. H. Niebyl, 'The Non-Naturals', *Bulletin of the History of Medicine*, 45 (1971), 486–92; and C. R. Burns, 'The Nonnaturals: A Paradox in the Western Concept of Health', *Journal of Medicine and Philosophy*, 3 (1976), 202–11.

manipulation to ensure such well-being. Thus in the eighteenth century the classical doctrines became a convenient platform for launching a comprehensive programme of health conservation.[4]

Rational measures to maintain an appropriate balance of all bodily functions could be initiated by any person alone or with help from the medical professionals. Needed was a good knowledge of one's own individual constitution and reaction to the non-naturals before charting a desirable lifestyle which would preserve the state of health. 'There does not exist a definition of health applicable to everyone', declared Arnulfe d'Aumont, the French physician who wrote an article on the subject for Diderot's *Encyclopédie*, 'each has his own state of well-being.'[5]

As a positive value, health was attached to the 'satisfaction one feels in his physical and moral existence', a condition of bodily and psychological well-being conducive to a more enjoyable and longer life. Such an existence could be sustained if the daily dispersion of natural forces, especially nervous energy, was properly replenished by nourishment and rest. 'The more vital the nature of these forces and the less they are dissipated, the more durable and strong health will be,' wrote D'Aumont.[6] Wasting or using more than one's daily quota of such energies eventually threatened to enfeeble the body and thus invite disease.

By contrast, sickness was seen as an avoidable evil that endangered both the individual and the community. Aside from personal suffering, many authors also stressed the economic drain of sickness both for the afflicted, their families, as well as the state. Here again, a number of prophylactic measures, grouped under the term 'hygiene', were recommended to prevent the occurrence of disease. 'Hygiene,' wrote D'Aumont, also author of an article in the *Encyclopédie* by the same name, 'is a term that serves to designate the first of two medical procedures, the one concerning the conduct necessary to follow for maintaining the state of existing health.'[7] Fresh air, personal cleanliness,

---

[4] W. Coleman, 'Health and Hygiene in the "Encyclopédie": A Medical Doctrine for the Bourgeoisie', *Journal of the History of Medicine*, 29 (1974), 399–421.

[5] Arnulfe d'Aumont, 'Santé', in D. Diderot (ed.), *Encyclopédie ou dictionnaire risonné des sciences, des arts et des metiers* (Paris, 1751–65), XIV, p. 629. This passage and others have been translated from the French by G. B. Risse. For details, see Frank A. Kafker, *The Encyclopedists as Individuals: A Biographical Dictionary of the Authors of the Encyclopédie* (Oxford, 1988).

[6] d'Aumont, 'Santé', in *Encyclopédie*, XIV, p. 630.

[7] Arnulfe d'Aumont, 'Hygiène', in *Encyclopédie*, VIII, p. 385. For further details, consult L. J. Jordanova, 'Earth Science and Environmental Medicine: The Synthesis of The Late Enlightenment', in L. J. Jordanova and R. Porter (eds.), *Images of the Earth* (Chalfont St Giles, Bucks, 1979), pp.

sufficient exercise and rest, and control of the passions were recommended. Interestingly, it was now decided that individuals would have
to assume a measure of blame if they fell ill since society apparently
provided the means for keeping well.

However, this goal of staying healthy could prove elusive since 'it is
extremely rare that when feeling or believing to be feeling well, one
could ask advice on the best behaviour for continuing to enjoy such
well-being'.[8] Here lay reluctance to seek counsel from the medical
profession was matched by the physician's earlier aversion to dealing
with non-therapeutic issues. Health manuals written by experts were
therefore needed to serve as popular guides for self-help whenever health
practitioners were unavailable or disinclined to abandon their more
profitable curative chores. The traditional assumption was that medicine
and physicians were almost solely employed for the purpose of healing
established diseases rather than counsel on health maintenance or the
prevention of sickness.

Indeed, the role of medicine was to re-establish lost health by dealing
with the 'contra-naturals,' meaning diseases, their symptoms and causes.
The aim of therapeutic measures was to aid and supplement the healing
power of nature inherent in all human organisms. This was to be
accomplished through the employment of time-honoured strategies
aimed at the restoration of bodily fluid balances. While both lay and
professional authors took different positions with respect to the
appropriate degree of therapeutic activism, and expressed their own
doubts about the effectiveness of specific drugs, all of them seemed quite
optimistic about future developments. Surely medicine would prosper
and improve the treatment of diseases if physicians could enhance their
understanding of how human bodies functioned in health and sickness.
Eventually diseases could be more specifically treated as their clinical
characteristics became better known through systematic observation and
classification.

Not surprisingly, the majority of Europeans making up the lower
classes of society did not entirely share such cheerful views of wellness,

---

119–46; and J. C. Riley, 'The Medicine of the Environment in Eighteenth-Century Germany', *Clio Medica*, 18 (1983), 167–78; and C. C. Hannaway, 'From Private Hygiene to Public Health: A Transformation in Western Medicine in the Eighteenth and Nineteenth Centuries', in T. Ogawa (ed.), *Public Health: Proceedings of the Fifth International Symposium of the Comparative History of Medicine – East and West* (Tokyo, 1981), pp. 108–28.

[8] d'Aumont, 'Hygiène', in *Encyclopédie*, VIII, p. 385.

disease prevention, and medical intervention.[9] Their concepts of health and illness were not generally linked to biological models and functions espoused by professional medicine. Since the Fall in the Garden of Eden, man's imperfections were reflected in his fragile earthly frame, surrendering to periodic trials of disease. For many, sickness remained a mysterious, often unpredictable and mostly unavoidable event, the result of blind fate or divine punishment. To neutralize it, one could consult the stars, wear protective talismans, ingest herbal remedies, or find persons believed to possess special skills for warding off trouble.

Often, however, such an activist stance gave way to resignation. Health was too fragile, its preservation utopian. For some, to actively interfere with destiny or disease as punishment was considered useless and even sinful, a defiance of divine providence that might well spell greater tragedy. Others tended to accept human impotence realistically in the face of disease and epidemics, humbly interceding with God and the saints for a possible reversal of the conditions. Total resignation was not uncommon. As one French physician reported in 1785, 'the peasants do not appeal to anyone. They believe there is nothing to be done. Moreover the priests tell them that their hour is decided and that it is useless to spend money for remedies that will not help.'[10]

In popular healing, however, prayers were often supplemented by the use of home-made remedies designed to ameliorate bothersome symptoms. These treatments were based on concoctions prepared from time-worn, orally transmitted recipes, available in families or provided by local herbalists. If the circumstances allowed it, local priests, self-proclaimed folk healers, or travelling drug peddlers were primarily consulted, revealing a pragmatic eclecticism present in most historical periods. This attitude sought a certain measure of relief without challenging the ultimate causality of sickness.

[9] For details about conditions in France, see W. Coleman, 'The People's Health: Medical Themes in 18th-Century French Popular Literature', *Bulletin of the History of Medicine*, 51 (1977), 55–74; and John McManners, 'Defences against Death: Eighteenth-Century Medicine', in *Death and Enlightenment* (Oxford, 1981), pp. 24–58.

[10] Quoted from H. Mitchell, 'Rationality and Control in French Eighteenth-Century Medical Views of the Peasantry', *Comparative Study of Society and History* 21 (1979), 105. For an overview, C. C. Hannaway, 'Medicine and Religion in Pre-Revolutionary France', *Social History of Medicine*, 2 (1989), 315–20; and J. Barry, 'Piety and the Patient: Medicine and Religion in Eighteenth-Century Bristol', in R. Porter (ed.), *Patients and Practitioners, Lay Perceptions of Medicine in Pre-Industrial Society* (Cambridge, 1985), pp. 145–75. These letters were among the correspondence generated by the Royal Society of Medicine, an institution which after 1778 periodically received reports about epidemics and medical activities. See C. C. Hannaway, 'La Société Royale de Médecine and Epidemics in the Ancien Régime', *Bulletin of the History of Medicine*, 46 (1972), 257–73.

A similar pragmatic stance brought the popular sector of society increasingly into contact with the professional healers, including physicians when available, and their services, free of charge. It was often a last resource to be tapped under the threat of death and accordingly the results were not always encouraging. Peasants often viewed prescribed remedies with the utmost suspicion, frequently failing to follow medical advice or blaming any untoward developments in their ailments on such professional interventions. Writing in 1779 about dysentery in certain regions of France, one practitioner complained that 'the disobedience of the peasant and his frequently unsurmountable aversion for any kind of remedy administered by doctors are such that it is ordinarily impossible to make him continue a methodical treatment'.[11]

At the heart of most activities promoted by representatives of Enlightenment medicine was the displacement of such pessimistic concepts of sickness for more hopeful outlooks enshrined within new biomedical models of health and disease. Fatalism and ignorance in health-related matters had to be overcome. Much unnecessary suffering would thus be avoided.

Happiness could be promoted if physical health was protected and restored. According to Enlightenment ideology, society therefore had to be 'medicalized' through the employment of professionals who could deal expertly with health-related problems. By contrast, all other individuals in the popular sector claiming healing roles were to be branded as quacks and discredited as obstacles on the road to better collective health.[12] Previous self-sufficiency in treatment based on superstition or lack of knowledge was to be transformed into dependency on qualified physicians and surgeons. From superior knowledge about bodily processes in health and sickness to familiarity with measures for the prevention of epidemics, from expertise in individual wellness programmes to responsibility for care in hospitals and dispensaries, a new

---

[11] Mitchell, 'Rationality', *Comparative Study of Society and History*, 21 (1979), 96.

[12] A view of the relationships between professional and popular healing in France and the problems of so-called 'quackery' are contained in J. P. Goubert, 'The Art of Healing: Learned Medicine and Popular Medicine in the France of 1790', in R. Foster and O. Ranum (eds.), *Medicine and Society in France* (Baltimore, 1980), VI, pp. 1–23. The article appeared originally in French in the *Annales, Economies, sociétés, civilisations*, 30 (Sept.–Oct. 1977), 908–26. See also M. Ramsey, 'The Repression of Unauthorized Medical Practice in Eighteenth-Century France', *Eighteenth-Century Life*, 7 (1982), 118–35; and more recently by the same author, 'Property Rights and the Right of Health: The Regulation of Secret Remedies in France, 1789–1815', in W. Bynum and R. Porter (eds.), *Medical Fringe and Medical Orthodoxy* (London, 1987), pp. 79–105.

medical elite took charge and increasingly played a more prominent role in European society.[13]

Medical systems

The ebb and flow of medical systems during the eighteenth century deserves attention. Enlightenment physicians eagerly followed the Newtonian model and searched for simple and general laws pertaining to the functions of living beings in health and sickness.[14] 'Nature delights in simplicity and uniformity,' wrote the Scottish physician Robert Whytt (1714–66) in 1751, 'and general laws applied to particular bodies produces a vast variety of operations; nor is it all improbable that an animal body is a system regulated much after the same manner.'[15]

Such striving for first principles in medicine was certainly not new. Since Hippocratic times healers had sought to discover the fundamental laws governing all phenomena of health and disease. This quest was prompted by the belief that reality was orderly, and had an underlying regular pattern. Recognition of such schemes, and specifically in medicine the circumstances and mechanisms conducive to illness, resulted in the elaboration of theories of balanced and corruptible bodily fluids. For nearly two thousand years classical humoralism explained all of physiology and pathology. Yet, in the seventeenth century obsolescence of these theories under the onslaught of new iatromechanical and iatrochemical insights clearly demanded a total reconstruction of medical theory.[16]

Thus Enlightenment physicians followed in the tradition established since Greek antiquity: elaborate a rational theory of medicine which could provide comprehensive explanations of disease causation and effect, while simultaneously supplying a firm foundation for medical practice. As a result, eighteenth-century medical system-makers examined available facts of contemporary experience regarding the

[13] See also D. Roche, 'Talent, Reason, and Sacrifice: The Physician during the Enlightenment', in *Medicine and Society in France*, pp. 66–88.
[14] In the preface to the first edition of his *Principia*, Newton wrote in 1686: 'I wish we could derive the rest of the phenomena of Nature by the same kind of reasoning from mechanical principles.' Isaac Newton, *Newton's Philosophy of Nature*, ed. H. S. Thayer (New York, 1953), pp. 9–10.
[15] Robert Whytt, *Essay on the Vital and other Involuntary Motions of Animals* (Edinburgh, 1751), p. 4.
[16] For a comprehensive background of seventeenth-century medicine, consult King, *Medical Enlightenment, 1650–1695*; and A. G. Debus (ed.), *Medicine in Seventeenth-Century England* (Berkeley, 1974).

functioning of living beings, and using their own judgements, established a number of new generalizations and definitions. Once in possession of a somewhat coherent theoretical framework, medical authors worked mostly deductively, fashioning sets of explanations – some highly speculative – which covered virtually all possible clinical situations.[17]

Most medical systematists during the eighteenth century tended to be prominent physicians affiliated with famous European universities such as Leyden, Halle, Edinburgh, and Montpellier. As teachers in the classroom and at the bedside, these men explained their doctrines to scores of medical students who flocked to the lectures. Often from as far away as the American colonies, the listeners then helped diffuse the new schemes to others upon return to their hometowns or countries of origin. The prestige of such system-makers was further buttressed by appointments to royal households, private practice among upper-class members, and extensive professional consultation through the mails. Their famous creations – the systems – were often zealously defended in print through sweeping indictments of rival theories. Bitter professional controversies and personal feuds involving the authors and their devoted followers were common.

One of the motivations for system-building by eighteenth-century physicians was the intellectual goal of achieving a simple and logical synthesis of medical knowledge designed to replace increasingly obsolete humoral conceptions inherited from antiquity. Newer models of physiology and physiopathology based on Vesalian anatomy, Harvey's circulation of the blood, recent laws of motion, and microscopical findings all demanded integration and placement into an updated scaffolding. Boundless optimism and confidence in the powers of human reason made the task seem easier. To be sure, these endeavours remained largely exercises in armchair speculation. Indeed, most authors lacked the necessary experience and methodology to ensure precision in their empirical observations, while failing to conduct a rigorous analysis of their findings before establishing far-reaching conclusions.[18]

The wish for a rational synthesis often led to the establishment of just

[17] L. S. King, 'Some Problems of Causality in Eighteenth-Century Medicine', *Bulletin of the History of Medicine*, 37 (1963), 15–24. The topic has received more attention by the same author in 'Rationalism and Empiricism', in *The Philosophy of Medicine* (Cambridge, MA, 1978), pp. 233–58, ch. 10.

[18] L. S. King, 'Evidence and Its Evaluation in Eighteenth-Century Medicine', *Bulletin of the History of Medicine*, 50 (1976), 174–90; and by the same author 'Attitudes towards "Scientific" Medicine around 1700', *Bulletin of the History of Medicine*, 39 (1965), 124–33.

one single principle regulating both physiology and pathology. For Enlightenment physicians a monistic system of medicine confirmed the inherent simplicity of the natural biological world. The pitfalls of such a venture lay in the selection and inadequacy of the available data. Careless use of analogies and mathematical–deductive reasoning compounded the errors. Eventually, some new anatomical, physiological, and pathological discoveries could no longer be accommodated within the rigid frameworks. As a result, time and again entire medical schemes began to crumble when challenged by the emergence or recognition of new or previously overlooked information. As the eighteenth century wore on, such increased vulnerability and turnover of medical systems reflected the accelerated acquisition of new facts concerning health-related subjects, as well as a more critical approach towards the methods previously used in gathering knowledge.[19]

Another inducement to system-building and the employment of logically deduced explanations resided in their capacity to confer higher professional status and a mantle of intellectual respectability to medical practitioners devising and employing them. At a time when patient patronage was usually drawn from the upper classes of society, physicians strenuously competed among themselves for financial security and upward social mobility in patient–doctor relationships largely controlled by their wealthy clients.[20] Physicians are always under considerable social pressures to apply all known measures for the benefit of their patients. Being able to rationalize the causes and manifestations of disease within contemporary cosmologies shared by the educated elite, however, helped to firm up the necessary bonds between healer and patient. More importantly, to avoid the impression of any gulf between the new viewpoints in medicine and their traditional practices, practitioners were forced to overhaul their therapeutic rationales. Physicians thus continued

---

[19] Richard H. Shryock, *The Development of Modern Medicine* (New York, 1947), pp. 26–30, ch. 2. A more detailed treatment of medical systems is contained in Guenter B. Risse, 'Eighteenth-Century Medical Systems', in 'The History of John Brown's Medical System in Germany During the Years 1790–1806' (University of Chicago Ph.D. thesis, 1971), pp. 3–67.

[20] N. D. Jewson, 'Medical Knowledge and the Patronage System in 18th Century England', *Sociology*, 8 (1974), 369–85; and Malcolm Nicolson, 'The Metastatic Theory of Pathogenesis and the Professional Interests of the Eighteenth-Century Physician', *Medical History*, 32 (1988), 277–300. A further analysis of the various professional levels is contained in B. Hamilton, 'The Medical Professions in the Eighteenth Century', *Economic History Review*, 4 (1951), 141–70; and T. M. Brown, 'The Changing Self-Concept of the Eighteenth-Century London Physician', *Eighteenth-Century Life*, 7 (1982), 31–40. The Porters have recently described the dynamics of the medical market place in Georgian England: see Dorothy and Roy Porter, *Patient's Progress: Doctors and Doctoring in Eighteenth-Century England* (Cambridge, 1989), esp. parts I and III.

to employ traditional remedies by linking them rationally to their novel theories, thereby infusing the old therapy with new logic and authority.

Early systematists such as Herman Boerhaave (1668–1738) of Leyden and Friedrich Hoffmann (1660–1742) of Halle adhered to ideas derived from the mechanical philosophy. Both borrowed extensively from iatrophysical conceptions of physiology elaborated during the seventeenth century under the influence of Descartes. The body was regarded as a machine and the Cartesian duality of matter and mind maintained.[21] Rejecting the view that there were occult or 'hidden' forces operating in nature, these physicians created medical systems based on the assumption that human bodies were made up of elementary particles in motion susceptible to observation and measurement.

Boerhaave, the leading medical figure in Europe during the early eighteenth century, created an eclectic medical system which sought to incorporate the most important physical and chemical advances made during the preceding century.[22] His ideas were initially published in 1708 under the title of Institutes of Medicine, followed by the extensive Commentaries of his system by Gerhard van Swieten (1700–72), a favourite student and assistant. For Boerhaave the solid portions of the human frame joined to form small fibres which then combined to build membranes and cylindrical blood vessels making up the bodily tissues. In turn, the less cohesive and hence fluid components constantly flowed in mixtures along the vessels according to the laws of hydrodynamics.[23] Blood particles, for example, were impelled by the heart through a network of vessels of decreasing size which selectively trapped them at various locations in the body. Motion, temperature, and secretions were all explained mechanically through circulation, flow resistance, and a constant mixture of corpuscles. Disease occurred when the normal interactions between circulating fluids and their elastic vessels became disturbed, and blood particles were sent into the wrong vessels and organs or accumulated dangerously in front of totally occluded channels.

[21] The best discussion of Boerhaave's system is in Lester S. King, 'Hermann Boerhaave, Systematist', in The Medical World of the Eighteenth Century (Chicago, 1958), pp. 59–93, ch. 3. For Hoffmann see by the same author, 'Medicine in 1695: Friedrich Hoffmann's Fundamenta Medicinae', Bulletin of the History of Medicine, 43 (1969), 17–29.

[22] For a biographical sketch, consult G. A. Lindeboom's article in Charles C. Gillispie (ed.), Dictionary of Scientific Biography (New York, 1970), II, pp. 224–28. The same author has written a complete biography titled Hermann Boerhaave, The Man and his Work (London, 1968).

[23] For more details, G. A. Lindeboom, 'Boerhaave's Concept of the Basic Structure of the Body', Clio Medica, 5 (1970), 203–8. Boerhaave's ideas were translated into English: Dr Boerhaave's Academical Lectures on the Theory of Physic, 2nd correc. edn, 6 vols. (London, 1751). For the physiological ideas consult especially vol. I.

To such a speculative pathogenesis of fluid changes and circulatory disorders, Boerhaave effectively linked the clinical symptomology observable in his patients. Fevers, for example, arose from friction between solids and fluids compacted because of blockages in vascular channels. Significantly, the author also made the time-worn therapeutics inherited from humoralism appear to be logical derivations from his theoretical schemes. Bloodletting, for example, was designed to reduce both the flow and volume of blood, thereby reducing its deleterious pressure on certain obstructed vessels. Purging caused a beneficial reduction of bodily fluids in cases of excessive circulation and actual flooding of critical organs.[24]

In Germany, Boerhaave's contemporary, Friedrich Hoffmann, promoted his own medical system with publication of a monograph titled *Fundamenta Medicinae*, (1695) followed by *Medicina Rationalis Systematica* (1718).[25] The author placed greater emphasis on the role of nerves in physiology and pathogenesis, subordinating Boerhaavian hydrodynamics to an integrative control of the nervous system. In Hoffmann's view, finely structured particles of an ethereal quality flowed through the nerves, creating a degree of tension in all bodily fibres that ensured healthy functions. Through the actions of the nervous system, certain 'sympathy' linked all bodily organs allowing for the proper coordination of motions and other organic functions.[26] Disease for Hoffmann was the result of abnormal bodily motions precipitated by changes in the nervous system. An increase in tension or tone of said fibres caused spasms, especially in the blood vessels. An opposite loss of tension created fibre atony and paralysis. According to such a pathogenesis, traditional therapeutic measures were explained as either relieving spasms or contributing to an increase in fibre tension.

Like Boerhaave's theories, Hoffmann's medical system was still primarily based on hydrodynamic schemes and digestive chemistry.[27] However, Hoffmann was forced to recognize the importance of nervous

[24] L. S. King, 'Medical Theory and Practice at the Beginning of the 18th Century', *Bulletin of the History of Medicine*, 46 (1972), 1–15.

[25] For a biographical sketch of Hoffmann, see G. B. Risse, 'Friedrich Hoffmann', *Dictionary of Scientific Biography* (New York, 1972), VI, pp. 458–61. A good secondary source is E. Rothschuh, 'Studien zu Friedrich Hoffmann', *Sudhoffs Archiv*, 60 (1976), 163–93, 235–70.

[26] Hoffmann's early work was translated into English by Lester S. King: *Fundamenta Medicinae* (London, 1971).

[27] Wrote Hoffmann in his preface to *Fundamenta Medicinae*: 'I work hard to reduce the basic principles of medicine into a brief system and into a structure arranged by the easiest method, according to the precepts of sound modern mechanical–chemical philosophy. From this the whole science of medicine may be properly acquired in a short time', King, *Fundamenta Medicinae*, p. 3.

actions and their coordinating capacity. Unable to further explain the well-integrated and goal-directed action of the entire organism with the help of mechanical analogues, he asserted that all unexplained organic phenomena responded to a higher form of physics hitherto unrecognized by scientists. The speed of nerve messages suggested a transmission by means of subtle ether particles.

Hoffmann's colleague at the University of Halle, Georg Stahl (1660–1734), tried to remedy the apparent inadequacies of iatromechanism in explaining living beings.[28] In a work entitled *Theoria Medica Vera* and published in 1707, Stahl adopted a theoretical framework that subordinated previous mechanical explanations of bodily functions to the activity of an immaterial soul or 'anima'. While agreeing that the body was composed of fibres and fluids, Stahl postulated the need for a vital motion provided by the soul to prevent the spontaneous dissolution and corruption of matter. The unity exhibited by living organisms, their ability to integrate diverse functions, regulate and control growth, resist decay, and react to environmental stimuli suggested to Stahl the existence of a plan of action and foresight totally absent from purely mechanical models.[29]

To be sure, both Boerhaave and Hoffmann had accepted the Cartesian premise that the mind could influence and somehow communicate with the bodily machine, but these systematists had carefully avoided speculating about the possible nature of this connection.[30] By contrast, Stahl took on the problem directly with his proposal to recognize the existence of a supreme director – the soul – executing the necessary vital motions in accordance with specific blueprints. Stahl saw the 'anima' as the sole agent ensuring normal circulation, body heat, muscular movements, and the chemical mixture of particles by imposing the proper degree of tension to fibres which constituted the blood vessels and tissues.

[28] A biographical sketch of Stahl by L. S. King appeared in the *Dictionary of Scientific Biography* (New York, 1975), XII, pp. 599–606.
[29] A summary of Stahl's views is contained in B. J. Gottlieb (ed. and trans.), *Über den Unterschied Zwischen Organismus und Mechanismus* (Leipzig, 1961). See J. Geyer-Kordesch, 'Georg Ernst Stahl's Radical Pietist Medicine and Its Influence on the German Enlightenment', in *Medical Enlightenment*, pp. 67–87.
[30] For further reading see L. S. King, 'Basic Concepts of Early Eighteenth-Century Animism', *American Journal of Psychiatry*, 124 (1967), 797–802. The differences between Hoffmann and Stahl are outlined in L. S. King, 'Stahl and Hoffmann: A Study in Eighteenth-Century Animism', *Journal of the History of Medicine*, 19 (1964), 118–30. See also J. M. Lopez Piñero, 'Eighteenth-Century Medical Vitalism: The Paracelsian Connection', in W. R. Shea (ed.), *Revolutions in Science: Their Meaning and Relevance* (Canton, MA, 1988), pp. 117–32.

Disease for Stahl was a temporary disruption of the otherwise harmonious regulation exerted by the soul. Under the influence of environmental challenges or inner emotional turmoil, Stahl's anima could trigger abnormal motions with unfavourable effects on the tone of most bodily fibres. This was followed by secondary circulatory disturbances and ended in humoral stagnation and corruption. Healing, however, was possible, since the same anima which caused the disease could be trusted to restore health by commanding the necessary compensatory movements which culminated in the elimination of all accumulated particles harmful to the body.[31]

Stahl's medical system profoundly influenced all subsequent medical theory because it stressed the basic functional unity of the human organism as well as the interactions between mind and body which the Cartesian model had generally avoided. Iatromechanical and chemical explanations for bodily functions were retained but deemed insufficient in explaining by themselves the more complex interrelationships occurring in health and disease.[32] The existence of a first cause or principle operating within the organism and directing its actions emerged as a plausible interpretation of the observable phenomena. It seemed rather obvious that such a principle could not just simply be the product of random corpuscular mixtures. Therefore, Stahl's system became the forerunner and inspiration for a number of subsequent vitalistic theories in Germany, France, and England.[33]

After the Swiss physician Albrecht von Haller (1708–77) presented his experimental findings in 1752, the impact of his report for physiology and medicine was momentous.[34] Bodily motions had increasingly been considered essential manifestations of vitality. Haller devoted his

[31] One of the few secondary sources on Stahl is L. J. Rather, 'G. E. Stahl's Psychological Physiology', *Bulletin of the History of Medicine*, 35 (1961), 37–49; and R. Koch, 'War Georg Ernst Stahl ein selbstständiger Denker?', *Sudhoffs Archiv*, 18 (126), 20–50.

[32] For further details regarding the mind–body question consult Lelland J. Rather, *Mind and Body in Eighteenth Century Medicine* (Berkeley, 1965); and J. P. Wright, 'Metaphysics and Physiology: Mind, Body and Animal Economy in Eighteenth-Century Scotland', in M. A. Steward (ed.), *Studies in the Philosophy of the Scottish Enlightenment* (Oxford, 1990), pp. 251–302.

[33] The shift to vitalistic concepts has been extensively examined by T. M. Brown, 'From Mechanism to Vitalism in 18th Century English Physiology', *Journal of the History of Biology*, 7 (1974), 179–216; and B. J. Gottlieb, 'Bedeutung und Auswirkungen des hall. Prof. und kgl. Leibarztes Georg Ernst Stahl auf den Vitalismus des 18. Jahrhunderts', *Nova Acta Leop*, 12 (1943), 444–70.

[34] Albrecht von Haller, 'De partibus corporis humani sensilibus et irritabilibus', in *Commentarii Societatis Regiae Scientarum Gottingensis ad Annum 1752*, II. Haller's work was translated into English and reprinted: 'A Dissertation on the Sensible and Irritable Parts of Animals – 1755', *Bulletin of the History of Medicine*, 4 (1936), 651–99.

attention to the problem of irritability, a property which seemed peculiar to living beings enabling them to respond with movements to certain external influences. While this topic had already received recognition since the time of Galen and more recently by the English physician Francis Glisson (1597–1677), Haller subjected irritability to systematic experimental scrutiny.[35]

In his conclusions, Haller postulated the existence of a local property, irritability, directly residing in the muscular structures of the body and therefore independent from the nervous system. A second immanent quality which he called sensibility was defined as the capacity to perceive outside stimuli, and Haller located it in the inner core of the nerves. Bodily tissues exhibiting a rich network of nerves were considered to possess sensibility. By placing the newly discovered properties in the fibres of muscles and nerves, Haller implicitly stressed the functional importance of the solid components of the body. Moreover, both irritability and sensibility manifested themselves independently from the soul, a rebuke to the followers of Stahl's animism. However, these attributes could not be materially explained with the help of existing mechanical and chemical principles, inflicting another disconcerting blow to iatrophysical models.[36]

After Haller's publication a major reorientation occurred in medical theory. Henceforth greater emphasis was to be placed on the role played by the neuromuscular system in the phenomena of health and disease. Indeed, every medical system proposed after 1752 had to take Haller's physiological discoveries into account.[37] Among them were the theories of Jerome D. Gaub (1705–80), the German disciple and successor of Boerhaave, who published his work in 1758, followed by the physiological treatise of his compatriot, Johann A. Unzer (1727–99),

[35] For the background consult O. Temkin, 'The Classical Roots of Glisson's Doctrine of Irritation', *Bulletin of the History of Medicine*, 38 (1964), 297–328.

[36] A summary of Haller's concepts is G. Rudolph, 'Haller's Lehre von der Irritabilität und Sensibilität', in K. E. Rothschuh (ed.), *Von Boerhaave bis Berger* (Stuttgart, 1964), pp. 14–34. For a detailed examination of Haller see Richard Toellner, *Albrecht von Haller* (Wiesbaden, 1969). The same author has also written 'Anima et irritabilitis, Haller's Abwehr vom Animismus und Materialismus', *Sudhoffs Archiv*, 51 (1967), 130–44. See also W. D. Keidel, 'Albrecht von Haller's Reizbarkeit und Erregbarkeit in der experimentellen Neurophysiologie der Gegenwart', In R. Janzen (ed.), *Die Bedeutung der klinischen Neurologie für die allgemeine Medizin* (Stuttgart, 1988), pp. 23–43.

[37] See G. Rath, 'Neural Pathology: A Pathogenetic Concept of the Eighteenth and Nineteenth Centuries', *Bulletin of the History of Medicine*, 33 (1959), 526–41; and H. Buess, 'Albrecht von Haller and His *Elementa Physiologiae* as the Beginnings of Pathological Physiology', *Medical History*, 3 (1959), 123–31.

written in 1771, and above all the theories of the Scot William Cullen (1710–90), professor of medicine at the University of Edinburgh and the most celebrated British physician of the century.[38]

In his system, Cullen incorporated Boerhaave's and Hoffmann's mechanical schemes concerning the behaviour of bodily fluids. He reinforced the importance of solids in human physiology and pathology announcing that he considered them to be chemical mixtures susceptible to constant recombinations. The actions of both fluids and solids were placed under the direction of the nervous system. In attempting to explain the 'nervous power' responsible for the transmission of sensations to the brain and voluntary as well as involuntary motions to the muscles, the Scottish physician rejected the presence of an immaterial force. Instead he suggested that the Newtonian ether was the medium of nervous conduction.[39]

With his publication of the *Institutions of Medicine* in 1772 and later the *First Lines of the Practice of Physic* in 1776–78, Cullen based his system of medicine on neuromuscular physiology and physiopathology. A proper degree of tension or 'excitement' in the nerves assured the normal transmission of impulses necessary for suitable blood circulation, skeletal posture and locomotion, as well as chemical combinations. For Cullen, maintenance of this excitement depended on sufficient sensory stimulation derived from environmental stimuli plus enough internal incitement provided to the brain by the mind. An immaterial thinking principle was also located within the brain.

Disease was bound to occur when the amount of excitement was altered. Cullen believed that all outside agents either stimulated or depressed the nervous system. Excessive excitement in the nervous system increased the muscular tone, produced vascular spasms with

---

[38] There was a great deal of support for the system of Boerhaave among the early members of the medical faculty of Edinburgh: D. Guthrie, 'The Influence of the Leyden School upon Scottish Medicine', *Medical History*, 3 (1959), 108–22. See also A. Cunningham, 'Medicine to Calm the Mind: Boerhaave's Medical System and Why It Was Adopted in Edinburgh', in *Medical Enlightenment*, pp. 40–66. The relationships have been further examined by E. A. Underwood, *Boerhaave's Men at Leyden and After* (Edinburgh, 1976); and more recently by Christopher J. Lawrence, 'Medicine as Culture: Edinburgh and the Scottish Enlightenment' (University College London Ph.D. thesis, 1984).

[39] There is no comprehensive biographical study of Cullen. For more information see R. W. Johnstone, 'William Cullen', *Medical History*, 3 (1959), 33–46; and more recently R. Stott, 'Health and Virtue: Or How to Keep out of Harm's Way. Lectures on Pathology and Therapeutics by William Cullen *c.* 1770', *Medical History*, 31 (1987), 123–42. The standard secondary source for Cullen is John Thomson, *An Account of the Life, Lectures and Writings of William Cullen*, 2 vols. (Edinburgh, 1859). See also Inci A. Bowman, 'William Cullen (1710–90) and the Primacy of the Nervous System' (Indiana University Ph.D. thesis, 1975).

subsequent circulatory disturbances, and chemical abnormalities in the bodily solids. Depression tended to create muscular debility, vascular paralysis, and the eventual collapse of all body functions.[40]

Cullen's therapeutic procedures followed along traditional lines but were also readily explained within his theoretical scaffolding. All healing efforts were designed to restore normal functions in the neuromuscular system through measures that could augment or decrease the degree of nervous excitement. Stimulating agents such as exercise, fresh air, animal foods and wine, warm baths and the employment of tonic drugs were said to increase excitement. By contrast, a depleting regimen consisting of rest, a meatless diet, bloodletting, purging and the use of antispasmodic and sedative drugs accomplished a decrease in excitement.[41]

Cullen's medical system was not highly original. The author had carefully combined mechanical explanations elaborated by Boerhaave and especially Hoffmann, supplementing them with a neuro-physiological design based on the researches of Haller and Whytt.[42] This new synthesis carefully steered away from Stahlian animism without completely avoiding the issue of organismic integration and purposeful activities. Cullen posited a material explanation – ethereal vibrations – for the functions of sensation and volition, and selected the brain as the key organ in charge of bodily actions. This flexible scheme was posited because of the author's conviction that medicine needed a theoretical framework. According to Cullen, medical systems had heuristic and practical value, giving students and physicians a coherent albeit somewhat speculative set of explanations. Cullen was under no illusions

[40] For an assessment of these ideas in Scottish culture see C. Lawrence, 'The Nervous System and Society in the Scottish Enlightenment', in B. Barnes and S. Shapin (eds.), *Natural Order: Historical Studies of Scientific Culture* (Beverley Hills, CA, 1979), pp. 19–40. A survey of the term 'tonus' appeared in C. S. Sherrington, 'Note on the History of the Word "tonus" as a Physiological Term', in *Contributions to Medical and Biological Research*, 2 vols. (New York, 1910), I, pp. 261–68. For background consult the following: David Daiches, *The Scottish Enlightenment: An Introduction* (Edinburgh, 1986); and Roger L. Emerson, 'Science and the Origins and Concerns of the Scottish Enlightenment', *History of Science*, 26 (1988), 333–66.

[41] For details consult William Cullen, *First Lines of the Practice of Physic*, 2 vols. (Edinburgh, 1776–78). See also G. B. Risse, 'Dr William Cullen, Physician, Edinburgh: A Consultation Practice in the Eighteenth Century', *Bulletin of the History of Medicine*, 48 (1974), 338–51; and his *Hospital Life in Enlightenment Scotland. Care and Teaching at the Royal Infirmary of Edinburgh* (Cambridge, 1986); especially pp. 177–227, ch. 4: 'Hospital Care: State of the Medical Art'. Also check C. Lawrence, 'Ornate Physicians and Learned Artisans: Edinburgh Medical Men, 1726–1776', in W. F. Bynum and R. Porter (eds.), *William Hunter and the Eighteenth-Century Medical World* (Cambridge, 1985), pp. 153–76.

[42] For a summary of Whytt's ideas see R. K. French, 'Sauvages, Whytt and the Motion of the Heart: Aspects of Eighteenth-Century Animism', *Clio Medica*, 7 (1972), 35–54; and his book, *Robert Whytt, The Soul and Medicine* (London, 1969).

concerning the permanence of his theories. These were working ideas subject to debate and revisions with the help of new observations and experiments.[43]

Such professional debates reached a high level of personal vituperation and led to the establishment of another medical system by a disciple of Cullen, the Scottish physician John Brown (1735–88). His 'Brunonian' theory also accepted the existence of one fundamental principle, the excitability, a basic quality now assigned to all living matter instead of being restricted to the neuromuscular system as Cullen had postulated. Brownian excitability was portrayed as the ultimate cause of life and, like Newtonian gravity, incapable of further definition.[44]

In Brown's scheme every human being at birth was endowed with a fixed quantity of excitability which through continuous interactions with environmental and internal impulses generated the necessary energy to live called excitement. Opposing Stahlian animism, Brown stressed that life was neither a spontaneous nor independent phenomenon but the product of constant reactions between stimuli consuming specific amounts of excitability. Health was merely the balance between adequate amounts of stimulation and normal levels of excitability.[45]

Brown sought to provide his system with a mathematical certainty comparable to that of Newton's gravity. He therefore divided the excitability into 80 degrees with the half mark, 40 degrees, reflecting the ideal state of health. When stimuli become either deficient or excessive, Brown's excitability suffers opposite fluctuations above or below the 40 degrees line, indicating an unhealthy state. Two basic abnormal conditions characterize human pathology: 'asthenia', when the body receives inadequate stimulation, lacks excitement and therefore is weak, and 'sthenia' when too many stimulants created a surplus of excitement while dangerously dissipating the body's excitability.

Therefore, one must distinguish with Brown two opposing roads to disease and death, both resulting from an imbalance of stimuli and

[43] Wrote Cullen: 'it is necessary from time to time, to reform and review the whole system, with all the additions and amendments which it has received and is capable of', Cullen, *First Lines*, preface to 1784 edition, I, p. 5.

[44] See T. S. Hall, 'On Biological Analogs to Newtonian Paradigms', *Philosophy of Science*, 35 (1968), 6–27.

[45] G. B. Risse, 'The Brownian System of Medicine: Its Theoretical and Practical Implications', *Clio Medica*, 5 (1970), 45–51. Further details are covered in various contributions contained in W. F. Bynum and R. Porter (eds.), *Brunonianism in Britain and Europe* (London, 1988). For a view of Brown's system in Germany, see G. B. Risse, 'Scottish Medicine on the Continent: John Brown's System in Germany 1796–1805', *Proceedings of the XXIII International Congress on the History of Medicine* (London, 1974), I, pp. 682–87.

excitement. Even contagion was believed to have a stimulant power. Thus, there is but one single pathophysiology underlying all general disease. In fact, in one of Brown's clinical record studies, ninety-seven out of every one hundred cases were ascribed to asthenia. He eschewed the usual disease nomenclature preferring instead to characterize the various illnesses according to their intrinsic causes.

Brown urged physicians seeing patients to translate their clinical observations into concrete levels of excitement according to the previous table. To accomplish this, practitioners were encouraged by Brown to make an inventory of the stimulants, both environmental and internal, to which their individual patients had been exposed prior to the onset of illness. Once arrived at a specific grade of excitability which provided the diagnosis of asthenia or sthenia, physicians were encouraged to take therapeutic actions designed to re-establish health through a mathematically titrated regimen of stimulants.[46]

Brown's ideas first appeared in his work titled *Elementa Medicinae* (1780). They represented the culmination of all eighteenth-century efforts at medical system-building. At last a simple theoretical scheme based on one fundamental principle, excitability, explained both human physiology and pathology. No lengthy disease classifications were needed, and the uncertainties at the bedside were suddenly eliminated by making clinical events measurable. Like physics, medicine had finally become an exact science, all of its phenomena logically deduced from first principles. In this scheme, therapy was equally predictable and similarly computed. However, the appealing simplicity and precision of Brownianism could not be applied at the bedside. Physicians attracted to Brown's system found it near impossible to implement in their daily practices. Not even the most skilled clinicians could detect specific grades of excitability among the protean manifestations of sickness.

In the end, the stability furnished by eighteenth-century medical systems was short lived, their turnover and downfall inevitable. After Brown, sustained hopes for simple theoretical frameworks providing medical certainty faded. Most physicians gradually recognized that much more basic and clinical knowledge was needed before a genuine synthesis could be attempted. With biology and sciences such as microscopical anatomy, physiology, biochemistry, pathology, pharmacology and others largely undeveloped, all systematizing efforts were

---

[46] An English translation of Brown's work appeared in 1788: *The Elements of Medicine*, 2 vols. (London, 1788). For details concerning this therapeutic approach see G. B. Risse, 'Brunonian Therapeutics: New Wine in Old Bottles?', in *Brunonianism in Britain and Europe*, pp. 46–62.

premature. Fortunately, the spirited polemics and repeated disappoint-
ments surrounding system-building not only helped strip away the
rationalistic naïveté fuelling these speculations, but encouraged further
clinical observations as well as therapeutic scepticism. In ever increasing
numbers, physicians abandoned the armchair and returned to the sickbed
to obtain knowledge. For many, collection of clinical facts became the
proper road towards medical certainty.[47]

Nosology
Eighteenth-century physicians also attempted to overcome the uncertainties in medicine by establishing systematic classifications of disease
or 'nosologies'. Often, this movement was associated with rational
system-building, but some nosologists remained sceptical about the
value of medical theories exclusively based on iatrophysical and
iatrochemical models. If scrupulously carried out, the nosological
approach could, in the eyes of some proponents, provide generalizations
and eventually furnish useful theoretical frameworks.[48]

The roots of nosology can be found in the programmatic statements
of the English physician Thomas Sydenham (1624–89) who considered
the remote causes of diseases both inscrutable and inexplicable, urging
physicians to establish instead the 'natural history of every disease.'
Sydenham's plan had the support of his disciple and friend, the
philosopher John Locke (1632–1704). Locke had also concluded that the
acquisition of useful medical knowledge was being thwarted by
hypothetical systems concerned with providing the hidden causes of
diseases.[49]

The first task for nosologists was to clinically define each disease by
enumerating its essential and constant symptoms and signs. This
undertaking meant that physicians had to carefully observe individual
patients and abstract from particular cases those occurrences believed to
be common to them all. For this purpose, particular symptom sequences

[47] See G. B. Risse, 'The Quest for Certainty in Medicine: John Brown's System of Medicine in
France', *Bulletin of the History of Medicine*, 45 (1971), 1–12. For other contemporary efforts to
quantify in medicine see Ulrich Tröhler, '"To Improve the Evidence of Medicine"': Arithmetic
Observation in Clinical Medicine in the 18th and Early 19th Centuries,' *History and Philosophy of
Life Science* 10 (1988), suppl. 31–40.
[48] The basic work on this subject is Knud Faber, *Nosography, The Evolution of Clinical Medicine
in Modern Times*, 2nd edn (New York, 1930). The original edition appeared in 1919. See also O.
Temkin, 'The History of Classification in the Medical Sciences', in M. M. Katz (ed.), *The Role and
Methodology of Classification in Psychiatry and Psychopathology* (Washington, DC, 1965), pp. 11–20.
[49] For the statements of Sydenham and Locke see E. Fischer-Homberger, 'Eighteenth-Century
Nosology and Its Survivors', *Medical History*, 14 (1970) 397–403.

or clusters were lifted out of the confusing array of clinical events and defined as independent diseases. Such complex judgements first took into consideration the subjective reports of patients obtained in the form of clinical histories. Next the physician searched for objective signs of the disease at the sickbed, in the eighteenth century a rather undeveloped art restricted to inspection and palpation. At the end, the practitioner had to discriminate between a number of seemingly similar clinical manifestations and recognize distinctive, so-called pathognomonic events which at times were considered specific for certain diseases.[50]

According to the Italian physician Giorgio Baglivi (1668–1707), the primary obligation of the physician was to be a witness of nature, faithfully observing the course of individual illnesses.[51] The emphasis on obtaining 'natural' histories of diseases reflected a widespread contemporary belief that all sickness evolved in predetermined patterns reflective of their individual natures. To preserve the original markings of disease, practitioners were cautioned about the premature administration of medicines which could in effect blur essential features and thereby jeopardize diagnosis. More importantly, the therapeutic interference could actually transform one sickness into another of greater magnitude.[52]

If the disorganized healing efforts hitherto employed distorted or obscured the natural evolution of diseases, current nosological efforts would outline, as Baglivi put it, a 'pure and exact history of diseases...such as flows from the very nature of things'. Against this 'natural' backdrop future physicians would be in a better position to arrive at diagnoses and gauge the success of their treatments. Moreover both the timing and mode of therapeutical intervention could be dramatically improved. As Sydenham observed, 'we should have known the cures of many diseases before this time if physicians...had not been deceived in their disease and not mistaken one species for another'.[53] For nosologists, then, distinguishing and defining particular diseases was the first step physicians needed to take in their search for specific cures.

[50] Further details are in Lester S. King, 'Nosology', in *The Medical World*, pp. 193–226, ch. 7.
[51] Giorgio Baglivi, *The Practice of Physick* (London, 1704), pp. 210–24.
[52] 'Diseases went through their periods, not by their natural and constant laws, but according as they were variously treated in the divers courses of practice...the progress, exit and symptoms of such diseases were more owing to the respective methods of practice than to the immutable and individual nature of the distemper', *ibid.*, p. 214.
[53] Thomas Sydenham, *The Works of Thomas Sydenham, M.D.*, R. G. Latham (Trans.), 2 vols. (London, 1849), I, p. 17. The passage is from Sydenham's preface to the third edition.

The next phase in disease classification demanded that practitioners compare the various sicknesses among themselves, determining similarities as well as differential features. Wrote Sydenham in 1676: 'It is necessary that all diseases be reduced to definite and certain species ... with the same care which we see exhibited by botanists in their phytologies.'[54] Thus, eighteenth-century nosologists followed Sydenham and Baglivi in also expressing their conviction that natural diseases were beholden to the same organization and order already recognized in plants and animals. Borrowing extensively from such taxonomic efforts in botany and zoology, medical men tried to introduce similar orderliness into clinical medicine. Diseases were eagerly collected into families, classes, species, and genera on the basis of anatomical, symptomatic, and pathological criteria established by those particular physicians attempting the classifications.

The first important nosological arrangement was prepared by the French physician François B. de Sauvages (1706–67), a professor of medicine at the University of Montpellier with strong botanical interests. His work, *Nouvelles Classes de maladies* was published anonymously around 1731, and in the prologue its author reiterated Sydenham's scepticism about the usefulness of theoretical speculations. By contrast nosology was seen by Sauvages as a pragmatic discipline providing practitioners with a compass to chart their voyages through the complex sea of symptoms. This new handle was to be especially beneficial to inexperienced younger members of the profession just entering the bewildering world of clinical medicine.[55]

To carry out his task, Sauvages rejected a classification simply based on the anatomical location of symptoms. Moreover, since the causes for most diseases remained unknown, the arrangements were based on phenomena readily available for observation: symptoms and signs. Thus, in an expanded version of his earlier work, the *Nosologia Methodica* of 1763, Sauvages began with ten classes of disease, establishing 44 species, 315 genera, and a total of approximately 2,400 separate disease entities entirely based on clinical symptoms. Not surprisingly his enormously detailed classification scheme contained a great number of inconsistencies and duplications.

A somewhat less complex system was presented by Carl Von Linné (1707–78), the famous Swedish naturalist whose botanical system had

---

[54] *Ibid.*, I, p. 13.
[55] L. S. King, 'Boissier de Sauvages and 18th Century Nosology', *Bulletin of the History of Medicine*, 40 (1966), 43–51.

already appeared in 1735. A practising physician and university professor, Linné published in 1763 a work titled *Genera Morborum* with eleven classes of diseases and 325 separate entities. Many of Linné's so-called diseases were simply symptoms such as fever, itch, cough, swellings, and others.[56]

Later in the century William Cullen published his own nosology specifically designed to guide medical students. Originally printed in 1769, the *Synopsis Nosologiae Methodicae* was a much more simplified arrangement no longer intended to be an all-encompassing taxonomic exercise but rather a didactic and practical index of clinical reality as experienced by the author himself. Indeed, Cullen reproached his predecessors for attempting comprehensive classifications not based on personal experience. In his view, lack of first-hand knowledge had made these authors include virtually every symptom as a separate disease.

Cullen was also concerned with establishing a universally acceptable nomenclature for the disease entities to be classified. He criticized Linné for introducing an excessive number of new and quite arbitrary terms. If nosology was to become a truly scientific enterprise and important pedagogical tool, precision in language was imperative and all classification efforts had to be made without recourse to hypothetical views of causality. Finally, for Cullen nosology was also the key for an improvement in therapeutics. 'It is well known to be necessary in order to successful practice, that remedies be adapted not only to every genus, but to every species, and even to every variety of a disease'.[57]

Eighteenth-century nosology, therefore, represents an important effort by contemporary physicians to discern separate disease states and systematically survey the perceived panorama of clinical pathology. Physicians saw the various classifications as true reflections of an established natural order. This was absolutely necessary to achieve an overview and attain successful diagnoses and treatments. To this effect practitioners were urged to abandon useless theoretical speculations and return to the bedside for comprehensive observations and descriptions.

In the true Baconian sense, Cullen's nosology was considered to be a scientific enterprise, a heuristic device especially useful to students. Although insufficient clinical data and changing criteria for classification also discredited successive nosological efforts, many physicians continued

[56] Lester S. King, 'Nosology', in *The Medical World*, pp. 198–204. Further information by the same author is available in 'Eighteenth-Century Nosology', in *Medical Thinking, A Historical Preface* (Princeton, NJ, 1982), pp. 117–23.

[57] William Cullen, *Nosology, Or a Systematic Arrangement of Diseases* (Edinburgh, 1800), pp. 16–17.

to classify diseases. As more patients were seen, especially in hospital and dispensary practice, and additional criteria obtained from autopsy findings, definitions and classifications of disease improved. For most Enlightenment physicians nosology became central to the study and practice of medicine. Concluded Cullen: 'it would make the study of physic absolutely impossible for if we cannot arrive at some distinction of diseases, we must act at random'.[58]

Implementation

Early in the eighteenth century, medicine dramatically expanded the scope of its activities under the influence of powerful social and political forces. The so-called 'medicalization' of society not only allowed physicians to reach new sectors of the burgeoning middle class but for the first time in history make significant contact with sectors of the lower classes of society.[59]

Hitherto most medical activities had followed the classical Graeco-Roman models of private health care, restricted to the individual demands of sick persons usually belonging to the upper social strata. As already mentioned, a preventative regimen advocating a moderate life style based on the so-called 'six things non-natural,' and a curative strategy based on the restoration of basic humoral balances constituted the boundaries of such medical intervention.

To be sure, European physicians especially since the Middle Ages had from time to time played prominent roles in public health efforts launched during the onslaught of deadly epidemics, notably the plague.[60] However, such activities had been mostly sporadic and local in scope, organized in response to the temporary assaults of mass disease. Not until the advent of effective political and bureaucratic organizations of national scope associated with the rise of the modern European states during the seventeenth and eighteenth centuries could medicine expect

[58] William Cullen, 'On Nosology', one of his introductory lectures reprinted in John Thomson (ed.), *The Works of William Cullen, M.D.*, 2 vols. (Edinburgh, 1828), I, p. 447.

[59] The concept of society's 'medicalization' has been advanced by Michel Foucault, among others, and members of the 'Annales' school in France. See for example his 'La politique de la santé au XVIIIe siecle' in M. Foucault et al. (eds.), *Les machines à guerir* (Paris, 1976), pp. 11–21; and J. P. Goubert, 'The Medicalization of French Society at the End of the Ancien Regime', in L. G. Stevenson (ed.), *A Celebration of Medical History* (Baltimore, 1982), pp. 157–79.

[60] Carlo M. Cipolla, *Public Health and the Medical Profession in the Renaissance* (Cambridge, 1976). See also by the same author, 'A Plague Doctor', in H. A. Miskimin, D. Herlihy, and A. L. Udovitch (eds), *The Medieval City* (New Haven, 1977), pp. 65–72; and A. G. Carmichael, 'Plague Legislation in the Italian Renaissance', *Bulletin of the History of Medicine*, 57 (1983), 508–25.

to play a greater role in society. In fact, the ideology of European mercantilism with its new biopolitical strategies radically changed the limited focus of earlier medical actions thereby propelling questions of health and disease to the forefront of social policy.[61]

Among the newly perceived requirements of national power was the need for a growing population capable of furnishing enough manpower for the production of crops and goods, consumption of taxable items, and maintenance of significant armies designed to implement geopolitical objectives. Such an expanding citizenry had to be properly organized and their material welfare improved, including attention to health-related issues. Thus, medicine experienced nearly a quantum leap in the range of its mission. Greater emphasis on environmental health and its relation to epidemiology,[62] infant and maternal welfare,[63] military and naval medicine,[64] as well as mass treatment of certain sectors of the population in newly erected hospitals and dispensaries[65] were among the new concerns. The underlying premise, of course, was that disease could be controlled, removed, and perhaps prevented by the conscious and deliberate application of 'enlightened' views about health hitherto individually employed in the private sector of both middle and upper classes.

Medical police

The most comprehensive theory of administration designed to 'medicalize' society during the eighteenth century was the *medical police*, a vague term encompassing not only programmes of public health and hygiene, but also notions of professional power and control and the regulation of medical education. The new governmental concept was most clearly articulated within the framework of German mercantilism – the so-called cameralism – assuming a paternalistic and comprehensive cradle-to-grave approach especially attractive to the exercise of absolute power by enlightened despots. Indeed, the term 'medical police' was first employed by the German municipal physician Wilhelm Rau

[61] For a general overview see A. Deutsch, 'Historical Interrelationships between Medicine and Social Welfare', *Bulletin of the History of Medicine*, 11 (1942), 485–502.

[62] Riley, *The Eighteenth-Century Campaign to Avoid Disease*.

[63] A. Wilson, 'The Enlightenment and Infant Care', *Society of the Social History Medicine Bulletin*, 25 (1979), 44–7; and Judith Schneid Lewis, *In the Family Way: Childbearing in the British Aristocracy, 1760–1860* (New Brunswick, NJ, 1986).

[64] See, for example, John J. Keevil, *Medicine and the Navy, 1200–1900*, 4 vols. (Edinburgh, 1961), especially vol. III.

[65] For an overview see I. Waddington, 'The Role of the Hospital in the Development of Modern Medicine, A Sociological Analysis', *Sociology*, 9 (1973), 221–24.

(1721–72) in his 1764 book. To supervise the health of an entire population, the medical profession also needed to be regulated and better trained. Ordinances to supervise apothecary shops and hospitals, as well as measures designed to restrict the brisk business of quacks were also components of the new policy.[66]

At its centre, the new programme aimed at furnishing a coherent policy with regards to health care, especially for the poorer segments of society. Plans were based on Lockeian notions of social contract between the state and its people in which the latter relinquished a measure of freedom in exchange for government ensuring social order and affording protection from foreign intrusion. Such protection was now extended to include the cure of existing diseases as well as prevention of those environmental factors responsible for epidemics. The advantages of medical care, hygiene, and healthier living conditions already enjoyed by the upper and middle classes were to be made available to the lower social order for the benefit of the poor themselves and the nation as a whole.

The most influential personality in the German-speaking movement of medical police was Johann P. Frank (1745–1821) whose work *A Complete System of Medical Police* became the most important document on public health in the century.[67] As Frank asserted in his introduction, 'the internal security of the state is the subject of general police science. A very considerable part of this science is to apply certain principles for the health care of people living in society.'[68] The author was quite explicit about the goal of preserving the population in the face of epidemic diseases such as smallpox, syphilis, and typhus.[69]

Frank envisioned a need for government to take on unprecedented regulatory functions which extended from choice of marriage to transportation networks, from personal hygienic measures to public water supplies. The new measures were designed to break down class barriers restricting the more optimistic view of health held by the educated elite. Thus at the root of the medical police schemes promulgated by Frank lay the task to also persuade the lower classes to achieve better health by following the governmental rules imposed on their individual lives.

[66] G. Rosen, 'Cameralism and the Concept of Medical Police', *Bulletin of the History of Medicine*, 27 (1952), 21–42; and L. Jordanova, 'Medical Police and Public Health: Problems of Practice and Ideology', *Society of the Social History of Medicine Bulletin*, 27 (1980), 15–19.
[67] E. Lesky, 'Johann Peter Frank and Social Medicine', *Annales Cisalpines d'Histoire Sociale*, 4 (1973), 137–44.
[68] Johann P. Frank, *A System of Complete Medical Police*, selections with an introduction, ed. E. Lesky (Baltimore, 1976), p. 12. [69] *Ibid.*, p. 23.

Moreover governments were called to suppress some of the health hazards generated by society itself. The innocence and primordial health which the Enlightenment associated with early man living in a natural state supposedly had given way to corrupt and sickly humans subjected to the harmful effects of civilized life. Frank and other reformers thus called for the protection of women and children already being exploited in pre-industrial societies with detrimental effects on the nation's demography and their own physical well-being. Occupational diseases affecting miners, millers, sailors, construction workers, and many others, pointed towards the need for environmental reforms and 'defensive', protective measures to ameliorate the problems. At the core of all the people's misery, of course, was their socio-economic status, the ultimate form of sickness demanding profound political reforms which most rulers Frank was addressing in his proposals were unwilling to consider, especially after the French Revolution. Thus in the end, Frank's medical police remained more of a programmatic statement only imperfectly and partially executed, a lofty goal too difficult to achieve given its scope and the political and demographic realities of post-Napoleonic Europe.

The authoritarian character of Frank's model of medicalization found few adherents beyond the boundaries of political systems identified with enlightened despotism such as in Germany, Austria, and Italy. While Frank defended his ideas suggesting in 1783 that nobody could 'retain natural freedom in social life without curbs', his far-reaching measures proved impossible to implement elsewhere. Political and social conditions prevailing in both France and Britain favoured the creation of other bureaucratic structures to accomplish the new goals of public medicine.[70]

In France mercantilist ideals of population expansion and welfare similarly meshed with Enlightenment goals of human progress.[71] Health-related matters had traditionally been the domain of French local communities, but the increasing centralization of administrative functions during the reign of Louis XIV resulted in important changes. By the early eighteenth century the provincial representatives of the royal administration had begun to take responsibility for the control and consequences of human and cattle epidemics occurring in their districts. A variety of relief measures, including the appointment of medical

[70] G. Rosen, 'The Fate of the Concept of Medical Police, 1780–1890', *Centaurus*, 5 (1957), 97–113.

[71] G. Rosen, 'Mercantilism and Health Policy in Eighteenth Century French Thought', *Medical History*, 3 (1959), 259–75.

personnel, sometimes from the medical faculty at Paris and Montpellier, were instituted.

Sustained by physiocratic principles advocating increased agricultural wealth, the central French government not only created two veterinary schools at Lyon (1762) and Alfort (1766), but began planning in the 1770s a more formal network of information and assistance.[72] Following a severe outbreak of rinderpest in parts of France that caused severe economic losses, a central Commission on Epidemics was created in 1776. Its purpose was to regularly and systematically collect information about local epidemics, including details concerning environmental variables possibly implicated in the outbreaks. Climate, season, geographical location, quality of soil, winds, precipitation, and other factors previously considered part of Sydenham's 'epidemic constitution' were to be transmitted together with knowledge about the measures employed in halting the disease.[73]

The Commission, which two years later became known as the Royal Society of Medicine, was empowered to collect, compare, and judge the data while also issuing suggestions to local authorities and practitioners about appropriate actions deemed necessary to control the problems. Thus, until the Revolution, the Society gradually expanded its activities and de facto became the top-level consulting organization for the French government in all matters related to outbreaks of epidemic disease.[74]

Increased concern about high infant mortality and maternal welfare and their combined demographic impact also brought the French government into the field of midwife regulation. In 1730 a series of royal statutes were issued requiring midwives to undergo a two-year apprenticeship at a provincial hospital. While the national requirements may not have been always implemented, there is enough evidence to show that local governments and even the Catholic church played important roles both in the selection and regulation of the midwives.[75]

---

[72] C. C. Hannaway, 'Veterinary Medicine and Rural Health Care in Pre-Revolutionary France', *Bulletin of the History of Medicine*, 51 (1977), 431–47.

[73] See Michel Foucault, *The Birth of the Clinic, An Archeology of Medical Perception*, trans. A. M. Sheridan Smith (New York, 1975), pp. 25–8. Some of the information about diseases has been examined by Jean-Pierre Peter, 'Disease and the Sick at the End of the Eighteenth Century', in *Biology of Man in History, Selections from the Annales*, R. Forster and O. Ranum (eds.), (Baltimore, 1975), pp. 81–124.

[74] For details, C. C. Hannaway, 'The Société Royale de Médicine and Epidemics in the Ancien Régime', *Bulletin of the History of Medicine*, 46 (1972), 257–73.

[75] R. L. Petrelli, 'The Regulation of French Midwifery during the Ancien Régime', *Journal of the History of Medicine*, 26 (1971), 276–92. Also useful for the French practices is J. Gelis, 'L'accouchement au XVIII siècle; pratiques traditionnelles et controle médical', *Ethnologie Française*, 6 (1976), 325–38.

In the British Isles mercantilist efforts to improve the health and size of the population relied largely on private initiatives. A tradition going back at least to the seventeenth century sought to achieve a climate for social and medical reforms through the publication of vital statistics. Beginning with John Graunt's *Natural and Political Observations upon the Bills of Mortality*, first published in 1662, and William Petty's *Essays in Political Arithmetic* of 1687, an important movement was launched in British society. It was designed to gather pertinent demographic data as a first step towards improving the size and health of the population.[76]

A typical representative of this voluntary reform movement in the eighteenth century was John Bellers, a powerful Quaker and merchant of London whose 1714 *Essay towards the Improvement of Physick* was highly influential. Based on his studies of mortality statistics in the city, Bellers concluded that about half of the inhabitants perished from what he believed to be curable diseases. When the London figures were extrapolated to the rest of Great Britain, Bellers calculated that the kingdom was losing approximately one hundred thousand inhabitants per year 'for want of timely advice and suitable medicines,' a most significant loss of human resources to the entire nation since in his computations every lost worker was worth two hundred pounds to the British economy.[77]

Thus, Bellers presented a twelve-point programme for legislative action that included the construction of hospitals for the destitute, blind, and incurable, as well as appointment of physicians and surgeons at the parish level to treat the sick poor. A national institute to carry out research with the goal of obtaining new medicines was also envisioned. Although such a plan failed to elicit a favourable governmental response, private philanthropy provided the necessary funds and institutional settings to at least carry out a number of improvements.[78]

In matters of maternal welfare, for example, the reformers were able to supply greater facilities for the study of midwifery by arranging after 1739 the admission of women in labour to the existing voluntary hospitals in London. A number of establishments exclusively devoted to

---

[76] G. Rosen, 'Medical Care and Social Policy in Seventeenth-Century England', *Bulletin of the New York Academy of Medicine*, 29 (1953) 420–37. Further details can be obtained from an article by J. H. Cassedy, 'Medicine and the Rise of Statistics', in A. G. Debus, *Medicine in Seventeenth-Century England* (Berkeley, 1974), pp. 283–312.

[77] John Bellers, *Essay towards the Improvement of Physick* (London, 1714), pp. 1–3. The economic arguments are repeated throughout the essay.

[78] For more details see G. Rosen, 'An Eighteenth Century Plan for a National Health Service', *Bulletin of the History of Medicine*, 16 (1944), 429–36.

this task were created in the British capital between 1749 and 1757, including the British Lying-In Hospital, City of London, Queen Charlotte, and Royal Maternity. All of them together dramatically expanded the facilities devoted to the study and the practice of midwifery, especially by males. Under the direction of the Scottish physician, William Smellie (1697–1763), such teaching improved significantly, aided by pelvic models, clinical records, and use of the forceps. Although midwifery remained unregulated, both male and female attendants acquired greater experience. With the creation of the London Lying-In Charity in 1757, poor women were also delivered in their own homes by visiting midwives, a practice which by the 1770s involved about a third of all the registered births in the city. Such upgrading of maternal care was slowly imitated in the provinces.[79]

Medicine's gradual encroachment on childbirth through the activities of physician– or surgeon–midwives also brought practitioners face to face with the care of infants.[80] Some beginnings had already been made since the opening of the London Foundling Hospital in 1741, where attending physicians realized the nefarious effects of the so-called 'dry feeding' – the common practice of starving newborns for several days after delivery.[81] With the 1748 publication of William Cadogan's (1711–97) *Essay on Nursing and the Management of Children* a decisive turning point in neonate feeding and care occurred with subsequent decreases in infant mortality directly ascribable to the newer practices.[82]

[79] For an overview consult Mabel C. Buer, 'General Hygiene and Midwifery', in *Health, Wealth and Population in the Early Days of the Industrial Revolution* (London, 1926), pp. 137–150, ch. 11. See also J. Schneid Lewis, 'Maternal Health in the English Aristocracy: Myth and Realities, 1790–1840', *Journal of Social History*, 17 (1983), 97–114; and her recent book, *In the Family Way*. The professional struggles between male and female midwives is summarized in B. Brandon Schnorrenberg, 'Is Childbirth Any Place for a Woman? The Decline of Midwifery in Eighteenth-Century England', in H. C. Payne (ed.), *Studies in Eighteenth-Century Culture* (Madison, WI, 1981), x, pp. 393–408.

[80] For a complete view of this subject in Britain consult Ernest Caulfield, *The Infant Welfare Movement in the Eighteenth Century* (New York, 1931). The contemporary health conditions are illustrated in: G. Rosen, 'A Slaughter of Innocents: Aspects of Child Health in the Eighteenth-Century city', in *Studies in Eighteenth Century Culture*, 5 (1976), 293–316. See also Bogna W. Lorence, 'Parents and Children in Eighteenth Century Europe', *History of Childhood Quarterly*, 2 (1974), 1–30.

[81] For details of the diseases encountered there as well as medical practice, see R. K. McClure, 'Pediatric Practice at the London Foundling Hospital', in H. C. Payne (ed.), *Studies in Eighteenth-Century Culture* (Madison, WI, 1981), x, pp. 361–71. Further details can be obtained from her recent book, *Coram's Children: London Foundling Hospital in the Eighteenth Century* (New Haven, 1981). For more information consult Albrecht Pieper, *Chronik der Kinderheilkunde*, 4th edn (Leipzig, 1966).

[82] V. Fildes, 'Neonatal Feeding Practices and Infant Mortality during the 18th Century', *Journal of Biosocial Science*, 12 (1980), 313–24. More information is available in her book, *Breasts, Bottles, and Babies, a History of Infant Feeding* (Edinburgh, 1986). For a general overview see also S. Wilson, 'The Myth of Motherhood a Myth: The Historical View of European Childrearing', *Social History*, 9 (1984), 181–98.

Moreover, in 1761, the British Parliament passed an Act designed to register at the parish level all poor children under the age of four. The intention of its chief sponsor, the philanthropist Jonas Hanway (1712–86), was to collect data about the deficiencies of infant and child care while helping to create greater public awareness concerning their plight. This effort in furthering the British infant welfare movement was particularly successful, and the cause gained additional momentum with the establishment of a London Dispensary for the Infant Poor in 1769 by George Armstrong (1720–89), the author of a classical text on children's diseases.

After centuries of neglect, the upper and middle classes in Europe became more conscious about the physical and emotional needs of children while realizing the economical impact of their wasteful mortality. Spurred by Enlightenment ideals of education and progress, the new approach towards child care gradually resulted in improved sets of rules governing their feeding, clothing and learning. The experience gained in foundling hospitals and dispensaries decisively contributed not only to lower institutional death rates but helped significantly in reducing the total infant and child mortality in several countries.[83]

Hospitals and dispensaries

A pivotal factor fostering the process of medicalization was the development of hospitals. Hitherto more a refuge for the poor and homeless, hospitals gradually shed their medieval welfare function becoming instead institutions for the care of sick people. Development of a primarily medical role for hospitals took a somewhat different course in the various European countries.[84]

In Britain only five so-called hospitals functioned in the early eighteenth century, all of them located in the city of London.[85] With the typical medieval hospices abolished by Henry VIII in 1545, the secular authorities in London operated these hospitals under royal auspices and financed by private donations. Sick, old, and infirm people from the

[83] For conditions in France and Germany see N. Senior, 'Aspects of Infant Feeding in Eighteenth-Century France', *Eighteenth-Century Studies*, 16 (1983), 367–88; and M. Lindemann, 'Love for Hire: The Regulation of the Wetnursing Business in Eighteenth-Century Hamburg', *Journal of Family History*, 6 (1981), 379–95.

[84] For a useful survey consult John D. Thompson and Grace Goldin, *The Hospital: a Social and Architectural History* (New Haven, 1975). See also G. B. Risse, 'Hospital History: New Sources and Methods', in Roy Porter and Andrew Wear (eds.), *Problems and Methods in the History of Medicine* (London, 1987), pp. 175–203.

[85] For an overview consult W. H. McMenemey, 'The Hospital Movement of the Eighteenth Century and Its Development', in F. N. L. Poynter (ed.), *The Evolution of Hospitals in Britain* (London, 1964), pp. 43–71.

lower classes of society were housed in these institutions.[86] In the face of growing urbanization with its detrimental effects on the poor, the available facilities in London proved totally inadequate, prompting leading citizens and influential physicians to vigorously lobby for the erection of more infirmaries – establishments solely devoted to treatment of the sick and wounded.

Britain's voluntary reform movement was fuelled by religious and secular philanthropic motives, protection of the social order, and the opportunity of personal rewards for the charitable patrons.[87] It also took into consideration the interests of the medical profession. Indeed physicians and surgeons progressively realized that they could markedly improve their knowledge and education through mass observation of sick people congregated in hospital wards. The first new hospital to open its doors in 1720 was the Westminster Infirmary of London, closely followed by Guy's Hospital (1724), St George's (1733), London Hospital (1740), and finally the Middlesex (1745).

Such London foundations were readily imitated in the British provinces where a number of local infirmaries and county institutions were created with the help of private donors. Notable among them was the Royal Infirmary of Edinburgh.[88] By the end of the eighteenth century the whole country could boast thirty general infirmaries in the provinces and five in the city of London with an estimated total number of four thousand beds, half of them located in larger establishments of the capital with a population of about nine hundred thousand persons. While the growth was impressive by contemporary English standards, and the foundations fully devoted to patients requiring medical attention, such a small number of beds could only serve a fraction of the total population.[89]

[86] Conditions and events prior to the eighteenth century are detailed in B. G. Gale, 'The Dissolution and Revolution in London Hospital Facilities', *Medical History*, 11 (1967), 91–6; and C. Rose, 'Politics and the London Royal Hospitals, 1683–92', in L. Granshaw and R. Porter (eds), *The Hospital in History* (London, 1989), pp. 123–48.

[87] Details can be obtained from David Owen, *English Philanthropy 1660–1960* (Cambridge, MA, 1965), especially pp. 36–61, ch. 2: 'The Philanthropy of Eighteenth-Century Humanitarianism'. See also R. Porter, 'The Gift Relation: Philanthropy and Provincial Hospitals in Eighteenth-Century England', in *The Hospital in History*, pp. 149–78.

[88] Risse, *Hospital Life*, especially pp. 7–59, ch. 1; and by the same author, 'Medicine and Charity: The Social Roles of a British Hospital, Edinburgh 1750–1800', in M. Nicolson (ed.), *Practice, Pedagogy and Politics: The Changing Face of Scottish Medicine* (in press).

[89] Brian Abel-Smith, 'The Sick and Lame Poor', in *The Hospitals 1800–1948, A Study in Social Administration in England and Wales* (Cambridge, MA, 1964), p. 1, ch. 1. See also W. B. Howie, 'The Administration of an Eighteenth-Century Provincial Hospital: The Royal Salop Infirmary, 1747–1830', *Medical History*, 5 (1961), 34–55.

Unlike other European countries, the British voluntary hospital strictly limited admission to the so-called 'deserving' poor – working-class people who could secure an official upper-class sponsor and bring a signed letter of recommendation from him or her to be hospitalized. It follows that because of their restrictive admission criteria and limited numbers of beds, these institutions failed to exert any noticeable influence on the reduction of mortality rates in the areas where they had been established.[90] Most of the patients admitted to the voluntary hospitals were young people suffering from self-limited, non-life threatening ailments, leading to exceptionally low mortality rates, often less than 5 per cent, for most of these establishments. However, coming to the hospital often meant a welcome shift in the burden of care from busy or even non-existing relatives, isolation of contagious persons, and relief from soiled garments, wretched living quarters, and deficient diets.[91]

Perhaps of greater demographic impact was the establishment of free *dispensaries*, outpatient clinics totally independent from the hospitals providing for the ambulatory sick poor. Beginning with the General Dispensary in Aldersgate Street, London, founded in 1770 according to plans designed by John C. Lettson (1744–1815), leader of Britain's dispensary movement, these establishments rapidly multiplied in the capital and provinces. By 1800, the country had thirty-eight general dispensaries with approximately one hundred thousand yearly admissions.[92]

Dispensaries formed part of the private philanthropic efforts which had helped create British voluntary hospitals half a century earlier. More economical to operate and providing as part of their mission home visits to sick patients among the 'deserving' poor, dispensaries played a significant role in the process of medicalization. Wider segments of the health professions were sensitized to problems of the lower classes, especially the relationship between unhealthy environments and con-

---

[90] A recent study concerning this subject is S. Cherry, 'The Hospitals and Population Growth: The Voluntary General Hospitals, Mortality and Local Populations in the English Provinces in the Eighteenth and Nineteenth Centuries', *Population Studies*, 34 (1980), 59–75 and 251–65.

[91] For a detailed review of the diseases seen in the hospital and patient care see Guenter B. Risse, 'Patients and Their Diseases', and 'Hospital Care: State of the Medical Art', in *Hospital Life*, pp. 119–239, chs. 3 and 4.

[92] I. S. L. Loudon, 'The Origins and Growth of the Dispensary Movement in England', *Bulletin of the History of Medicine*, 55 (1981), 322–42. For a glimpse at actual treatment in a Scottish dispensary, see L. S. King, 'The Practice of Medicine in 1787', *Illinois Medical Journal*, 130 (1955), 130–5.

tagious fevers. In turn, populations hitherto totally neglected from a medical standpoint became acquainted with rules of person hygiene, medical models of disease, and a host of therapeutic measures.[93]

In sharp contrast, eighteenth-century France boasted an estimated 1,961 'hospitals' during the pre-Revolutionary period. However most of these institutions were small welfare establishments at the parish level with only a few beds, taking care of old people, abandoned children, and the sick poor. A second category of institutions were the so-called *hôtels-Dieu*, often of medieval origin and located in larger towns, which also took in the sick and abandoned but excluded incurables, the insane, and those suffering from venereal diseases. Finally there was a seventeenth-century newcomer usually located in urban centres: the general hospital. Initially founded by religious and humanistic philanthropy to confine vagrants and beggars, general hospitals also became repositories of persons excluded from the *hôtels-Dieu*, and therefore housed a variety of individuals including foundlings, prostitutes, and the truly sick.[94]

Paris, the capital city with about seven hundred thousand people, had a total of forty-eight charitable establishments called 'hospitals' prior to the Revolution with an estimated population of over 35,000, including 42 per cent foundlings, 40 per cent aged, infirm, widows, and transients, and only 18 per cent persons who were labelled sick. Many of these hospitals were municipal institutions with significant outpatient facilities where the ambulatory poor could receive free medical advice and medications.[95]

While the French poor appeared to have had greater availability and access to hospital services, especially if one compares large urban centres such as London and Paris, severe overcrowding of these facilities

[93] Z. Cope, 'The Influence of the Free Dispensaries upon Medical Education in Britain', *Medical History*, 13 (1969), 29–36; and W. F. Bynum, 'Physicians, Hospitals, and Career Structures in Eighteenth-Century London', in *William Hunter*, pp. 105–28; and U. Tröhler, 'The Doctor as Naturalist: The Idea and Practice of Clinical Teaching and Research in British Policlinics, 1770–1850', *Clio Medica*, 21 (1987/88), 21–34. See also C. Webster, 'The Crisis of the Hospitals during the Industrial Revolution', in E. G. Forbes (ed.), *Human Implications of Scientific Advance* (Edinburgh, 1978), pp. 214–23; and J. V. Pickstone, S. V. F. Butler, 'The Politics of Medicine in Manchester, 1788–1792: Hospital Reform and Public Health Services in the Early Industrial City', *Medical History*, 27 (1984), 227–49.

[94] For an overview, see M. Joergen, 'The Structure of the Hospital System in France in the Ancien Régime', in R. Foster (ed.), *Medicine and Society in France*, pp. 104–36; and Colin Jones, *The Charitable Imperative: Hospitals and Nursing in Ancien Régime and Revolutionary France* (London, 1989). For an interesting case study see C. Jones, M. Sonenscher, 'The Social Functions of the Hospital in Eighteenth-Century France: The Case of the Hôtel-Dieu of Nimes', *French Historical Studies*, 13 (1983), 172–214.

[95] L. S. Greenbaum, 'Measure of Civilization: The Hospital Thought of Jacques Tenon on the Eve of the French Revolution', *Bulletin of the History of Medicine*, 49 (1975), 43–56.

jeopardized personal care and possible recovery from illness. A typical example was the infamous thousand-year-old Hôtel-Dieu in Paris which housed over 3,500 patients but only had slightly over 1,000 beds. With the sick and needy indiscriminately packed together, generally at least three persons in every bed except those suffering from smallpox, hospital contagion was rampant. Moreover, lack of cleanliness and inadequate support staff hampered recovery. Hospital routines were still more attuned to the spiritual rather than physical needs of those hospitalized, leading to harmful feeding practices and insufficient administration of remedies. Attempts at conversion and reinforcement of the Catholic faith occupied the religious orders running the wards.[96]

On the positive side, the abominable conditions in the Hôtel-Dieu – its mortality variously reported around 22 per cent – served as a stimulus for wide-ranging hospital reforms promulgated by a number of philanthropists, architects, and ultimately physicians as well as surgeons.[97] While the Hôtel-Dieu itself only partially benefited from the proposals, other city institutions old and new adopted some of the suggestions derived in part from visits to British voluntary hospitals.[98] Separate beds for each inmate, division of patients according to diseases, improved meal and medication schedules, and better medical record-keeping were among the most notable improvements.[99] As their medically oriented routines improved, certain establishments became centres for teaching and research, such as the Hospice of the Paris College of Surgery, founded in 1774.[100]

Early in the century the situation in the German states was somewhat similar to that of France. A fair number of undifferentiated welfare institutions housed the infirm, mentally ill, those suffering from

[96] P. A. Richmond, 'The Hôtel-Dieu of Paris on the Eve of the Revolution', *Journal of the History of Medicine*, 16 (1961), 335–53. Also consult A. Thalamy, 'La medicalisation de l'hôpital', in M. Foucault et al. (eds.), *Les machines a guerir*, pp. 43–53.

[97] The various hospital reform proposals are described in: L. S. Greenbaum, 'Jean Sylvain Bailly, the Baron de Breteuil and the Four New Hospitals of Paris', *Clio Medica*, 8 (1973), 261–84; and by the same author, 'Health-Care and Hospital Building in Eighteenth-Century France: Reform Proposals of Du Pont de Nemours and Condorcet', in T. Besterman (ed.), *Studies on Voltaire and Eighteenth Century* (Oxford, 1976), CLII, pp. 895–930; and 'Jacques Necker and the Reform of the Paris Hospitals on the Eve of the French Revolution', *Clio Medica*, 19 (1984), 216–30.

[98] L. S. Greenbaum, 'The Commercial Treaty of Humanity. La tournée des hôpitaux anglais par Jacques Tenon en 1787', *Revue d'Histoire des Sciences*, 24 (1971), 317–50.

[99] L. S. Greenbaum, 'Nurses and Doctors in Conflict: Piety and Medicine in the Paris Hôtel-Dieu on the Eve of the French Revolution', *Clio Medica*, 13 (1978), 247–67.

[100] T. Gelfand, 'The Hospice of the Paris College of Surgery (1774–1793), A Unique and Invaluable Institution', *Bulletin of the History of Medicine*, 47 (1973), 375–93. For further details about teaching, see M. J. Imbault-Huart, 'Concepts and Realities of the Beginning of Clinical Teaching in France in the Late 18th and Early 19th Centuries', *Clio Medica*, 21 (1987/8), 59–70.

contagious diseases, and the injured. Inadequate facilities also caused crowding with several inmates sharing one bed. Lack of hygiene, inadequate ventilation, and problems with the disposal of human wastes were common.[101]

After mid-century, however, expansion of existing physical facilities, construction of new buildings surrounded by extensive gardens, and stricter segregation of patients suffering from infectious diseases occurred in selected institutions. Prominent examples were the Charité Hospital in Berlin, founded in 1727, and the 1776 expansion of the Juliusspital in Würzburg. The former had a capacity of nearly four hundred beds. The facilities were not only open to the sick poor, but also included the aged, infirm, and soldiers. At mid-century, confinement of non-medical cases averaged between two and five years. Overall mortality rates at the Charité Hospital during the years 1731–42 fluctuated between 8 and 10 per cent, with higher deaths in the adult sick wards (24–30 per cent) than in the obstetrical and military sections. Such statistics coincide with the mortality figures for a typical German town in that period, leading to the conclusion that hospitals with both welfare and medical aims had no demographic impact but served useful functions of shelter and rehabilitation.[102]

Following similar philanthropic and mercantilist motives, Joseph II of Austria opened in 1784 a 186-room, 2,000-bed hospital in the Viennese capital, built in accordance with the most advanced contemporary notions of salubrity and ventilation. With separate facilities for the insane, pregnant women, and orphans, the Allgemeines Krankenhaus quickly became a model for subsequent foundations and renovations elsewhere in German-speaking countries. Affiliated with the Viennese medical school, the new hospital gradually became a world-renowned mecca for clinical training.[103]

[101] Alfons Fischer, 'Krankenanstalten', in *Geschichte des Deutschen Gesundheitswesens*, 2 vols. (Berlin, 1933), II, pp. 73–93. For greater details about German hospital architecture in the eighteenth century, consult Dieter Jetter, 'Barock-Spitäler des 18-Jahrhunderts', in *Geschichte des Hospitals, Westdeutschland von den Anfängen bis 1850* (Wiesbaden, 1966), pp. 93–116.
[102] A. E. Imhof, 'The Hospital in the 18th Century: For Whom?' in P. Branca (ed.), *The Medical Show* (New York, 1977), pp. 141–63. A slightly expanded version in German is 'Die Funktion des Krankenhauses in der Stadt des 18 Jahrhunderts', *Zeitschrift für Stadtgeschichte, Stadtsozologie und Denkmalpflege*, 4 (1977), 215–42. For further information regarding the Charité Hospital see A. H. Murken, 'Die Charité in Berlin von 1780 bis 1830', *Arzt und Krankenhaus*, 3 (1980), 20–36, and more recently Gerhard Jäckel, *Die Charité*, 2nd edn (Bayreuth, 1987).
[103] E. Lesky, 'Das Wiener Allgemeine Krankenhaus. Seine Gründung und Wirkung auf deutsche Spitäler', *Clio Medica*, 2 (1967), 23–37; and P. P. Bernard, 'The Limits of Absolutism: Joseph II and the Allgemeines Krankenhaus', *Eighteenth-Century Studies*, 9 (1975), 193–215. Similar developments occurred in Pavia, Italy under Austrian rule. See G. B. Risse, 'Clinical Instruction in

For members of the medical profession the rise of hospitals and dispensaries was a truly momentous event. Physicians and surgeons quickly realized that the opportunity to observe large numbers of patients allowed them to dramatically increase their understanding of diseases. Gradual experimentation with traditional treatments for the first time yielded hints about their iatrogenic potential, eventually forcing many young practitioners to acquire a salutary therapeutic scepticism. Verification of clinical data through numerous autopsy findings stimulated pathology and provided better criteria for nosological arrangements.[104]

More importantly, physicians and surgeons practising in hospitals found their activities progressively exposed to scrutiny by their peers and the lay public in general. Reputations could be made or even destroyed in hospital settings since ward journals and ledgers documented the success and failure of prescribed treatments. Increasingly the newly acquired knowledge filled more pages in medical journals and books, thereby shifting the focus away from purely theoretical disputes. Description of clinical cases and the use of observational data for statistical analyses readily followed. Such information was eagerly communicated in articles to those physicians practising in more isolated rural areas. Ultimately, the extensive clinical experience in hospitals was shared with successive waves of students, greatly improving the education of physicians, surgeons, and in Britain the apothecaries.[105]

Before the proliferation of hospitals, practitioners could only acquire a limited knowledge of medical matters and exert partial control over

Hospitals: The Boerhaavian Tradition in Leyden, Edinburgh, Vienna, and Pavia', *Clio Medica*, 21 (1987/88), 1–19. For another study of hospitals in Italy consult S. Cavallo, 'Charity, Power, and Patronage in Eighteenth-Century Italian Hospitals: The Case of Turin', in *The Hospital in History*, pp. 93–122.

[104] J. F. Kett, 'Provincial Medical Practice in England 1730–1815', *Journal of the History of Medicine*, 19 (1964), 17–29. See also L. M. Zimmerman, 'Surgeons and the Rise of Clinical Teaching in England', *Bulletin of the History of Medicine*, 37 (1963), 167–77; and Russell C. Maulitz, *Morbid Appearances. The Anatomy of Pathology in the Early Nineteenth Century* (Cambridge, 1987), especially pp. 9–35, ch. 1.

[105] W. S. C. Copeman, 'The Evolution of Clinical Method in English Medical Education', *Proceedings of the Royal Society of Medicine*, 58 (1965), 887–94; and S. C. Lawrence, 'Entrepreneurs and Private Enterprise: The Development of Medical Lecturing in London, 1775–1820', *Bulletin of the History of Medicine*, 62 (1988), 171–92. For similar information about France consult T. Gelfand, 'Gestation of the Clinic', *Medical History*, 25 (1981), 169–80. Further details can be obtained from two other articles by the same author: 'A Clinical Ideal: Paris 1789', *Bulletin of the History of Medicine*, 51 (1977), 397–411; and 'A Confrontation over Clinical Instruction at the Hôtel-Dieu of Paris during the French Revolution', *Journal of the History of Medicine*, 28 (1973), 268–82. Information about the German-speaking countries is available in Gernot Roth, *Die Entwicklung des klinischen Unterrichts* (Göttingen, 1965); E. Lesky, 'Johann Peter Frank als Organisator des medizinischen Unterrichts', *Sudhoffs Archiv*, 38 (1955), 1–30.

their treatments. Dependent on sporadic house calls by willing patients, restricted by poor roads and long distances to a few consultations, physicians could not expect to gain a better understanding of the diseases they were entrusted to heal. Such discontinuity forced healers to only focus on the patients' most bothersome symptoms responsible for the call while the need to impress the clients often prompted 'heroic' measures of antiphlogistic practice, especially bleeding and purging, without proper follow up.

In the hospital, by contrast, physicians had considerable authority and control over patients. This shift of power in the doctor–patient relationship allowed for more continuity of observation and care as well as compliance with the prescribed therapeutic regimen. Sydenham's earlier call for establishing the 'natural history of diseases' – meaning their complete clinical development – could now take place in an institutional setting which virtually imprisoned poor patients while empowering physicians to observe their suffering at all times, under any conditions, without even the need to intervene prematurely with dramatic therapeutic strategies.[106]

Lastly, Enlightenment physicians and surgeons working in hospitals, dispensaries, or making house calls to the poor, were quick to assess the importance of personal and environmental factors in the epidemiology of several infectious diseases, notably typhus or jail fever. Being controlled environments, hospitals thus became the ideal laboratories for testing the tenets of a new hygiene already formulated on the basis of observations carried out in army camps, ships, prisons, and other crowded hospitals. Once accepted by the growing urban middle class, such principles as personal cleanliness, proper home ventilation, and adequate nutrition were repeatedly preached to the lower class seeking admission to hospitals. By the end of the century, in fact, medical authors began considering such environmental factors of more importance in the recovery of the sick, especially those suffering from infectious diseases, than all the available medical and surgical measures combined.[107] Generally unable to sustain the previous ratio of inpatients to inhabitants in the face of late eighteenth-century population explosion, many hospitals experienced a degree of crowding and contagion similar to or

[106] O. Keel, 'The Politics of Health and the Institutionalization of Clinical Practices in Europe in the Second Half of the Eighteenth Century', in *William Hunter*, pp. 207–56.

[107] Such environmental progress is mentioned in J. H. Woodward, 'The British Voluntary Hospital Movement – Success or Disaster?', *Annales Cisalpines d'Histoire Sociale*, 1 (1973), 233–54; and repeated in his book, *To Do the Sick No Harm: A Study of the British Voluntary Hospital System to 1875* (London, 1974).

worse than conditions already present in lower-class urban districts. Thus institutionally based diseases quickly spread among the unfortunate inmates transforming many hospitals into establishments of last resort, the feared 'gateways to death'.[108]

Health manuals

Another example of eighteenth-century medicalization was the attempt to disseminate health-related knowledge and practices hitherto restricted to professional healers. Such endeavours to popularize medicine took the form of health manuals expressly written for laypersons. Often composed by physicians, in the vernacular, these publications embodied the Enlightenment ideals of human progress and popular education.[109] Their explicit goal was the improvement of community health through the transformation of medicine from an exclusively professional effort into a programme of curative and preventative guidelines for direct use by the public. As the author of the most popular work of this genre, William Buchan (1729–1805), asserted in his *Domestic Medicine* (1769): 'there certainly cannot be a more necessary, a more noble and a more god-like action than to administer to the wants of our fellow creatures in distress'.[110]

Previously outlined mercantilist motives also loomed large in the work of the Swiss practitioner Samuel A. A. D. Tissot (1728–97). His *Advice to the People in General with Regard to their Health* (1761) was a very popular book originally written in French and translated like Buchan's work into all the major European languages. Tissot's motives for sharing

[108] Concerning the harmful effects of hospitalization, see T. McKeown and R. G. Brown, 'Medical Evidence Related to English Population Changes in the Eighteenth Century', *Population Studies*, 9 (1955–6), 125. Similar statements appeared subsequently in K. F. Helleiner, 'The Vital Revolution Reconsidered', in D. V. Glass and D. E. C. Eversley (eds.), *Population and History* (London, 1965), p. 84; and Phyllis Deane, *The First Industrial Revolution* (Cambridge, 1965), p. 29. McKeown's conclusions were first questioned by E. M. Sigsworth, 'Gateways to Death? Medicine, Hospitals, and Mortality, 1700–1850', in P. Mathias (ed.), *Science and Society 1600–1900*, pp. 97–110.

[109] For an introduction to domestic medicine consult G. B. Risse, 'Introduction', in G. B. Risse, R. L. Numbers and J. Walzer Leavitt (eds), *Medicine Without Doctors* (New York, 1977), pp. 1–8. A number of articles dealing with the subject can be found in R. Porter (ed.), *Patients and Practitioners, Lay Perceptions of Medicine in Pre-Industrial Society* (Cambridge, 1985). A recent overview was written by Roy Porter, 'Lay Medical Knowledge in the Eighteenth Century: The Evidence of the *Gentleman's Magazine*', *Medical History*, 29 (1985), 138–68.

[110] William Buchan, 'Introduction', in *Domestic Medicine*, 14th edn (Philadelphia, 1795), p. 24. This work went through numerous editions, the last one in 1913, and was probably the most popular manual in English-speaking countries. For a complete analysis see C. J. Lawrence, 'William Buchan: Medicine Laid Open', *Medical History*, 19 (1975), 20–35; and C. E. Rosenberg, 'Medical Text and Social Context: Explaining William Buchan's Domestic Medicine', *Bulletin of the History of Medicine*, 57 (1983), 22–42.

medical knowledge with the public were primarily based on his concern that the inadequate or incorrect treatment of diseases in the countryside significantly contributed to rural depopulation and thus the agricultural decline of France.[111]

One of the fundamental reasons for new efforts to popularize medical knowledge was a widely perceived shortage of qualified health professionals, especially in rural areas. Notions of hygiene and proper life style would indeed 'trickle down' to the masses. Authors of these manuals made it clear that they were writing for literate, 'well-disposed' people as Buchan called them, who would employ and share this knowledge with the lower strata of society.'I have principally calculated it for the perusal of intelligent and charitable persons who live in the country', explained Tissot.[112]

Clergy figured prominently among the authors and recipients of medical advice. In his proposals Johann P. Frank already had given priest–physicians an important role in rural health-care schemes.[113] Moreover in Britain, John Wesley (1703–91), the famous founder of Methodism, contributed with his *Primitive Physic* (1747), a health manual containing much useful information derived from the works of the British physician George Cheyne (1671–1743).[114]

In addition to curative efforts by clergy, landowners, teachers, and other knowledgeable persons, the books and pamphlets were designed to furnish suitable materials for health education and prevention. Given the positive value of health fostered by the Enlightenment, medicine, broadly interpreted, needed to become part of the general education envisioned for everyone. For reformers, questions of diet, life style, and personal hygiene loomed important. Not only would such learning ensure health and prolong life, but in cases of children, facilitate their upbringing in the home and avoid disease or death. Wrote Buchan: 'no part of medicine is of more general importance than that which relates to the nursing and management of children'.[115]

[111] Samuel A. A. D. Tissot, *Avis au peuple sur sa santé* (Lausanne, 1761).

[112] Samuel Tissot, 'Introduction', in J. Kirkpatrick, *Advice to the People in General With Regard to Their Health*, 3rd edn (London, 1768), p. 16. Further information on Tissot can be obtained from Antoinette S. Emch-Deriaz, 'Towards a Social Conception of Health in the Second Half of the Eighteenth Century: Tissot (1728–1797) and the New Preoccupation with Health and Well-Being' (University of Rochester Ph.D. thesis, 1983).

[113] For details see R. Heller, 'Priest-Doctors as a Rural Health Service in the Age of the Enlightenment', *Medical History*, 20 (1976), 361–83.

[114] For more information consult G. S. Rousseau, 'John Wesley's Primitive Physic (1747)', in *Harvard Library Bulletin*, 16 (1968), 242–56; and S. J. Rogul, 'Pills for the Poor: John Wesley's Primitive Physick', *Yale Journal of Biological Medicine*, 51 (1978), 81–90.

[115] Buchan, *Domestic Medicine*, p. 23.

Buchan's ideas were echoed by other authors bent on popularizing medical concepts. In his *Catechism of Health*, published in 1794, the German physician Bernhard C. Faust (1755–1842) promoted similar views. Using a simple question-and-answer format in his work, this author portrayed the positive value of bodily health by closely linking it to spiritual happiness and insisting that it was a divine duty to preserve them both since they represented God's supreme gift to mankind. Readers were especially enjoined to watch out for the health of their children for which they received from Faust a number of useful tips regarding nutrition and clothing.[116]

Another important motive for 'laying open' the secrets of professional medicine was the growing alienation experienced by an increasingly better-educated public concerning recent developments in the cure and prevention of disease. Most of the information, including drug prescriptions, was still written in Latin, scattered among numerous specialized publications, and formulated in excessively technical or philosophical language. Sharing the knowledge, it was hoped, would foster a better patient–physician relationship since the former would be in a better position to understand the aims and activities of the latter. There was also, in Buchan's view at least, the possibility that informed laypersons might well contribute with discoveries of their own to the growing knowledge of health-related matters.[117]

Lastly, in the view of professionals, the demystification of medicine was to be the most effective antidote educated people could acquire against the perils of quackery. Knowledge of general medical principles was seen as a barrier 'against the destructive influences of ignorance, superstition, and quackery'.[118] Possessing the means for checking out 'pretenders to medicine' would unmask the impostors and charlatans plying their craft especially among the ignorant country folk. In his book, Faust portrayed quacks as persons who were ignorant about human anatomy, made quick diagnoses by only examining the urine of the sick, and promised immediate relief and cures in all diseases. He also

---

[116] Bernhard C. Faust, *Gesundheits-Katechismus, zum Gebrauche in den Schulen und beym häuslichen Unterrichte* (Buckenburg, 1794). Selected portions of Faust's work were translated into English and appeared as *The Catechism of Health* (Edinburgh, 1797).

[117] Buchan, *Domestic Medicine*, p. 18.

[118] Buchan, *Domestic Medicine*, pp. 17, 21. 'No laws will ever be able to prevent quackery...a very small degree of medical knowledge; however, would be sufficient to break this spell, and nothing else can effectually undeceive them.' For more details, consult W. F. Bynum and R. Porter (eds), *Medical Fringe and Medical Orthodoxy 1750–1850* (London, 1987); and more recently Roy Porter, *Health for Sale, Quackery in England, 1660–1850* (Manchester, 1989).

cautioned his readers against itinerant operators who promised to cure hernias and eliminate cataracts, as well as wandering peddlers of secret nostrums for human and animal consumption. Pointing to the dangers of losing one's health and even life through the utilization of such dubious remedies, Faust insisted that the best remedies for domestic consumption were fresh air and cold water.[119]

Smallpox inoculation

Finally, Enlightenment medicine organized the first extensive immunization programme in history by inoculating thousands of people with smallpox.[12] Bubonic plague had virtually disappeared from western Europe by the early 1700s, and the water-borne scourges characteristic of large unsanitary metropolitan areas were still in the future. Thus, smallpox was indeed a highly visible disease during the eighteenth century. Comprising about 10 per cent of all deaths, it was especially feared because of contagiousness, mortality and disfiguring consequences. Estimates indicate that perhaps sixty million people perished from the disease between 1700 and 1800. Suggestions that smallpox inoculations not only aided in the decline of mortality from the disease but saved enough lives in the British countryside to meaningfully contribute to the contemporary demographic expansion remain controversial.[121]

Long before the eighteenth century, popular measures to 'buy the pox' existed in the form of empirical procedures scattered among many cultures in Europe, Africa, and Asia. The numerous and varied techniques reported by Europeans in the late seventeenth and early eighteenth centuries all used material from the smallpox pustules of an active case in the form of fresh lymph or dried crusts. These substances were rubbed, scratched, or blown into the skin or nose of healthy individuals with the purpose of transferring or 'grafting' the smallpox. Such a

[119] Faust, *Gesundheits-Katechismus*, pp. 66–7.

[120] For an overview see W. L. Langer, 'Immunization against Smallpox before Jenner', *Scientific American*, 234 (1976) 112–17. A more detailed account is C. W. Dixon, 'The History of Inoculation for the Smallpox', in J. and A. Churchill, *Smallpox* (London, 1962), pp. 216–48, ch. 11. A general history of smallpox was written by Donald R. Hopkins, *Princes and Peasants* (Chicago, 1983).

[121] This thesis was first advanced in P. E. Razzell, 'Population Change in 18th Century England; A Reinterpretation', *Economic History Review*, 18 (1965), 312–32, and later appeared in more detail: Peter E. Razzell, *The Conquest of Smallpox: The Impact of Inoculation on Smallpox Mortality in Eighteenth-Century Britain* (London, 1977). See also B. Luckin, 'The Decline of Smallpox and the Demographic Revolution of the Eighteenth Century', *Social History*, 6 (1977), 793–7; and A. J. Mercer, 'Smallpox and the Epidemiological-Demographic Change in Europe: The Role of Vaccination', *Population Studies*, 39 (1985), 287–307.

procedure often resulted in a mild case of the disease, absence of residual scarring, and lifelong protection from further bouts of this sickness. However, the exclusively oral transmission of knowledge about inoculation and magico-religious explanation as disease-transference may have restricted diffusion of the method. More importantly, the hazards of acquiring a serious case of smallpox for a healthy individual and even starting an epidemic must have been significant deterrents for the wider employment of inoculation in those areas in which it was known.[122]

In England the death of prominent figures at the royal court from smallpox included Queen Mary (1694) and the Duke of Gloucester (1700). The latter's demise precipitated a constitutional crisis, and mobilized the Royal Society into investigating the disease and searching for ways to prevent it. Between 1700 and 1717, a series of reports from China and Turkey were presented to this scientific institution describing smallpox inoculation practices popular in those countries. The first English account of the method by a Greek physician living in Constantinople appeared in the *Philosophical Transactions* of 1714.[123]

By 1722, English medical circles had also received a number of communications from the American colonies, specifically New England, where a severe smallpox epidemic in Boston had prompted the inoculation of over two hundred persons.[124] Moreover, upon her return to London, Mary Wortley Montagu, wife of the English ambassador to Turkey, requested in 1721 that her daughter be inoculated during a smallpox epidemic afflicting the capital. Lady Mary, well acquainted in royal circles, had familiarized herself with the procedure several years prior while touring Turkey. Her wish was carried out by a Scottish surgeon, Charles Maitland (1668–1748), on condition that medical observers be allowed to follow the case. Success of the action did arouse a great deal of interest among members of the English aristocracy and the medical profession, the latter requesting permission in the same year to experiment with six condemned prisoners. Good results prompted several aristocrats to have their children similarly inoculated, a list of

[122] An extensive review of the reported popular measures appears in A. C. Klebs, 'The Historic Evolution of Variolation', *Bulletin of the Johns Hopkins Hospital*, 24 (1913), 69–83. Unfortunately the article lacks bibliographical references.

[123] Emanuel Timoni, 'An Account, or History of Procuring the Smallpox by Incision, or Inoculations', *Philosophical Transaction*, 29 (1714), 72–6.

[124] For more details consult J. B. Blake, 'The Inoculation Controversy in Boston: 1721–1722', *New England Quarterly*, 25 (1952), 489–506; and by the same author 'Smallpox Inoculation in Colonial Boston', *Journal of the History of Medicine*, 8 (1953), 284–300.

prominent offspring that eventually included the Prince of Wales. Numerous newspaper accounts quickly spread the information about variolation, as the practice was called, among other members of the upper and middle classes, not without creating a number of controversies since some fatalities occurred following the procedure.[125]

In accordance with the tenets of humoralism, physicians quickly transformed the rather simple folk method into a complex medical procedure. Patients had to be prepared for a period of three to six weeks to receive the presumed smallpox poison. the goal was to strengthen the bodily constitution and eliminate all harmful substances which could potentially contribute to the inflammatory state caused by inoculation. A regimen of fresh air, no alcoholic beverages, and a vegetable diet, coupled with repeated purgings and bloodletting was believed to be the most effective antidote against possible complications expected from the poison transfer. When patients were finally considered ready, physicians made a series of deep incisions into the skin before placing the smallpox lymph into such lesions. The wounds were deliberately kept open with linen threads to facilitate drainage, and a plaster applied over the wound. Individuals were isolated in special inoculation houses for several weeks until the incisions stopped draining and began healing, thereby minimizing the danger of contagion to others. During this period of convalescence, patients were subjected to the same regimen employed during the preparatory phase. The entire ordeal generally lasted about two months if no further complications ensued.[126]

Because of its length, complexity, and high cost, the practice of smallpox inoculation was until midcentury mostly restricted to the upper classes of society whose members had the necessary time and resources to afford it. Furthermore, the procedure was hampered by the frequent severity of the infection associated with inoculation; others contracted a severe case of the disease. Because of the inherent risks, physicians were somewhat reticent to proceed, and unable to properly explain to their clients the unpredictable effects of variolation. On the other hand, lower-class fatalism, fear of accidental contagion, and religious scruples based on the argument that the procedure attempted to interfere with God's work, were all barriers to its popularization. Perhaps more damaging were charges by opponents that in sporadic

[125] For the latest review of the evidence, see G. Miller, 'Putting Lady Mary in Her Place: A Discussion of Historical Causation', *Bulletin of the History of Medicine*, 55 (1981), 2–16. A full biography of Lady Wortley Montagu was written by Robert Halsband, *The Life of Lady Mary Wortley Montagu* (Oxford, 1956).

[126] See, for example, *Mr Maitland's Account of Inoculating the Smallpox* (London, 1722).

cases persons already inoculated had subsequently contracted the disease and died, a reflection of the uncertainties still surrounding the technique.[127]

During an outbreak of smallpox in Charleston, South Carolina, in 1738, a local physician, James Kirkpatrick (d. 1770), developed a simplified arm-to-arm inoculation method that dramatically lowered the mortality rate from the procedure to one case in a hundred. His report, first published in 1743, was later translated into various European languages, broadening the interest in variolation.[128] Buoyed by what appeared to be favourable statistics, the authorities of the London Foundling Hospital decided in 1747 that all children admitted to the hospital without previous exposure to smallpox were to be inoculated. Three years later, the Smallpox and Inoculation Hospital opened its doors in the capital with a special building reserved for the inoculation and isolation of the poor.

After 1750 the practice of inoculation spread rapidly in Britain among the middle and even lower classes of society. The simplified procedures, their cost significantly reduced, caused fewer complications, especially contagion, and also demanded less time. Their popularity was greatest in rural areas and small towns where smallpox was always epidemic and inhabitants periodically decimated by visitations of the scourge. The high toll in personal suffering and death was compounded there by the severe economic losses resulting from the imposition of quarantines and subsequent interruption of commerce.

In certain market towns various charitable organizations at the parish level took up the responsibility of systematically inoculating large segments of the population with smallpox. Given the paucity of trained medical professionals, these programmes were forced to employ an army of amateur inoculators drawn from the ranks of country surgeons, apothecaries, clergymen, and interested laypersons. Among them were Robert (1707–77) and Daniel Sutton (1735–1819) of Suffolk, a father-and-son team of surgeons whose variolation technique soon attracted a great number of paying customers, especially in London. By 1796 Daniel claimed to have inoculated 40,000 persons with only five fatalities.[129]

While smallpox inoculation developed mainly in Britain, other European countries also gradually introduced the techniques. In France

---

[127] W. Wagstaffe, *A Letter to Dr. Friend, Shewing the Danger and Uncertainty of Inoculating the Smallpox* (London, 1722).

[128] James Kirkpatrick, *An Essay on Inoculation* (London, 1743).

[129] D. van Zwanenberg, 'The Suttons and the Business of Inoculation', *Medical History*, 22 (1978), 71–82.

the procedure won strong endorsements from the *philosophes* and the Royal Academy of Sciences despite religious opposition and resistance from the conservative medical establishment. In the 1760s, however, both parties engaged in vigorous debates about the merits of inoculation. Frightened by the death of Louis XV, King of France, who succumbed to smallpox in 1774, members of the upper classes demanded to be variolated and in the face of official indecision and a temporary ban in Paris the method was carried out in several private clinics. Similar smallpox inoculations of members belonging to the royal households of Prussia, Austria, and Russia were performed, often by experienced British variolators.[130]

While a bitter war of pamphlets and newspaper articles between those advocating and rejecting the procedure raged in most European countries, inoculators went about their now lucrative task, primarily among the upper classes. However, only in Britain did the procedure gain wider acceptance, especially in the countryside. Both at Newcastle and Chester inoculation dispensaries were established later in the century, and the measure advocated in infants. Smallpox, however, remained endemic in the larger metropolitan areas where its destruction was elusive and methods of isolating the sick impossible to implement in the face of urban crowding and the continuous influx of new susceptible inhabitants.[131] Despite inoculation, therefore, mortality statistics for the disease were generally on the upswing in many cities, suggesting that the procedure was a failure in stemming the tide of this sickness. Yet inoculation fulfilled the Baconian principles of empiricism and utility, contributing to the taming of natural events for the benefit of humankind. Mathematical analysis in the form of comparative mortality statistics could be employed to demonstrate its advantages. First fuelled by upper-class fears of smallpox, variolation gradually broadened its appeal as other medicalization schemes developed under the banner of mercantilist and political ideals.

[130] For France see the detailed work of Genevieve Miller, *The Adoption of Inoculation for Smallpox in England and France* (Philadelphia, 1957), especially pp. 180–240, chs. 7 and 8. See also A. S. Emch-Deriaz, 'L'inoculation justifiée – Or Was It?', *Eighteenth-Century Life*, 7 (1982), 65–72. The story of Jenner's vaccine is depicted in Derrick Baxby, *Jenner's Smallpox Vaccine* (London, 1981).

[131] 'Whatever share of smallpox mortality takes place in London amongst persons turned twenty years of age, is almost solely confined to the new annual settlers or recruits who are necessary to repair the waste of London', William Black, *Observations Medical and Political on the Smallpox*, 2nd edn (London, 1781), p. 100.

Epilogue

Historians have recently begun to debate the meaning and place of medicine within Enlightenment society.[132] Gone are the days when solely 'optimistic' accounts celebrated the rationalism which lead to system-building or the growing empiricism responsible for nosologies and clinical experimentation. As noted, while providing temporary coherence to medical activities, the individual systems successively crumbled under the weight of new discoveries thereby discrediting their zealous followers. Moreover, systems and clinical activities remained linked to traditional medical treatments of dubious efficacy.

Nevertheless, historians should not embrace purely negative views about Enlightenment medicine. The charge that hospitals merely became 'gateways to death' has been put to rest by recent historical studies.[133] Indeed many of these institutions consistently reported very low mortality rates among their inmates. Others, of course, because of overcrowding and understaffing, created less favourable environments for recovery. Efforts to provide institutional assistance to the sick, mad, mothers to be, and young children were laudable. Such care, rendered in hospitals, dispensaries, and asylums provided segments of the lower class with some measure of rest and nourishment decisive for the recovery of countless patients.

On balance, the record of Enlightenment medicine remains mixed, its strategies of medical mercantilism and police equally problematic. Although providing new roles for health professionals, such cradle-to-grave health programmes in central Europe endured largely on paper. Others resulted in repressive measures by the state spilling over into matters of morality and education. Some resulted in useful public health schemes concerned with improved water supplies and sewage disposal. Plans to collect new data about epidemics flourished side by side with governmental shipments of useless drugs. Even smallpox inoculation, an old folk measure imported from Asia, remained a double-edged sword as often ready to start as protect against another epidemic.

The rise of population during this time was in part a function of decreased mortality from infectious diseases because of diminished epidemics of plague and perhaps smallpox, both a function of complex

[132] R. Porter, 'Was There a Medical Enlightenment in Eighteenth Century England?', *British Journal of Eighteenth-Century Studies*, 5 (1982), 49–63.
[133] See especially Risse, 'Eighteenth-Century Hospitals: For Better or Worse?', in *Hospital Life*, pp. 287–91.

changes in the ecology of disease rather than due to direct medical intervention. At the same time, European populations displayed a higher birth rate principally based on changes in family structure and economics rather than new infant feeding practices.

What then can one conclude about the importance of medicine during the Enlightenment? At the core there was a gradual change in values and perception regarding health as a positive tenet which could be attained, preserved, and even recovered with the aid of a proper life style, public and personal hygiene, and the aid of medicine. Indeed the health of nations became an integral part of European geopolitics and education of the masses in such matters a high priority. Such beliefs were essential components of Enlightenment ideology striving for human progress and perfectibility and they have survived into our own days forming the backbone of current health policies.

The rise of the modern hospital in Britain

LINDSAY GRANSHAW

Hospitals today are central to health care in the West. Most people are born in hospital, many die there. Many will experience hospital treatment at some point in their lives. Hospitals are not only crucial for patients: they are vitally important for doctors as well. It is the medical elite that is hospital-based. It is the hospitals, too, with their technical, building and staff needs, that largely account for rising costs in medical care, even though non-hospital doctors, pharmacists, patients themselves and their relatives cope with most illness.[1] However, the development of hospitals as the centrepoint of medical care is a recent phenomenon. Hospitals today may very well play a central role, but in 1700, certainly in Britain, they were peripheral. They were few in number, employed few people, used few resources, were financed on a largely voluntary basis and, above all, treated a very restricted social group of patients for a very restricted range of complaints.

The shift of hospitals from the margins to the centre in health care has become an expanding interest to social historians of medicine. Past histories of hospitals were mostly written by doctors from the institutions themselves. Fired by interest in their own hospital, they usually focused on it alone, and rarely sought to establish how far its history was part of a wider pattern. They usually adopted a positivist approach, seeing the history of medicine as the epitome of progress. Medicine seemed to fit the pattern so very well: medical knowledge, it was argued, had vastly progressed, becoming more accurate, specialized and technological. Hospitals grew as a natural response to this. They were founded for

---

[1] In Britain, GPs cope with 90 per cent of medically treated illness. Most illness is not medically treated.

humanitarian reasons by lay men and women who recognized and responded to the needs of the poor. Hospitals were staffed by medical men who served patients without payment out of a sense of philanthropic duty. Such histories tended to concentrate on the doctors, rarely mentioning nurses or other staff, except perhaps in the wake of the 'Nightingale Revolution'. Patients hardly figure, except in an occasional anecdote.[2]

After long disregard, however, hospitals are now being more systematically investigated by historians. A general questioning of social structures in the last two decades has stimulated examination of a range of institutions, from prisons and schools to business and government, and, as medicine too has come under scrutiny, hospitals have received increased attention. Social historians of medicine have begun to investigate the structure and place of the hospital. They have looked beyond the doctor – sometimes, it is said, with new distortions – to the governors, administrators, nurses, paramedics, ancillary staff and patients. They have sought to understand the nature of hospitals – what they represented to those who supported them, worked for them or were treated in them.[3]

Increasingly, too, historians of medicine do not assume that hospitals are the necessary, natural and obvious places in which to treat patients:

[2] See, for example, various histories of British institutions including C.T. Andrews, *The First Cornish Hospital* (Penzance, 1975); S. T. Anning, *The General Infirmary at Leeds. Vol 1: The First Hundred Years 1767–1869* (Edinburgh and London, 1963); H. C. Cameron, *Mr Guy's Hospital, 1726–1948* (London, 1954); E. W. Dormer (ed.), *The Story of the Royal Berkshire Hospital 1837–1937* (Reading, 1937); Sir P. Eade, *The Norfolk & Norwich Hospital 1770–1900* (London, 1900); A. G. Gibson, *The Radcliffe Infirmary* (London, 1926); Eric C. O. Jewesbury, *The Royal Northern Hospital 1856–1956* (London, 1956); O. V. Jones, *The Progress of Medicine* (Llandysul, 1984); G. Munro Smith, *A History of the Bristol Royal Infirmary* (Bristol, 1917); J. B. Penfold, *The History of The Essex County Hospital, Colchester* (Colchester, 1984); P. Rhodes, *Doctor John Leake's Hospital* (London, 1977).
  Many such histories are very useful, providing a great deal of information, even if they may lack a sense of overall context. Perhaps the best history of a hospital by a medical man is A. E. Clark-Kennedy, *London Pride. The Story of a Voluntary Hospital* (London, 1979).
  Occasionally a history has been written by another member of staff. A nurse, Janet Gooch, was the author of *A History of Brighton General Hospital* (London, 1980). One of the histories of St Thomas's Hospital was written by its archivist: E. M. McInnes, *St Thomas' Hospital* (London, 1963). A hospital administrator, E. J. R. Burrough, was the author of *Unity in Diversity: The Short Life of the United Oxford Hospitals* (Abingdon, 1978).
[3] See, for example, Morris Vogel, *The Invention of the Modern Hospital* (Chicago, 1980); David Rosner, *A Once Charitable Enterprise: Hospitals and Health Care in Brooklyn and New York, 1885–1915* (Cambridge, MA, 1982); Lindsay Granshaw, *St Mark's Hospital, London: A Social History of a Specialist Hospital* (London, 1985); John V. Pickstone, *Medicine and Industrial Society: A History of Hospital Development in Manchester and its Region, 1752–1946* (Manchester, 1985); Charles Rosenberg, *The Care of Strangers. The Rise of America's Hospital System* (New York, 1987); Hilary Marland, *Medicine and Society in Wakefield and Huddersfield, 1780–1870* (Cambridge, 1987).

they therefore question why the hospital became an important medical institution. For some, epistemological changes explain the rise of the hospital. The major significance of modern hospitals is seen as dating from the French Revolution, in common with other features of modern European and North American society. A radically new approach was taken to medicine, which placed the hospital at the centre of health care.[4]

But epistemological reasons for the changed position of the hospital have been challenged more recently, as a more empirically based social history has become a dominant force in the history of medicine. Historians have increasingly looked to social change, the growth of bourgeois philanthropy and professionalization in medicine as explanations for the rise of the hospital. Shifts in ideas are not seen as sufficient. It is no accident, it is argued, that the hospital developed as an important institution in the wake of economic and social changes. It was the growth of towns and increased social mobility which lay behind the rise of the hospital. The pursuit of social status – by both patrons and doctors – becomes a key to the growth of hospitals.[5]

The main focus here will be on Britain, but casting developments in the wider context of continental Europe and the United States. A theme which runs through the history of hospitals, across time and place, is the manner in which their function derived from their funders. It is usually thought that medieval hospitals were mostly founded by the church, especially the monasteries, and that they grew out of the hospices which accommodated travellers and the sick among local people. Recent historians have presented a more sophisticated picture.[6] Such institutions were normally funded by the laity as a means of buying grace. As in later times, establishing a hospital could be seen as a public way of demonstrating charity, with the social status that this brought. Often an intention to support a hospital barely outlived the founder, and the money would be diverted to other uses. Not all institutions went under rapidly, and some lasted through medieval times. Such hospitals reflected

---

[4] Michel Foucault, *The Birth of the Clinic. An Archaeology of Medical Perception*, trans. A. M. Sheridan (London, 1976); Erwin H. Ackerknecht, *Medicine at the Paris Hospital, 1794–1848* (Baltimore, 1967).

[5] Toby Gelfand, *Professionalizing Modern Medicine. Paris Surgeons and Medical Science and Institutions in the 18th Century* (Westport, CT, and London, 1980); Pickstone, *Medicine and Industrial Society*; Vogel, *Invention of the Modern Hospital*; Granshaw, *St Mark's Hospital*; Marland, *Medicine and Society*; Lindsay Granshaw and Roy Porter (eds.), *The Hospital in History* (London, 1989).

[6] See, for example, Martha Carlin, 'Mediaeval and English Hospitals', and Miri Rubin, 'Development and Change in English Hospitals: 1100–1500', in Granshaw and Porter, *The Hospital in History*; Katharine Park, *Doctors and Medicine in Early Renaissance Florence* (Princeton, NJ, 1985).

contemporary notions of Christian charity and the purchase of spiritual benefits through temporal acts. Their architecture illustrated their religious context: they were often designed on a cruciform pattern, with a chapel at the centre, to which patients might look and gain inspiration. To their endowers, hospitals were intended more for the cure of souls than of bodies.[7]

The development of hospitals on any scale in Europe accompanied the growth of trade, the expansion of towns, and increased geographical and social mobility among the continent's population. The converse can also be seen: as Britain lagged behind Italy and the Low Countries in the development of sizeable trading towns, so it lagged behind in the growth of hospitals. Since lay philanthropy was so important in their upkeep, it is perhaps not surprising that it was in larger towns such as Florence that hospitals tended to be significant and numerous. There has also been the suggestion that hospitals served trading groups by caring for employees when sick. The kind of continuity in the workforce which was increasingly important was more easily guaranteed if merchants could rely on a hospital to take the burden of care at times of crisis. Hospitals have also been seen as part of a pattern of social control in towns. Merchant families could ensure that their expanding town or city did not become too unruly: town vagrants would be swept up at night and into the hospital, while those from outside the town might be despatched home.[8]

In Britain many small hospitals and leprosaria came and went in medieval times, serving a variety of functions. Some remained through the Reformation, despite designs on their property, and, as in the case of St Thomas's or St Bartholomew's, have lasted through to modern times.[9] However, it was in the eighteenth century, and more particularly the nineteenth, that significant expansion in the number and position of hospitals occurred, as towns and cities grew. In London in the first half of the eighteenth century five general hospitals were founded. The founders were laymen. They might recruit supporters from among the

[7] J. D. Thompson and G. Goldin, *The Hospital: A Social and Architectural History* (New Haven, CT, and London, 1975); Rubin, 'Development and Change' in Granshaw and Porter, *The Hospital in History*.

[8] John Henderson, 'The Hospitals of Late-Mediaeval and Renaissance Florence: A Preliminary Survey'; and Sandra Cavallo, 'Hospitals in Turin in the Eighteenth Century', in Granshaw and Porter, *The Hospital in History*.

[9] Carlin, 'Mediaeval English Hospitals' in Granshaw and Porter, *The Hospital in History*; Brian Abel-Smith, *The Hospitals, 1800–1948. A Study in Social Administration in England and Wales* (London, 1964).

clergy, but the church was usually not the main initiator. In a few early foundations, in fact, minority rather than establishment voices predominated: members of a religious group or a group lacking in political clout bound themselves together by establishing a hospital.[10]

The pattern of establishment was quickly set. A leading lay figure or group would decide on the need for a hospital; the support of a few aristocrats would then be enlisted, and their names published prominently to encourage those of lower social standing to make donations as well. Friends, relatives and other contacts were also tapped for their support. Donors were given certain benefits. According to the sum contributed, they had the right to admit patients. A guinea donation might, for example, buy the donor one admission ticket for an in-patient for the year and one for an out-patient. A more sizeable donation would bring multiple rights. In addition, benefactors became hospital governors: they elected a dozen or so of their number to supervise the hospital and they voted for members of staff, an important right as it meant that doctors had to seek lay approval if they wished to work at the hospital.[11]

Many replicas of the early-eighteenth-century London foundations were established in other British cities, the first in England being the Winchester County Hospital (1723) and the first in Scotland the Royal Infirmary of Edinburgh (1729).[12] They all aimed to take in the same type of patient – the 'deserving' poor. Their *raison d'être* was their charity function: they were certainly not regarded as appropriate places for the treatment of better-off patients. Hospitals carried a charity stigma with them well into the twentieth century: the middle and upper classes sought their own treatment at home. Neither though did hospitals aim to care for the very poor in society. The destitute were to be returned to their parish of origin when sick. The 'deserving' poor were seen as labourers, from 'respectable' families, where the men would be conscientiously trying to support their families by employment. The

---

[10] The Westminster was established in 1719, Guy's in 1721, St George's in 1733, the London in 1740 and the Middlesex in 1745. See Abel-Smith, *The Hospitals*, p. 4. For minority groups, see Adrian Wilson, 'The Early History of the Westminster Hospital', Paper given to the Wellcome Unit for the History of Medicine, University of Cambridge, October 1983.

[11] See hospital *Annual Reports* and histories of hospitals.

[12] John Woodward, *To Do the Sick No Harm. A Study of the British Voluntary Hospital System to 1875* (London, 1974), pp. 12, 16; David Hamilton, *The Healers. A History of Medicine in Scotland* (Edinburgh, 1981), p. 105. Institutions for the destitute were set up by parishes, for example Glasgow's Town Hospital in 1733 and Aberdeen's Poor Hospital in 1739. Both were poorhouses in which some space was allocated for the sick.

benefactors did not want to give charity to the destitute (who were considered to be largely responsible for their own plight) or to others whom they regarded as undeserving, such as criminals or prostitutes.[13]

Patients received treatment free of charge, but had to find a benefactor first from whom to secure an admission ticket before attending the hospital. Thus, it was the governors, not the doctors, who decided who should and who should not be admitted to hospital. It was not just socially 'undeserving' patients who found themselves excluded: children, pregnant women, fever cases, lunatics and incurables, were all regarded as cases to be kept out. The patient population in eighteenth-century British hospitals consisted mostly of accident cases or minor medical problems.[14]

When admitted, an in-patient had to agree to a strict set of rules, and governors visited to make sure that these were kept. These rules implicitly assumed that patients were not desperately ill and, far from being bed-ridden, needed to be constrained from wandering out of the hospital and coming back drunk. Disobedience of the rules could result in summary dismissal from the hospital – and it happened, whatever the stage of recovery of the patient. Patients who were convalescing, especially the women, were expected to make themselves useful, mending sheets and tending to other patients.[15]

For some historians a significant disjunction occurred between the patterns in eighteenth- and nineteenth-century hospitals. Michel Foucault, for example, argued that medicine changed radically in Revolutionary France, with major consequences for hospitals. Although he agreed that students had already been learning by direct experience on the wards in Edinburgh, he saw a conceptual shift between the Edinburgh and Paris models. While previous medical 'knowledge' – including that in Scotland – had been based on book learning and theory, the French Revolution liberated medical thinking: blinkers fell from medical eyes and doctors suddenly saw clearly.[16] Foucault spoke of a 'free garden where by common consent doctor and patient met, observation took place, innocent of theories, by the unaided brightness

---

[13] See Abel-Smith, *The Hospitals* and other more recent hospital histories.

[14] *Ibid.* However, Cavallo found exceptions to this in Turin, where benefactors competed to support beds for incurables. Cavallo, 'Turin hospitals', in Granshaw and Porter, *The Hospital in History*.

[15] See, for example, Lindsay Granshaw, 'St Thomas's Hospital, London, 1850–1900' (Bryn Mawr College, USA, Ph.D. thesis, 1981), pp. 104–5.

[16] Foucault, *The Birth of the Clinic*, p. 39.

of the gaze, where from master to disciple, experience was transmitted beneath the level of words.'[17] The new medicine was reductionist and analytical: one of its features was the use of post-mortems to correlate appearances after death with pathology in the living. Foucault argued that 'the living night is dissipated in the brightness of death'.[18] The essential locus of the new anatomico-clinical medicine which replaced the old classificatory medicine was not the lecture theatre but the hospital, where real experience was to be gained. The clinic became central to the ideas and practice of medicine as it had not been before.[19] There was also the greater ease of trying out the new medicine on hospital patients. They were seen as 'the most suitable subjects for an experimental course'.[20] Poor and unable to complain, lessons learned from them could be applied to better-off patients. The new clinical medicine united the hospital and teaching in an instructive and profitable manner.

Erwin Ackerknecht also wrote of changes in the conception of disease and methods of treatment as vitally important to the development of the hospital. The Revolutionary period saw the rise of a 'quite specific and unique type of medicine' – hospital medicine. It was typified by observation rather than book learning, by physical examination, pathological anatomy, statistics and the concept of the lesion. After identifying pathological conditions in cadavers through physical change in the organs, the same condition was to be recognized in the living, if possible through signs which were independent of symptoms. Important in the rise of the hospital, though, this type of medicine had come to an end by 1848, to be replaced by laboratory medicine.[21]

Others do not see these changing ideas in quite the same way, arguing that many of the patterns in European hospitals were established long before developments in Paris medicine. In Italy the use of hospitals as places of research, teaching and medical practice was well established by the eighteenth century, and possibly much earlier.[22] The professional and ideological developments were well underway, as also were the social changes which supported the hospitals. Even in France, for some historians it was professional developments which were most influential in the rise of the modern hospital, rather than epistemological changes.

---

[17] *Ibid.*, p. 52.   [18] *Ibid.*, p. 146.   [19] *Ibid.*, p. 17.
[20] John Aikin, quoted in *ibid.*, p. 83.
[21] Ackerknecht, *Medicine at the Paris Hospital*, p. xi.
[22] Park, *Doctors and Medicine*; Cavallo, 'Turin Hospitals', in Granshaw and Porter, *The Hospital in History*.

Professionalization perhaps followed and justified an extended use of hospitals that was already beginning to occur.[23]

Neither would social historians accept Foucault's ideas that humoral notions of disease were simply blind classifications based on book learning, explanations which were swept away by clear-thinking in the nineteenth century.[24] However, it is agreed that these notions were indeed changing in the nineteenth century. Illness was coming to be seen not so much as particular to an individual as a unique whole in his or her own setting, but rather the result of specific disease entities which showed common traits regardless of the individual sufferer. Under the new schema, diseases were localized first to the organ, and later to tissue and cell. The focus therefore shifted from the whole body to the diseased part. The emphasis was less on symptoms reported by the patient, now seen as subjective, and more on signs that could (in theory) be objectively measured, often with the use of instruments, by the doctor.

However important such changing ideas might be, it is difficult to see them dictating the rise of hospitals in Britain. A closer correlation can be found with social mobility, the growth of towns and the professionalization of doctors. The growth in number and size of the hospitals tended to follow immigration to towns: London grew from half a million in the early eighteenth century, to one and a half million in 1800, to five million by 1900, and the number of its hospitals multiplied.[25] The patterns for supporting hospitals were already in place: as the middle classes in Britain expanded, benefitting from industrialization and the growth of trade, they were just as anxious to demonstrate their position as any Florentine merchant had been. Hospitals were not the only beneficiaries of these developments. In nineteenth-century Britain libraries, parks, museums and schools were all set up by philanthropists for the benefit of local people. Providing such facilities became part of civic pride: any self-respecting town – and its leading figures – came to need a museum, a library, and, of course, a hospital.[26]

Besides benefactors and patients, the new hospitals attracted keen medical interest. By the mid-eighteenth century, doctors had come to see hospitals as increasingly important to their professional careers.

---

[23] See, for example, Gelfand, *Professionalizing Modern Medicine*.

[24] See, for example, Charles Rosenberg, 'The Therapeutic Revolution. Medicine, Meaning and Social Change in Nineteenth-Century America', *Perspectives in Biology and Medicine*, 20 (1977), 485–506.

[25] H. J. Dyos and Michael Wolff (eds.), *The Victorian City: Image and Reality* (London and Boston, 1973). *Medical Directory* (London and the provinces), various years.

[26] Marland, *Medicine and Society*; Pickstone, *Medicine and Industrial Society*.

Hospital positions enabled doctors to become well known amongst leading lay people: medical men built up their private practice through their links with the hospital and its well-off governors. The profession as a whole respected those in hospital positions, and hospital surgeons and physicians found themselves at the top of the medical tree. The growing importance of teaching to doctors further encouraged the development of the hospital, given the increased emphasis on the bedside rather than the lecture theatre. Since significant income could be derived from students, hospital positions which afforded such teaching possibilities became ever more sought after.[27]

Variations in the pattern can be seen around Britain. Loudon has found less of a division between hospital doctors and general practitioners in country towns than in London. In Scotland rotas were often drawn up for the physicians and surgeons of a town to attend patients for a few months to a year. The lay domination of hospitals was apparently weaker there, too, with hospital managers often including medical men. The Royal Infirmary of Edinburgh charged a fee to some patients, a practice not usually found in the English hospitals. Servants, too, could be admitted for a fee. However, as elsewhere, those with hospital positions increasingly took their apprentices and students around the wards with them: holding a hospital position thus opened the door to lucrative fees from students.[28]

Medical men in Britain without hospital positions had every incentive to see new hospitals founded. In the second half of the eighteenth century a number of new hospitals were set up, mostly by medical men. The first were the lying-in hospitals, catering for one of the classes of patients excluded from the general hospitals, women in childbirth. Other specialized hospitals set up in the second half of the eighteenth century included lunatic asylums, smallpox hospitals and hospitals for venereal disease. Again these all served categories of diseases and groups of patients not admitted to the general hospitals – and their establishment could be justified on these grounds.[29]

Towards the end of the eighteenth century dispensaries for out-patients began to be established. The idea behind them – that patients should be treated in their own homes – was more in keeping with

[27] M. Jeanne Peterson, *The Medical Profession in Mid-Victorian London* (Berkeley, 1978), pp. 16, 138–93.
[28] Hamilton, *The Healers*, p. 106; Irvine Loudon, *Medical Care and the General Practitioner, 1750–1850* (Oxford, 1987).
[29] Abel-Smith, *The Hospitals*, pp. 22–3; Alistair Gunn, 'Maternity Hospitals,' in F. N. L. Poynter, *The Evolution of Hospitals in Britain* (London, 1964), 77–101.

contemporary ideas about disease (that illness was unique to an individual in his or her setting, and could not easily be understood outside that setting) than hospital treatment could be said to be. The first dispensary, in Aldersgate Street in London, was set up in 1770 by John Lettsom. Lettsom had found that London's closed social and medical world prevented him from securing a position at one of the general hospitals, a factor which also encouraged him and a number of other young Quaker medical men to set up the Medical Society of London. Their complaints of exclusion echoed down the nineteenth century – and not unexpectedly, once doctors established themselves, similar complaints were levelled against them and their institutions. Dispensaries and hospitals came to play their part in these battles.[30] Dispensaries were set up all over Britain, mostly by less established doctors. However, the first Scottish dispensary was opened in 1776 in Edinburgh by Andrew Duncan, Professor of the Institutes of Medicine. Home visits were carried by Duncan's students, and he used the dispensary for teaching purposes.[31]

It was in the nineteenth century that there was a really massive increase in the number of hospitals established in Britain. Again, the medical profession was the driving force behind the setting up of these institutions, rather than lay men. The growth in the numbers and power of hospitals reflected Britain's entrepreneurial nature in its first century of industrialization. The entrepreneurs were the medical men who sought to advance themselves through founding their own institutions. The extensive social mobility generated by the Industrial Revolution affected doctors just as much as other groups. Unwilling to accept the status quo if it worked to their disadvantage, some set up new institutions in opposition to traditional patterns. Assisting them were the expanding merchant classes as they themselves benefited from industrialization.[32] Setting up specialized institutions seemed an especial justification of their action. It could be argued that their hospital catered for patients otherwise excluded from general hospitals. Increasingly, too, it was stressed that specialized study enabled doctors to understand

[30] Zachary Cope, 'The History of the Dispensary Movement,' in Poynter (ed.), *Evolution of Hospitals*, pp. 73–6; Thomas Hunt (ed.), *The Medical Society of London 1773–1973* (London, 1972), pp. 47–8.
[31] Hamilton, *The Healers*, p. 107. Dispensaries were set up in Kelso in 1777, and Dundee and Montrose in 1782.
[32] A typical medical entrepreneur was Frederick Salmon, founder of St Mark's Hospital. Typical of his supporters was the nouveau riche Lord Mayor of London, William Taylor Copeland. See Granshaw, *St Mark's Hospital*, pp. 7–18.

specific complaints more fully – an argument which fitted the shift from humoral, holistic explanations of disease to the notion of disease as localized.[33]

The first of this new wave of specialist institutions in Britain was an eye hospital, later known as Moorfields or the Royal Ophthalmic Hospital. It was set up in 1804 by John Cunningham Saunders, who found his career ladder at the general hospitals in London blocked.[34] Despite opposition from the elite in the profession, the idea caught on rapidly and in the next two decades at least eighteen eye hospitals were founded, most of them in major towns, including Exeter, Bristol, Bath, Manchester, Birmingham, Liverpool, Glasgow and Edinburgh.[35]

From the 1830s there was a great expansion in the number and range of special institutions as well as general hospitals and dispensaries set up. By the 1860s there were at least sixty-six special institutions in London alone.[36] New hospitals were relatively easy to establish. The practitioner rented a part of a house and installed a few beds in the care of a residential matron and perhaps a house surgeon. There was greater difficulty in securing support and ensuring the expansion of the institution.[37] But the tide was running with specialization: patients and benefactors flocked to their doors. Patient demand dictated eventual professional acquiescence. The new generation at the teaching hospitals led the way: it became standard practice for any ambitious young surgeon or physician to seek a number of temporary positions at specialist hospitals.[38] Some retained a special hospital affiliation even when they were appointed to a general hospital position. They received status in the profession from the general hospital, but among potential well-off patients they were sought out often because of specialist expertise. The special hospitals began to have a great impact on the general hospitals, which, in competition with the newcomers, started to specialize, setting up eye departments in the 1850s,

---

[33] See, for example, the arguments given by Salmon on setting up St Mark's: 'Original Address', *List of Subscribers to the Infirmary for the Relief of the Poor Afflicted with Fistula and Other Diseases of the Rectum* (London, 1837).

[34] J. R. Farre, *A Treatise on Some Practical Points Relating to the Diseases of the Eye by the late John Cunningham Saunders...[and] A Short Account of the Author's Life* (London, 1811), pp. ix–xlii; Abel-Smith, *The Hospitals*, p. 26.

[35] Richard Kershaw, *Special Hospitals* (London, 1909), pp. 62–4.

[36] *Medical Directory* (London and provinces), 1860s.

[37] 'Hospital Distress', *British Medical Journal*, part 1 (1860), 458.

[38] See biographies of surgeons and physicians in *Plarr's Lives of the Fellows of the Royal College of Surgeons of England*, rev. D'Arcy Power, with A. G. Spencer and G. E. Gask, 2 vols. (Bristol, 1930); *Lives of the Fellows of the Royal College of Physicians, 1826–1925*, comp. G. H. Brown (London, 1955); Granshaw, '"Fame and Fortune by Means of Bricks and Mortar". The Medical Profession and Specialist Hospitals in Britain, 1800–1948', in Granshaw and Porter, *The Hospital in History*.

ear departments in the 1860s, and other special sections as the century wore on.[39] More importantly, perhaps, the new hospitals gave a further impetus to the medicalization of the general hospitals. In the special hospitals, it was the doctors who selected most of the medical staff and sorted patients for admission. Medical control was from the beginning far greater than in the older hospitals. This did not escape those at the general hospitals and fuelled their attempts to throw off the yoke of lay control.

The special hospitals were medicalized in other ways earlier than their general counterparts, with more medical intervention and doctors spending more time at the hospital. In the early nineteenth century doctors spent very little time indeed in the general hospital. The junior doctors lived in and looked after the patients, while the senior staff attended only occasionally. (In Scotland, apothecaries attended to most day-to-day medical affairs.) However, by mid-century, work within the hospitals was becoming more central to the medical profession. In some areas, such as London, this can be seen as partly due to the growth in medical schools. From the end of the eighteenth century private medical schools grew rapidly. However, with new emphases on clinical studies, it was argued that students needed to attend hospital wards in order to train properly. The shift to hospital-based medical schools gradually took place, undermining the older schools. To be licensed by the Royal College of Surgeons of England, a year's experience in walking the wards was required. In 1815 the Apothecaries' Act laid down that anyone applying for the licentiate of the Society of Apothecaries must walk the wards for six months. By the 1850s and 1860s hospital medical schools had become the central foci for medical education, a development which the 1858 Medical Act helped to consolidate.[40]

By the mid nineteenth century, then, voluntary hospitals were becoming increasingly important to doctors, benefactors and patients. However, the voluntary hospitals were not the only institutions catering for the poor by this time. Alterations in the way that poor relief was offered had led to the growth of workhouse infirmaries. From 1834, outdoor poor relief was no longer given: it was argued that topping up the wages of the poor encouraged pauperization. The semi-destitute now had to choose between supporting themselves with no recourse at

---

[39] Peterson, *Medical Profession*, pp. 278–80; Abel-Smith, *The Hospitals*, p. 159; histories of individual hospitals.

[40] Charles Newman, *The Evolution of Medical Education in the Nineteenth Century* (London, 1957); Granshaw, 'St Thomas's Hospital'; Hamilton, *The Healers*, p. 106.

all to the parish, or entering the workhouse. It tended to be the old and the sick who could not stay above absolute destitution, and found themselves institutionalized. Increasingly, infirmaries were built to accommodate such inmates, and by the last third of the nineteenth century workhouse infirmaries in London, for example, were being specially constructed under the Metropolitan Asylums Board. The workhouse infirmaries were, therefore, assuming a role that the voluntary hospitals had always been reluctant to take on, the support of incurables and the destitute.[41] This development had its effect on the voluntary hospitals. Potential lower-middle-class patients could now be reassured that the really destitute were in the workhouse infirmaries, not the voluntary hospitals.

In addition to these two groups there were the cottage hospitals, one of the first being set up at Cranleigh in Surrey in 1859.[42] Patients were treated on payment of a weekly sum: the cottage hospital was therefore geared slightly above the level of the voluntary hospital. Sir Henry Burdett of the British Hospitals Association, and a fierce critic of what he saw as 'charity abuse' of the voluntary hospitals by those who could afford to pay for treatment, was a strong champion of the cottage hospital. In his eyes the scheme:

provided against indiscriminate medical relief; secured justice for the medical profession as every member is allowed to follow his patients in the cottage hospital and put hospital patients for the first time in England in the position of having the privilege of being able to pay something for treatment.[43]

Burdett argued that the cottage hospitals gave country patients access to hospitals, and raised the professional status of the country general practitioner. The rich recognized the increased skill of the doctor: 'the peasant's misfortune...has been...the means of saving the life of the squire'.[44] As with the establishment of other hospitals, there was initial medical hostility. Burdett reckoned, in 1896, that, with several hundred cottage hospitals by then in existence, such medical opposition was declining.

Public attitudes to hospitals generally were changing as the century ended, a shift in which perceived reforms in nursing played a part.

---

[41] Ruth Hodgkinson, *The Origins of the National Health Service: The Medical Service* (London, 1967).

[42] The founder was Albert Napper. See Albert Napper, *On the Advantages Derivable by the Medical Profession and the Public from Village Hospitals* (1864).

[43] Sir Henry Burdett, *Cottage Hospitals, General, Fever, and Convalescent. Their Progress, Management, and Work in Great Britain and Ireland, and the United States of America*, 3rd edn (London, 1896), p. 7. [44] *Ibid.*

Nursing reformers in the second half of the nineteenth century – in particular Florence Nightingale – vehemently stressed the darker side of earlier nursing in order to emphasize the case for reform. They pointed to real and imagined cases of drunkenness, dishonesty, immorality, corruption and laziness among nurses, suggesting that all were like that. The picture they drew by contrast at the end of the century was of clean, neat, disciplined, uniformed nurses trained in the nursing schools.[45] Matrons in the early nineteenth century were usually respectable widows but the other nurses were generally recruited from the poorer classes, frequently from among the patients themselves. A gradual change in the social origins of the nurses over the century had its effect on the practice of nursing. Domestic service in the nineteenth century drew in many women, but some turned to nursing.[46] There were strong parallels between the two occupations. Nurses were required to do a great deal of housework in the hospital. As the Victorian sanitation movement progressed, cleanliness and discipline were stressed both in domestic service and in nursing. Literacy improved, especially after elementary education was made compulsory in 1876. The demand for nurses expanded as new institutions were established, and as the number of in-patients grew. Moreover, as medical intervention increased, more nursing work was demanded, and hospitals increased their nurse/patient ratios. The changes were slow to filter through, however, especially in small hospitals. Nurses still undertook menial tasks, their turnover was high, they were paid on a weekly basis, and they were sacked without notice. But the generally improved change in the image of nursing certainly helped to encourage the middle classes to look on hospitals with greater favour.

There were also other changes in the nineteenth century which brought hospitals from the periphery of medical care to its centre. Surgery changed almost beyond recognition. In the early nineteenth century very few operations were carried out, but by the twentieth century the amount of surgery was increasing very rapidly and came largely to dominate the business of hospitals. In the Paris hospitals there had been a greater emphasis on surgery, but further expansion followed the introduction in the late 1840s of general anaesthesia into medicine. At mid century, though, there was a crisis of confidence in hospitals themselves. To some they were considered to be 'gateways to

---

[45] Monica E. Baly, *Nursing and Social Change* (London, 1982), pp. 64–75; Monica E. Baly, *Florence Nightingale and the Nursing Legacy* (London, 1986); Abel-Smith, *A History of the Nursing Profession* (London, 1982), pp. 1–35.   [46] Abel-Smith, *Nursing Profession*, p. 17.

death': patients entered with one disease only to contract another and die. As Florence Nightingale remarked:

it may seem a strange principle to enunciate as the very first requirement in a Hospital that it should do the sick no harm. It is quite necessary nevertheless to lay down such a principle, because the actual mortality in hospitals, especially those of large crowded cities, is very much higher than any calculation founded on the mortality of the same class of patient treated *out* of hospital would lead us to expect.[47]

There had been increased concern since at least the 1830s about 'hospital diseases', so-called because they infected patients only after they entered hospital. Various studies were undertaken to see whether patients treated in country hospitals fared worse than those treated at home and whether those in city hospitals fared worst of all.[48] Whatever the disputes over the figures, it was generally agreed that hospital mortality was far too high. By the 1850s there was a movement among lay sanitary reformers to disband and close city hospitals or to move them to the country: they were seen as precisely the *wrong* places in which to treat the sick.[49]

In response, surgeons sought to bring down mortality and, in the 1850s and 1860s, there were energetic attempts to clean up hospitals in the hope of reducing infection.[50] As part of this general concern, in 1867 Joseph Lister published his work on antisepsis.[51] Since the germ theory itself was far from accepted, antisepsis proved very controversial. However, by the 1880s, antisepsis, or at least a combination of the earlier practice of emphasizing great cleanliness together with antisepsis, was securing widespread support. By the 1890s a combination of asepsis and antisepsis was used within most hospitals.[52]

As anaesthesia and antisepsis allowed surgeons to undertake more ambitious and more frequent operations the surgeons themselves began

[47] Florence Nightingale, *Notes on Hospitals*, 3rd edn (London, 1863), p. iii.

[48] See, for example, John P. Potter, 'Results of Amputations at University-College Hospital, London, Statistically Arranged,' *Medical and Chirurgical Transactions*, ser. 2 (1841), 155–76; J. H. James, 'On the Causes of Mortality after Amputation of the Limbs,' *Transactions of the Provincial Medical and Surgical Association*, 17 (1849), 49–51; and Thomas Bryant, 'On the Causes of Death After Amputation,' *Medical and Chirurgical Transactions*, ser. 2, 24 (1859), 67–90. See Lindsay Granshaw, 'The Development and Reception of Antisepsis in Britain', in John Pickstone (ed.), *Medical Innovations in Historical Perspective* (London, 1991), pp. 17–19.

[49] See, for example, the debate over St Thomas's Hospital: Granshaw, 'St Thomas's Hospital', pp. 110–90.

[50] One of the chief proponents of great cleanliness was George Callender, a surgeon at St Bartholomew's. See, for example, George W. Callender, 'Comparison of Death Rates after Amputations in Country Private Practice, in Hospital Practice, and on Country Patients in a Town Hospital,' *St Bartholomew's Hospital Reports*, 5 (1869), 243–63.

[51] Joseph Lister, 'On the Antiseptic Principle in the Practice of Surgery,' *The Lancet*, part 2 (1867), 353–6. [52] Granshaw, 'Antisepsis', pp. 130–40.

to play a more prominent part within the hospital. In addition, the extension of surgery further encouraged an expansion in the class of patients, since their surgeons increasingly wished to operate on them within hospital rather than in patients' homes. Gradually a referral system was building up which placed hospitals on a pinnacle. Other developments in scientific medicine also changed the hospital. From the 1850s hospitals set up laboratories to undertake chemical analyses; from the 1890s bacteriological work was included. Other procedures too began to be carried out in hospital. Roentgen developed x-rays in the mid 1890s, and by the 1920s, spurred on by the use of radiology in the First World War, x-ray equipment had been installed in many British hospitals. If patients, whatever their class, were to undergo such examinations they needed to come into hospital.[53]

The late nineteenth century also saw the introduction into the hospital of ideas from the wider administrative world. Since mid century the emphasis in the British and imperial civil services had been on meritocracy and efficiency. By the early years of the twentieth century, borrowing from ideas prevalent in the United States, 'scientific management' was increasingly seen as important. For administrative reformers hospitals became targets just as much as government departments, and were deemed to be in need of efficient, professional administration rather than relying on management by treasurers and secretaries drawn from lay governors. From the 1890s, hospital administrators began to be recruited from among those with experience in the Civil Service or the army. In the United States, in particular, hospital administrators banded together in their own Association, promoting the aims of scientific management within hospitals.[54]

Changes in practice in hospitals, but also in their voluntary ethos, had an impact on potential patients. The social changes of the nineteenth century were producing a class of clerks and other white-collar workers, sometimes unsupported by families in the cities. These were numbered among new applicants for hospital aid. Throughout the century out-patient demand had expanded. Towards the end of the century, in-

[53] Rosemary Stevens, *Medical Practice in Modern England: The Impact of Specialization and State Medicine* (New Haven, CT, and London, 1966), pp. 5, 11, 17, 32, 39. See also Joel D. Howell, 'Patient Care at Guy's and the Pennsylvania Hospital, 1900–1920', paper presented at British Society for the History of Science – History of Science Society Anglo-American Conference, Manchester, England, 11–15 July 1988.

[54] Rosner, *A Once Charitable Enterprise*; Vogel, *The Invention of the Modern Hospital*; Morris Vogel, 'Managing Medicine: Creating a Profession of Hospital Administration in the United States, 1895–1915' in Granshaw and Porter, *The Hospital in History*; Granshaw, 'St Thomas's Hospital', pp. 50–7.

patient demand, too, seemed to be on the increase. The system of patients having to seek a governor's letter of admission had by now largely fallen by the wayside, and for many years there had been talk of charity abuse. The establishment of cottage hospitals had of course been seen partly as a means of curbing such abuse, by putting both patients and ordinary general practitioners in a hospital setting, with re-muneration to the doctors. Towards the end of the century the voluntary hospitals began to head in a similar direction – not so much to allow in general practitioners (although the general practitioner/hospital doctor division was perhaps less rigid in most of Britain than in London[55]) but to realize a potential source of income – payments from patients. Rooms were set aside for private patients who paid both for treatment and for their hospital beds, and hospitals also reserved beds in the public wards for patients who were deemed able to contribute something towards their upkeep but not their treatment. Almoners appointed originally to screen out those who could afford to pay a general practitioner were now called upon to assess appropriate levels of contributions from such patients.[56]

In some ways an extension of the cottage hospital principle, the new institutions set up by medical entrepreneurs at the end of the century tended to be private nursing homes and hospitals, catering for the lower-middle classes. They continued nevertheless in many instances to seek some voluntary assistance so that fees could be subsidised in the more needy cases. Philanthropists, however, had a mixed view of them, assuming they were there to do little more than guarantee the medical staff's income.[57]

As the lower-middle classes as well as the working classes increasingly sought hospital care, insurance schemes came to be introduced. The Hospital Saturday Fund, set up in the early 1870s, collected a penny a week from workmen and in return secured admission tickets from hospitals to which it made contributions.[58] Some employers made similar contributions, or workers would group together to do so. Unions and Friendly Societies often did likewise. A more formalized

---

[55] Loudon, *Medical Care and the General Practitioner.*

[56] See hospital histories; Granshaw, *St Mark's Hospital,* pp. 413–15.

[57] For example, the Gordon Hospital, established in Vauxhall Bridge Road in London, in many ways reflected the pattern of earlier specialist hospitals, yet it charged fees to some of its patients from its foundation onwards, nevertheless also appealing for additional help from philanthropists. There are many other examples in the late nineteenth century of similar establishments.

[58] For London hospitals' financial positions, see Geoffrey Rivett, *The Development of the London Hospital System, 1823–1982* (London, 1986).

arrangement was worked out after the First World War, with the assistance of the King Edward's Hospital Fund for London, in the shape of the Hospital Savings Association. The lower-middle classes were encouraged to contribute, and in return became eligible for hospital care, with the Association reimbursing the hospital.[59]

The First World War served as a stimulus to hospital development. Those wounded in battle were conveyed to first-aid posts, casualty clearing stations and then down the line to hospitals in France or back in Britain. All, whatever their rank, were expected to be treated in hospital if their injuries necessitated it. It was partly to incorporate such patterns in peacetime care that Lord Dawson of Penn, commissioned to report on health care after the war, argued that there should be a network around the country of primary health centres, with groupings of general practitioners dealing with minor medical problems, and secondary health centres, based on hospitals. Although he did not address funding, he did argue for a health-care system, with a strong emphasis on hospitals, which would make available to all the advances in medical science which contemporaries identified with such optimism.[60]

The assumption that all would seek hospital treatment was gradually being borne out in practice: hospitals were losing their charity stigma. As patient demand increased, and costs rose as more staff were employed, hospitals all seemed to be in competition with each other for a seemingly declining slice of the philanthropic cake: the years after the First World War therefore saw many voluntary hospitals in acute financial crisis. They looked with some envy to the former workhouse infirmaries, in the hands of the local authorities from 1929, and receiving relatively stable support as a result. The workhouse still functioned by looking after the elderly and destitute, but increasingly now the infirmaries were seen as town hospitals, not just for the care of paupers but for a wider range of people. Such infirmaries remained lower status, however, than the voluntary hospitals, and although under the 1929 Local Government Act they were supposed to cooperate with the voluntary hospitals in coordinating provision, there was no similar instruction to their voluntary counterparts.

However, whereas the voluntary hospitals staggered through the twenties and thirties from one financial crisis to another, the local

[59] Frank D. Long, *King Edward's Hospital Fund of London. The Story of its Foundation and Achievements, 1897–1942* (London, 1942).
[60] Ministry of Health. Consultative Council on Medical and Allied Services. *Interim Report on the Future Provision of Medical and Allied Services.* Cmd. 693. (London, 1920).

authority hospitals seemed to have a more assured future. By 1939 the voluntary hospitals argued that some state support was going to be needed: what was not seen as part of the equation was that the state should have any rights in return. The intervention of the Second World War helped to change the way that voluntary hospitals viewed the state. In anticipation of the war, and in particular in expectation of huge civilian casualties from bombing, government plans were made for a comprehensive wartime health-care system. Under the Emergency Hospital Service, both local authority and voluntary hospitals were grouped into a regional structure, and classified according to which types of patient they were allowed to treat. In return they were given grants to cover the costs of reserving beds for casualties. Although bombing on the scale anticipated did not materialize, the voluntary hospitals became used to receiving state support, so much so that they feared for their future if they had to resort to fund raising alone after the war.[61]

A national health service had been discussed on and off for decades (as was foreshadowed by the Dawson Report), but it was firmly on the agenda by 1942. The Beveridge Report assumed that free health care at point of need would complement its proposed social security system.[62] How such a scheme would operate was subject to much discussion. The health service was in the end brought in by a Labour government, in 1948. Aneurin Bevan, as Minister of Health, rejected previous Labour arguments that the service should be local authority based: seeking to win over the doctors, he argued rather that it should be administered directly by the Minister of Health. The preservation of private practice, teaching hospital endowments, and the special place of hospitals within the service, all helped to reconcile the hospital doctors to a national health service. A major concern – that their hospitals would otherwise founder financially – was at least to be dealt with.[63]

In 1948 all hospitals became the property of the Ministry of Health. The National Health Service was divided into three branches, one of which was for hospitals. During war, the emphasis had been on the hospital treatment of casualties, and therefore hospitals had seemed – perhaps disproportionately for peacetime – crucially important. This position was enshrined in the service. Hospitals were funded separately,

---

[61] Charles Webster, *The Health Services Since the War. Vol. I. The Problems of Health Care: The National Health Service before 1957* (London, 1988); John F. Pater, *The Making of the National Health Service* (London, 1981).

[62] Sir William Beveridge, *Social Insurance and Allied Services. Report.* Cmd. 6604. (London, 1942).

[63] Webster, *National Health Service.*

and teaching institutions answered directly to the Ministry of Health
rather than to a hospital board. Hospitals were already high up in the
medical hierarchy, and consultants within them had long been the elite
in the profession. The health service now helped to perpetuate that.
General practitioners found that very few of them had access to hospital
beds.[64]

There had been some emphasis on medical research in hospitals, or at
least in hospital medical schools, since at least the end of the nineteenth
century. After the First World War, through support from the Medical
Research Council, the Rockefeller Foundation and other agencies,
greater stress had been placed on this, and although the Ministry of
Health did not support medical research, the pressures were there to
increase research, thus differentiating the hospitals further from other
areas of health care. Research was expected to be carried out even in the
new district general hospitals which were now appearing.[65]

Under the NHS attempts were made to ensure that every region was
autonomous, with each area and district within it able to offer a wide
range of services to the local population. In each district there should be
a general hospital which should deal with most medical problems. If
necessary, patients could be referred from the district general hospital to
more specialized hospitals in the region. Over the first twenty years of
the service, a number of new hospitals were built in order to extend the
district general hospital pattern. The divisions within the health service,
between general practice and hospitals and between both and community
medicine, came under fire within the first decade of the service's
existence. It was argued that better integration was required. In 1974 an
attempt was made to scale down the significance of hospitals or at least
to raise the importance of general practitioners. The NHS was
reorganized to try to integrate the three arms of the service more fully,
but with limited success.[66]

[64] Ibid.
[65] The Rockefeller Foundation was keenly interested in supporting medical research in Britain,
funding part of University College Hospital Medical School just after the First World War, and
cooperating with the Medical Research Council, in particular its Secretary, Walter Morley Fletcher,
in attempting to advance the cause of medical research in the United Kingdom. See, for example,
Thomas Bonner, 'Abraham Flexner as Critic of British and Continental Medical Education' and
Darwin Stapleton, 'Assessment and Decision: The Rockefeller Foundation in Great Britain in the
1920s', papers presented at British Society for the History of Science – History of Science Society
Anglo-American Conference, Manchester, England, 11–15 July 1988.
[66] Webster, The National Health Service; idem 'The National Health Service', Lectures, Oxford
University (1985); Ruth Levitt, The Reorganised National Health Service, 2nd ed (London, 1979), pp.
15–22, 213–20. On the hospital/general practitioner division, see Frank Honigsbaum, The Division
in British Medicine (London, 1979).

It is instructive to compare the development of health-care provision, and the hospital's place within that, in Britain and the United States in the twentieth century in seeking to cast light on what was common to both Western nations and what unique to one country alone. Close nineteenth-century parallels between the two countries can be seen, yet clear divergences a few decades later. The hospital/general practitioner divide was not to be found in the United States: most doctors had access to hospital beds, often contracting to the hospital to secure this. The hospitals themselves tended to divide into municipal institutions treating the poor and others that soon evolved in effect into profit-making organizations, despite charitable status. Supporting such business tendencies was a far wider development of insurance than in Britain. For this reason, American hospitals never ran into quite the same financial problems as their interwar British counterparts, perhaps helping to explain why American doctors more consistently and absolutely rejected any kind of government intervention than in the end did British hospital doctors. When federal involvement did manifest itself, with Medicare and Medicaid in the 1960s, it affected hospitals treating the poor and elderly. However, the development in the early 1980s of government attempts to regulate costs by introducing DRGs (Diagnosis Related Groups), according to which the costs of treating particular ailments were averaged and hospitals reimbursed on this basis, then had a knock-on effect on insurance companies, which were less than enthusiastic about paying much more than DRG levels for insured medical care.[67]

The pattern in the United States – of insurance rather than govern-ment-based funding – together with a legal system which encouraged rather than discouraged lawsuits which could result (with no cost to the plaintiff) in massive settlements in medical cases, encouraged the development of vast arrays of technical investigation as all possible avenues of diagnosis were explored.[68] Governmental involvement, when it finally came, began to act as a curb on such exponential growth. Nevertheless the comparative costs in Gross National Product terms of health care in the United Kingdom and United States to the mid 1980s reflected the different financial bases of the two systems: Britain's NHS over its history cost between about 4.5 per cent and 6 per cent of GNP, while America's health-care system ran at about double that, 10 per cent.

[67] Rosemary Stevens, *In Sickness and in Wealth: American Hospitals in the Twentieth Century* (New York, 1989); Daniel M. Fox, *Health Policies, Health Politics: The British and American Experience, 1911–1965* (Princeton, NJ, 1986).

[68] Stanley J. Reiser, *Medicine and the Reign of Technology* (Cambridge, MA, 1978).

Medical technology was highly rated in the United States, perhaps even more so than in Britain. However, possibly because leading doctors in the USA were based partly in their own clinics as well as having hospital beds, the hierarchy of hospital and general practice was not as pronounced as in the United Kingdom. Nevertheless, in both countries – as in the West generally – hospitals are seen as crucial to health care.

Thus, in Britain, hospitals remain by far the most highly valued part of health care – in the public's eyes, in terms of resources committed to them, and to the staff that serve in them. In 1700 hospitals were not numerous, and those that existed were peripheral to the health care of all. Today there are hospitals in most towns and in almost every city district, and they play a central role in health care. They are the centres of medical education and training, the places in which the elite of the medical profession is based, and the foci for medical technology and a whole range of investigative procedures. Other health-care workers are expected to provide primary health care; hospitals now provide secondary health care for the whole of the population.

Medical practitioners 1750–1850 and the period of medical reform in Britain

IRVINE LOUDON*

Important changes occurred in the medical profession in Britain between the late eighteenth and the middle of the nineteenth century which have earned it the title 'The period of medical reform'. Traditionally this period has been described as one of uninterrupted progress, confirmed by medical legislation in the Apothecaries Act of 1815 and the Medical Act of 1858. Those who have adopted the progressive view base it on advances in medical education and professional unity in this period. Educational advances were made possible by the growth of academic medicine and the development of the voluntary hospitals as centres of teaching, research and care. While the study of medicine in Oxford and Cambridge had scarcely emerged from the doldrums of the eighteenth century, the development of medical education at London University and the establishment of provincial medical schools were products of the movement for reform. The foundation of medical associations – especially the Provincial Medical and Surgical Association, the predecessor of the British Medical Association – are cited as evidence of the birth of a new spirit of professional unity. The introduction of the LSA (Licence of the Society of Apothecaries) in 1815 and the MRCS (the diploma of Membership of the Royal College of Surgeons)[1] – the dual qualification known colloquially as 'College and Hall' – provided the general practitioner with a broad education and formal certification. It is quoted not only as evidence of the rise of the lower ranks of the profession, but also of the protection of the public from unqualified medical

* The author is most grateful to Jonathan Barry, Michael Dols and Roy Porter for reading the draft and providing valuable advice. He also acknowledges with gratitude the support of the Wellcome Trust.

[1] Charles Newman, *Medical Education in the Nineteenth Century* (London, 1957); A. M. Carr-Saunders and P. A. Wilson, *The Professions* (London, 1964).

practitioners. Medical reform, moreover, has been presented as part of the general climate of social reform with parliament playing, for the first time, a central role in the politics of medicine. For example, public health measures were introduced by doctors and politicians working together to deal with the problems of health arising from increasing population and urbanization, while a new level of medical care for the poor was provided by the Poor Law Amendment Act of 1834.

The list of achievements is impressive. It is not surprising that the period rom 1794 to 1858 (which, for reasons which will appear, are the conventional boundaries of the period of medical reform), has been honoured as an important period of progress. A new and enlightened profession initiated a system of medical education and medical care based on scientific principles which ushered in medicine as we know it today.

Is it still possible to hold such a rosy view of medical reform? Recently a series of attacks has been mounted against the ways that scholars have traditionally described the history of medicine and the medical profession. Medical history has been too Whiggish, too deferential to the great men and great advances, too fond of stressing the myths of relentless medical progress, insensitive in its treatment of unorthodox practice and too fond of equating medical legislation with medical progress.[2] It is therefore not surprising that the traditional Whiggish description of the period of medical reform has been attacked. No critic denies that it was a period of extensive change, but there are serious reservations about motives, aims and the extent of change.

One view of the period of medical reform would be that it formed a watershed between a low plateau in the eighteenth century and the beginning of modern medicine. In other words there was a major step upwards, a discontinuity, separating the old from the new. The opposite view would suggest that the period of reform was only part of a continuous process of evolution, extending back at least to the first half of the eighteenth century and forwards to the late nineteenth.

What are the criteria by which advance and reform can be measured? Do we appeal to changes in methods and standards of medical education, the unification of the medical profession or to changes in the social and economic status of medical practitioners? How significant is evidence of changes in the doctor/patient relationship? Is effectiveness of care – the ability to prevent, cure or relieve – what really matters, or should we look for evidence of the growth of those analytical, statistical and critical

---

[2] See R. Porter, 'Introduction', in R. Porter (ed.), *Patients and Practitioners: Lay Perceptions of Medicine in Pre-Industrial Society* (Cambridge, 1985).

attitudes on which research and advances in medicine are dependent? How much weight should be given to the 'birth of the clinic' and the growth in the size, number and importance of medical institutions? Is medical legislation, which always receives attention, a sign of advance? Is the legislation of the period of medical reform, for instance, no more than an example of the manipulation of parliament by doctors, motivated by self-interest, for the purposes of the professionalization and monopolization of medicine? If we insist on the centrality of professional changes, are we in danger of forgetting the patient's point of view? Is a change in the demand for medical care and its availability to all sections of the population a forgotten criterion? This, for example, would be the basis for believing that the introduction of the National Health Service is the most important event in British medicine in the twentieth century. What, in other words, were the components of the dramatic change in this period of professional history?

All this is fertile ground for scholars from different backgrounds. Those with a clinical background tend to stress medical institutions and medical legislation and the history of the teaching hospitals and the medical corporations. Those with a historical background may take a more analytical approach to the economic and social significance of changes in medicine, placing them firmly within the context of the social and political changes of the period. Recently, contributors from the social sciences have found in certain aspects of medical reform an opportunity for testing sociological concepts concerned with occupations and group behaviour such as professionalization, monopolization and the changing position of the sick man in medical cosmology.[3]

These different viewpoints are, or certainly should be, regarded as complementary not competitive. Revisionary scholarship has given us a wider understanding of the origin and nature of medical reform. Indeed, the iconoclastic approach gains in authority when we realise that what I have called 'the traditional view' of medical reform was in fact a twentieth-, not a nineteenth-century celebration of medical progress. To those who practised medicine in the nineteenth century, medical reform was by no means an occasion for self-congratulation; on the contrary, most of the changes were accompanied by a sense of disappointment and frustration. Medical education had become much more expensive while

[3] I. Waddington, *The Medical Profession in the Industrial Revolution* (Dublin, 1984); N. D. Jewson, 'Medical Knowledge and the Patronage System in Eighteenth-Century England', *Sociology*, 8 (1974), 369–85, and 'The Disappearance of the Sick Man From Medical Cosmology', *Sociology*, 10 (1976), 225–44; Eliot Freidson, *Professional Dominance* (New York, 1970) and *Profession of Medicine* (New York, 1972).

medical incomes were falling. The universal demand for the outlawing of quackery had failed. The general practitioner had been relegated to a subordinate status and competition was appalling because 'the supply of medical practitioners is in fact not only very much beyond what is necessary to ensure a just and useful competition ... [it is] so great as to be actually mischievous'.[4] Bitter arguments, broken promises and endless delays accompanied the introduction of legislation. Initially, plans for reform were formulated in a spirit of high optimism. By the end of the period almost no one was content either with the Apothecaries Act or with the Medical Act of 1858.[5]

Indeed, one could argue that 'medical reform' is an unfortunate title. A better one, were it not so clumsy, would be 'the period of intra-professional strife', because it was a time when:

so strangely perverted and unharmonised has the whole medical profession become...that it is impossible to conceive any change that could be as productive of equal recriminations. The surgeon exclaims against the apothecary, the physician answers both, the apothecary retorts and thus they go on mutually exasperating each other by every vilifying epithet and opprobrious insinuation until they have rendered life such a scene of heart-burning animosity and contention, that the strongest feeling of every liberal mind must be a desire to escape for ever from the profession and its bickerings.[6]

Why were animosity and strife the key features of the period of medical reform? To answer this question we must say something about the state of medical practice which preceded it.

Medical practice 1750–1815

The rank-and-file practitioners of the eighteenth century have, on the whole, had a poor press. The famous are acknowledged, but only as giants amongst that race of pygmies, described as the 'quasi-irregular' apothecaries and surgeon–apothecaries of the back streets and villages,[7]

[4] Unsigned article by Sir Benjamin Brodie on medical reform in *Quarterly Review*, 47 (Dec. 1840), 53–79.

[5] 'Medical Reform', leading article, *Medical Quarterly Review*, 2 (1834), 233. Edwin Lee, *The State of the Medical Profession Further Exemplified* (London, 1863). 'We have got our protection [from the Medical Act], wrote a Dr Wilks, 'we have obtained our registration at last; but as for advantage it may be of to the profession, I value it at a straw.'

[6] 'A Disinterested Physician', letter to the *Medical and Physical Journal*, 30 (1831), 265–96. The author of this quotation, Dr Edward Barlow, recognized that the central feature of medical reform was the rise of the general practitioner. As a physician (and one of the founders of the Provincial Medical and Surgical Association) he was unusual in forecasting that this would lead to a fall in the number of physicians and he appeared to welcome the prospect. It is not surprising, therefore, that the earliest of his influential articles on medical reform were published anonymously.

[7] Richard H. Shryock, *The Development of Modern Medicine* (Madison, WI, 1979).

implying that the formation of a corpus of trained and respectable doctors for the great majority of the people only occurred with the arrival of the general practitioner in the nineteenth century.

This kind of assumption is part of a general tendency, noted by Porter, to treat medical developments in the eighteenth century not in their own right but as mere forerunners of what was to come later.[8] The general practitioner rose, it is assumed, from a base which was anything but professional, for his predecessors were ignorant, if not illiterate, shopkeepers who struggled to survive against the competition of numerous quacks whose existence is quoted as evidence of a widespread distrust of orthodox medicine. Who, then, were these ordinary practitioners of towns and villages who were regarded by their patients, friends and neighbours as typical of their time? What was their family background and their general and medical education? How much did they earn and what was their standing in society? How can they be identified when there was no clear distinction between the orthodox practitioner and the unorthodox or irregular? Is 'quasi-irregular' a fair description of what, in any case, is meant by a regular or orthodox practitioner?

One group of orthodox practitioners, the physicians, were identifiable by the possession of a medical degree, although some 'MD's were purchased through the post without any kind of examination. Other groups can be identified by their honorary appointments as physician or surgeon to a voluntary hospital or dispensary – a definite sign of orthodoxy – or by appointments as army or naval surgeons. A few were members of the Company of Surgeons or the Society of Apothecaries. Many students, realizing that medical education in Scotland was far advanced beyond anything in England, obtained a formal qualification from Edinburgh or Glasgow.[9] Apart from these, most of the rank-and-file practitioners such as the surgeon–apothecaries are recognizable as orthodox by having served an apprenticeship, and by the nature and manner of their practice.

The typical surgeon–apothecary of the second half of the eighteenth century was a grammar school, not a public school boy, leaving school somewhere between the age of thirteen and sixteen to take up an

[8] R. Porter, 'Laymen, Doctors and Medical Knowledge in the Eighteenth Century: the Evidence of the *Gentleman's Magazine*', in Porter (ed.), *Patients and Practitioners*.

[9] J. D. Comrie, *History of Scottish Medicine* (London, 1932); D. Hamilton, *The Healers: a History of Medicine in Scotland* (Edinburgh, 1981). See especially G. Risse, *Hospital Life in Enlightenment Scotland: Care and Teaching at the Royal Infirmary, Edinburgh* (Cambridge, 1986).

apprenticeship varying from three to seven years. Apprenticeship was often the only form of medical training, and the extent of training as opposed to servitude must have varied widely. At best it was an ideal training for an occupation which was as much a business as a profession, and a number of publications show the extent to which apprenticeship in the late eighteenth century was being organized into something resembling a structured form of medical education.[10] Instruction in pharmacy and the business side of practice was followed by the apprentice being sent out to visit the sick, first with his master and then on his own. Increasingly through the late eighteenth and early nineteenth century, however, the ambitious student would follow his apprenticeship by attending courses, demonstrations and ward rounds at hospitals and private medical schools which provided a reasonably comprehensive training in anatomy, physiology, medicine, surgery and midwifery. Many who attended the provincial infirmaries later spent a year at a London hospital. As hospital training increased, special ties and loyalties were built between the pupil and his hospital. Young men would then speak of themselves as a 'Guy's man' or 'Bart's man' with that common sense of identity and 'tribal' loyalty that one is apt to find amongst ex-members of regiments, schools and universities.[11] There is also a tenuous link between the growth of medical education and the foundation of provincial medical clubs and societies in the late eighteenth and early nineteenth century at which medical men of all ranks met to discuss their cases and often to establish medical libraries. These were small, local, and often ephemeral societies, social as well as academic. They were quite different in character from the strongly political associations established after 1820. It would be foolish to exaggerate their importance, but they were, nevertheless, indicators of a new sense of unity between all ranks of medical men where physicians, surgeons and surgeon–apothecaries met as equal members, taking the chair in succession.[12]

Many surgeon–apothecaries in the late eighteenth century were the

[10] J. Makittrick, *Commentaries on the Principles and Practice of Physick* (London, 1772).

[11] The education, apprenticeship and family background of eighteenth-century practitioners are explored more fully in I. Loudon, *Medical Care and the General Practitioner: 1750–1850* (Oxford, 1986), and I. Loudon, 'Provincial Medical Practice in Eighteenth-Century England', *Medical History*, 29 (1983), 1–32.

[12] Edward Jenner, for example, belonged to two such societies in Gloucestershire. Matthew Flinders recorded the formation of a medical society in Donington in Lincolnshire in 1796 which met regularly at the Red Cow Inn (see note 20 below). The Lincolnshire Benevolent Medical Society (see note 35 below) provides another example. In their constitutions and purpose these can all be seen as forerunners of the much more famous Provincial Medical and Surgical Association, established in 1832, which became the British Medical Association.

sons of medical practitioners. This conferred the advantages that there was no apprenticeship premium, and usually a ready-made practice to inherit. Practitioners from a medical family and others who were the sons of the clergy, attorneys, naval and army officers, 'gentlemen' and minor landed proprietors accounted for two-thirds of the total. The remaining third came from backgrounds which ranged from bank employees, musicians and schoolmasters to grocers, carriers and sailmakers. What is notable is that the general practitioners of the first half of the nineteenth century came from a similar social background.[13]

By the mid eighteenth century, medical practice at the rank-and-file level had become both a paying and respected occupation. Why it should have risen in status and prosperity at this time is unclear. It has been said that any historian of the modern or early modern period searching for the causes of social change can find handy if threadbare explanations in increasing urbanization and the birth of the consumer society. Nevertheless these do in fact provide the most convincing answer to our question. For instance, two books about the trades and professions, both published in 1747, stressed the recent improvement in the income and status of the lower grades of practitioners. The occupation of the apothecary was described in one of them: 'There is no Branch of Business in which a Man requires less Money to set him up than this very profitable Trade…His profits are unconceivable: Five Hundred per cent is the least he receives.' The other noted that the business of the apothecary had become 'a very genteel business *and in great vogue of late years* [my italics]'; apothecaries 'especially in the country, often become Men of large Practice and eminent in their way'.[14] To be an apothecary needed, as Adam Smith emphasized, 'a nicer and more delicate skill' than any other trade.[15] In fact, the surgeon–apothecary stood on the dividing line between the tradesman and the professional man. Partnership agreements of the period generally speak of the 'business or profession' of surgeon–apothecary, and, before the rise of gentility in the nineteenth century, there were fewer social overtones in the descriptions of occupations as trades, businesses or professions.

---

[13] This is based on an analysis of the parental occupation of eighty-three practitioners between 1760 and 1830 included in the 'Bristol Infirmary Biographical Memoirs', 14 vols., Bristol Record Office, and on a similar analysis of 149 entries between 1764 and 1781 in the apprentice binding book, MS 8207, the records of the Society of Apothecaries, the Guildhall Library, London. See also David van Zwanenberg, 'The Training and Careers of those Apprenticed to Apothecaries in Suffolk', *Medical History*, 27 (1983), 193–50.

[14] R. Campbell, *The London Tradesman* (London, 1747), Anon. *A General Description of all Trades* (London, 1747). [15] Adam Smith, *Wealth of Nations* (London, 1776).

Indeed, both the publications just quoted placed the physician unequivocally amongst the professional men but treated him with scant respect compared to the surgeon and apothecary.

While tradition attributes the rise of the rank-and-file practitioner (the apothecaries and surgeon-apothecaries) to the Apothecaries Act of 1815, and Holmes suggests that the rise took place much earlier (between 1680 and 1730),[16] a number of sources point to the mid eighteenth century as the most likely period for a significant rise in their social and economic status. High fees were paid for simple surgical procedures and large profits could be made, even in country areas, from the practice of pharmacy. In an age of conspicuous consumption medicine was often consumed in astonishing quantities.[17] Practitioners exploited the demand for medicine by supplying large amounts in small individual quantities, often delivered daily, to maximise profits. It is important to understand that pharmacy – the art of compounding and dispensing drugs – was the major source of income of all practitioners except the small number of elite physicians and surgeons in London and a few large cities. It explains why Richard Smith junior called the late eighteenth century 'The Golden age of Physic'.[18]

The riches of the famous physicians of the time are well recognized; what is not so well established is the relative wealth of the surgeon–apothecary. The Bristol apothecary William Broderip, for instance, achieved at the height of his practice an astonishing income of over £3,000 a year.[19] This, admittedly, was a city practice; but the records of country practitioners often reveal steady incomes of £400 to £500 a year.[20] Financially (and often socially) the surgeon–apothecary was on

[16] Geoffrey Holmes, Augustan England: Professions, State and Society, 1680–1730 (London, 1982).
[17] Medical records of the eighteenth century including ledgers, diaries, account books (private and poor law [overseers] accounts) and numerous bills in various County Record Offices form the basis for this statement. For example, a family in Somerset was supplied in one year (1754) with 687 items of medicine, as well as two 'blisters' and seven 'bleedings', and the bill was over one hundred pounds: Somerset County Record Office, Taunton, bill from Mr Bernard Baine, surgeon-apothecary, to Thomas Carew, DD/TB box 14/20. For further evidence see Loudon, 'Provincial Medical Practice'.
[18] 'Bristol Infirmary Biographical Memoirs', pp. 157–9. Richard Smith Junior (1772–1843) was a Bristol surgeon with an appointment as surgeon to the Bristol Infirmary from 1796. His life-long collection of material about medicine in Bristol and the West of England, consisting of memoirs, letters, anecdotes, advertisements and his inimitable biographies of medical men, has been preserved in fourteen large volumes known as the 'Bristol Infirmary Biographical Memoirs'.
[19] Ibid., I, 46.
[20] For example, Matthew Flinders, who practised as a surgeon–apothecary and man-midwife in Donington, Lincs., from 1775 to 1802, first achieved an income of over £400 in his fourteenth year in practice and his income averaged £450 per annum (except for a peak of £582 in 1798) until his death at the age of fifty-two. 'The Diaries of Matthew Flinders', Lincoln Archives Office.

a level with the attorney, the middle or upper ranks of the clergy, and the better-off farmers. Often he followed a second part-time occupation (usually farming) not from the inability to make a living from medical practice but, on the contrary, as a means of investing his earnings. These practitioners were entrepreneurs in a commercial age. Not all were brash and mercenary men, for there were educated and literary practitioners.[21] But most were probably hunting and shooting people and good judges of horse-flesh. As for their patients, people from a very wide range of social classes consulted them and paid their fees, not just for major illnesses, but also (and frequently) for minor self-limiting disorders.[22] There is little evidence that a substantial part of the fee-paying population shunned the regular practitioner in preference to the quack, although many have employed both, even for the same illness.

If, as I have suggested, the rank-and-file practitioners were on the whole making a reasonable living and occupying a comfortable niche in society, why did they not continue undisturbed? Why did such an explosive period of change and upheaval occur? In looking for the answer, one must recognize first of all that medical reform was not confined to Britain.

The beginnings of medical reform 1794–1815

In the eighteenth and nineteenth centuries, calls for reform and professional unity were heard throughout Europe. The 'academization'[23] of medicine together with a growing tendency for state involvement in medical affairs was evident, for example, in France, Spain, Holland and Germany, although it started at different times. France, where state involvement was substantial even before the revolution precipitated extensive changes, played an early and a leading part in the academization of surgery. In Holland the two significant dates

---

[21] There are many examples, but the best known is W. Brockbank and F. Kenworthy (eds.), 'The Diary of Richard Kay (1716–51) of Baldingstone, near Bury', *The Chetham Record Society*, 16 (1968). See also 'Notebooks of the Carr Family, Surgeons near Leeds (1780–1853)' (London, The Wellcome Institute for the History of Medicine, manuscript collection, MS 1916–17).

[22] The most persuasive evidence comes from such manuscript sources as 'the ledgers of William Pulsford', in the Somerset County Record Office, Taunton, DD/FS Box 48. This is described in Loudon, 'Provincial Medical Practice'.

[23] The term 'academization', which I have borrowed from E. H. Ackernecht and E. Fischer-Homberg (see note 24 below), is a shorthand description of the process by which there is a rise in the status of an occupation through the accumulation of a corpus of theoretical and practical knowledge which is taught in educational institutions in a regular and systematic manner. Thus in medicine it applies not only to university departments of medicine but also to medical academies, colleges, hospitals, societies or other institutions.

for medical legislation and medical reform – 1818 and 1865 – are close to the dates of the Apothecaries Act and the Medical Act in Britain. Throughout Europe, hospitals, growing in number and size, played an increasingly central role in medical education. In England the voluntary hospitals prevailed. On the continent, hospital provision in the late eighteenth and early nineteenth century was generally on a larger scale and financed partly or wholly by the state or local authorities.

In other words, reform of medical education and of the structure of the medical profession was a European phenomenon in which, broadly speaking, the similarities between different countries were more striking than the differences. In most countries the profession was divided into an elite group of university-trained practitioners, mostly in large towns and cities, and a lower level of apprenticed practitioners, often derived from the barber–surgeons, who were the mainstay of medical care in the provinces and country areas. Raising the educational status and competence of the lower orders of practitioners was one of the first objectives of reform. Narrowing the gap between the elite practitioners, trained at universities, and the rank and file was seen both as a means of meeting the medical needs of the whole population and as a means of achieving professional unity.

There were two notable differences between England and the continent. First, the role of the pharmacist. The merging of pharmacy with medical practice occurred in England through the rise of the apothecary. On the continent legislation prevented a similar evolution, and there seems to have been no equivalent to the English phenomenon, described below, where the dispensing druggist suddenly appeared and became the pharmacist of the nineteenth and twentieth centuries.[24]

Secondly, the status of obstetrics or 'man-midwifery'. On the continent obstetrics was usually granted equal status with medicine and surgery. In England it was the 'Cinderella' of medicine, ignored and excluded by the Royal Colleges of Physicians and Surgeons. For this reason obstetrics before 1850 was relegated almost entirely to the general practitioner.[25]

---

[24] See E. H. Ackernecht and E. Fischer-Homberg, 'Five Made It – One Not. The Rise of Medical Craftsmen to Academic Status During the 19th Century', *Clio Medica*, 12 (1977), 255–67. The one who failed to 'make it' was the midwife.

[25] The existence of a number of famous physician– and surgeon–accoucheurs during this period in no way invalidates this view. They were a small minority, conspicuous through authorship. But the attitudes of the two Royal Colleges remained adamant – neither would accept responsibility for teaching or examining students in obstetrics. This rejection had a profound effect on the development of obstetrics in Britain.

It may seem obvious to stress the need to see the reform of medicine in the broad European context of social change and scientific advance, but it is only too easy to mistake associations with causes. Thus medical reform in Britain was associated with, but not the direct result of, scientific advances in medicine. Likewise, there is no evidence that reform was in any way a response to the growing crisis in health associated with the increase in population and urbanization of the industrial revolution. Medical reform was in part a reflection of the rise of the middle classes, secondary education, and the growing importance of the professions; and parliament was increasingly involved in medical affairs. But legislation concerning professional structure and medical education (as opposed to public health legislation) was initiated by medical men, not by government.

Following the train of thought that medical reform might have originated from changes in society as a whole, it may be suspected that reform was a response to patient demand; in other words, that the consumer demanded the fruits of a real or perceived improvement in the effectiveness of medical care. But there is no evidence of this, either. From the patients' point of view, there was little their regular medical attendant could do for them when they were ill in 1840 that his predecessor could not have done in 1780;[26] and on the whole the public knew it. By far the most striking feature of medical reform was the extent to which it was inward-looking. It was more like a family quarrel than a public debate. Beneath the slogans of educational and scientific advance were the burning issues of rank, title and status, linked to questions of social and professional respectability, which in turn were linked to questions of fees and income. Such issues had preoccupied medical men for a long time. They were not new. But they reached new heights in the unstable atmosphere of medical reform. Why, then, did such matters come to a head at the end of the eighteenth century?

To a certain extent reform was the inevitable consequence of the growing success and expectations of medical practitioners at a time when medicine was outgrowing its institutions. By the end of the eighteenth century, eighteen medical corporations in the United Kingdom granted a medical diploma, licence or degree.[27] Many of them still possessed,

---

[26] It is difficult to think of any effective therapy introduced between these dates apart from digitalis and vaccination against smallpox.

[27] The universities of Oxford and Cambridge, the Royal College of Physicians of London, the Company of Surgeons and the Society of Apothecaries of London, the universities of Edinburgh, Glasgow and St Andrews, the two universities of Aberdeen, the Royal College of Surgeons of

even if they did not enforce, jurisdiction over practice in surrounding areas. The Royal College of Physicians still had the legal monopoly of the practice of physic in London and a seven-mile radius, but it was seldom enforced after the Rose case of 1704.[28] Glasgow graduates had, in theory, sole rights to practice in Lanark, Renfrew, Ayr and Dumbarton, and there were other instances. It was a chaotic system of separate and autonomous medical corporations which led, in the end, to the demand for a 'single portal of entry' – qualification through a single examination held simultaneously in different parts of the country, resembling the examination for the Registered General Nurse today.

But the establishment of a formal system of medical education and licensing was not just a question of producing better doctors. It was also a question of creating a clear distinction between the properly trained practitioner and the irregular. Until all practitioners received a regular medical education and a licence as proof of competence, how could the public tell the real from the false? Initially it was a specific part of irregular practice which acted as the trigger to reform. In the eyes of regular practitioners, irregulars included not only the traditional fly-by-night itinerant, and the local blacksmith or shopkeeper who practised as a part-time healer. These had existed openly for more than a century, and as long as the regular faculty prospered, irregular practice was not a major concern. It was a new form of irregular, the dispensing druggist, who brought matters suddenly to a head; and he did so because he posed a new and serious threat the rank-and-file practitioner.

Until the 1780s, druggists were, with few exceptions, wholesalers supplying practitioners with the raw materials for the practice of pharmacy. When, however, quite suddenly they began to open shops and supply the public over the counter, the effect on the surgeon–apothecary was devastating.[29] This new type of druggist differed from

Edinburgh, the Faculty of Physicians and Surgeons of Glasgow, the university of Dublin, the College of Physicians of Ireland, the Royal College of Surgeons of Ireland, the Apothecaries Hall of Ireland, the Lying-in Hospital, Dublin.

[28] William Rose, a London apothecary, was prosecuted by the Royal College of Physicians of London for practising physic. Information had been laid against him by a disgruntled patient, a butcher of Hungerford market who received a bill for £50 but claimed he was no better for Mr Rose's attentions. The College of Physicians won their case, but the Lords reversed the verdict in 1704. Thereafter an apothecary could visit patients and provide advice (previously the prerogative of the physician) but he could only charge for medicines. This decision merely confirmed a practice which had already become widespread. See Loudon, *Medical Care and the General Practitioner*.

[29] Accounts of the rise of the dispensing druggist can be found in J. M. Good, *The History of Medicine as Far as it Relates to the Apothecary* (London, 1796); Jacob Bell, *Historical Sketch of the Progress of Pharmacy* (London, 1843); 'Letters to the President of the Associated Apothecaries',

other irregulars in one important respect. The dispensing druggist was not a seller of quack remedies for which he made extravagant claims; usually he sold the same orthodox medicines that medical practitioners dispensed at a large profit, and he sold them cheaper. The public welcomed the druggist and flocked to him in increasing numbers. He was an inexpensive source of medical care when the expense of the regular practitioner had become notorious. 'I have a family of four' wrote 'C. H.' from Ipswich, 'and until I grew wiser by experience I annually paid 20 to 30 pounds for their little ailings, for which I now get medicine for about as many shillings at a neighbouring druggist.'[30] To medical men, however, druggists were the most dangerous form of irregular that ever existed, 'mere grocers and tea-dealers' with no knowledge of the properties of medicine and no ability to dispense them properly.[31] Worse still, as the druggists became established they started to visit the sick, dispensing medicine and advice, performing venesections and claiming to set fractured limbs. They could only be stopped, it was believed, by legal measures which licensed the regular and outlawed the quack.

In London it was estimated in 1794 that the rise of the druggists had already cost the average practitioner £200 a year. In Bristol, William Broderip, the rich apothecary noted above, lived in great style with a carriage and coachman, a large town house, and a country seat with expensive furniture and pictures. By the early 1800s, such was the competition of Bristol druggists that he was forced to sell medicines for pence instead of shillings, and soon he was bankrupt.[32] From the end of the eighteenth century, dispensing druggists sprang up all over England, in cities, towns and villages. Where the ratio of dispensing druggists to medical practitioners in the 1780s was about 1:20, by the 1840s they existed in equal numbers.[33]

An angry meeting of 200 surgeon–apothecaries in June 1794, protested at the 'depradations' of the dispensing druggist, and established the General Pharmaceutical Association of Great Britain. Politically the Association was a failure. Parliament was petitioned (unsuccessfully) and

Medical and Physical Journal, 43 (1820), 496–510, and especially in the 'Bristol Infirmary Biographical Memoirs', I, p. 94; II, p. 163; VI, p. 350.

[30] 'Increase of Medical Fees', *Monthly Magazine*, 44 (1817), 498–9.
[31] J. Power, letter, published in the introduction to *Medical and Chirurgical Review*, 13 (1806), clxxi–ii.   [32] 'Bristol Infirmary Biographical Memoirs', II, p. 164.
[33] Statistics derived from an analysis of various town and county directories of the eighteenth and early nineteenth century; data recorded in the 'Bristol Infirmary Biographical Memoirs'; and population census for 1841, PP, 1844, *xxvii*, 31–44, 48–51.

the Association faded out in 1795. There had been protests about quackery before; now the druggist was included in the 'vile race of quacks with which this country is infested'.[34]

In 1804, the first major step in medical reform was instituted by Dr Edward Harrison, a Lincolnshire physician and Edinburgh graduate who was not a member of the Royal College of Physicians for which he had scant respect.[35] As the first president of the Lincolnshire Benevolent Medical Society he was persuaded to undertake an investigation into the nature and extent of irregular practice. He showed that in many areas irregulars exceeded regular practitioners by ratios as high as 9 : 1.[36] What had started as a local initiative rapidly became a national one when Harrison published his first report with the title *Remarks on the Ineffective State of the Practice of Physic in Great Britain with Proposals for its Future Regulation and Improvement*. Published in 1806, the title displays the two purposes Harrison had in mind; first the exposure of quackery, secondly the measures for reform. An Act of Parliament was needed which would regulate the education, examination and licensing of physicians, surgeons and apothecaries. Henceforth, midwives and druggists would need to acquire a licence to practise, bringing them under the control of the medical profession.

Harrison's energy, and high-mindedness are not to be doubted, but he underestimated the power of the medical colleges and was shocked by the back-biting within 'the London faculty'. The Royal College of Physicians saw him and agreed to act only if he left matters in their hands. Harrison refused, and the College was furious with this upstart provincial physician who was not even a licentiate and not in the least deferential. The College knew that parliament would refuse to introduce legislation without their approval, and their opposition to Harrison's proposals was totally successful. Harrison failed not because his plans for reform were unacceptable, or because the outlawing of irregular practice

[34] Good, *History of Medicine* (1796) and Bell, *Historical Sketch* (1843), J. Forbes, editorial, 'On the Patronage of Quacks and Impostors by the Upper Classes of Society', *British and Foreign Medical Review*, 21 (1846), 533–40. See chapter by I. Loudon, 'The Vile Race of Quacks with Which This Country is Infested', in W. F. Bynum and R. Porter (eds.), *Medical Fringe and Medical Orthodoxy* (London, 1986).

[35] Edward Harrison, *Remarks on the Ineffective State of the Practice of Physio* (London, 1806), and *An Address to the Lincolnshire Medical Benevolent Society* (London, 1810).

[36] Harrison's survey of irregular practice was extensive and based on answers to a questionnaire sent to practitioners all over the country. Because it was the only attempt to establish the nature and extent of irregular practice at that time its importance can hardly be exaggerated. Some of the replies were published as an introduction to volume 13 (1806) of the little-known *Medical and Chirurgical Review* (1794–1808), no. 31 in LeFanu's *British Periodicals of Medicine, 1640–1899* (Oxford, 1984). A copy exists in the library of the Royal College of Surgeons in London.

was impractical; he failed because he trod on the toes of the powerful medical corporations; because

> those who believed themselves deprived of rights, and those who feared a change on the grounds that all change was dangerous, united into a phalanx, compact, formidable and impenetrable. Against this host...all looking to particular interests, fearing the loss of some good already possessed, or apprehending the demolition of some expectancy, it would have been unwise to contend; and Dr Harrison, judiciously perhaps, suspended his projected plan of reform.[37]

It was a foretaste of the attitude of both the College of Physicians and the College of Surgeons to the concept of medical reform.

The Association of Apothecaries and the Apothecaries Act of 1815

The term general practitioner had no legal sanction or definition. It replaced the clumsier title of surgeon–apothecary and man-midwife, but it remained a colloquialism, first mentioned in print as far as I can discover in 1809.[38] The older usage continued to appear in legal documents such as partnership agreements and government reports. 'General practitioner', however, was in common use throughout the medical profession by the second and third decades of the nineteenth century, although the public (and novelists) were slow to adopt the term. It was not universally popular. Some practitioners who held the MRCS as well as the LSA (and some who did not) preferred the more prestigious title of 'surgeon'.

The chronology of these changes is important. The existence of a remarkably comprehensive form of medical education based on teaching hospitals, the rise of the surgeon–apothecary and the introduction of the term general practitioner pre-dated the Apothecaries Act. Indeed, the Act would scarcely have been possible without the pre-existing educational structure. The regulation of medical education and the licensing of those who passed the examinations were seen as changes benefiting the public and the practitioners. Since it seemed that the needs of the public and medical self-interest went hand in hand, the new breed of general practitioners never doubted they would succeed in establishing for themselves a new and prestigious position in the profession and in society.

[37] Leading article, *Medical and Physical Journal*, 26 (1811), 2–5.
[38] 'H', untitled letter to the *Medical and Physical Journal*, 21 (1809), 382–5.

There was therefore a sense of determined optimism amongst the earliest general practitioners of London and the provinces. It was evident in the establishment of the Association of Apothecaries and Surgeon–Apothecaries (hereafter 'The Association' for brevity) on 3 July 1812 at a meeting held in London. Those who attended this meeting were no mere collection of 'discontented men without practice, or public estimation', but 'the first in rank, ability and character amongst the London practitioners.' The initial membership of 200 grew to over 3,000 in three years.[39]

The Association's initial plans were far-reaching. They included a system of education and licensing for the general practitioner based on a new London college with hints of a future 'fourth body' which would be a college or society of general practitioners. Midwives and druggists would be required to hold a licence and come under the control of the medical profession. Apprenticeship was retained because general practitioners had become dependent on their apprentices. This decision was later regretted. A committee that included physicians and surgeons, but containing a majority of general practitioners, would be appointed to administer the system of education and licensing.

Between 1812 and 1815 the physicians and surgeons, joined by the pharmacists, successfully opposed the Association's plans. The College of Physicians wanted to retain its position of eminence. The College of Surgeons, established in 1800, feared a fall in membership and the loss of examination fees (in modern terms the equivalent of about £1,000 per candidate) on which it depended. The druggists, or to be more specific a powerful group of London pharmacists, convinced parliament of their right to independent existence and self-regulation. It was only at the insistence of the Royal College of Physicians that the Society of Apothecaries reluctantly accepted responsibility for administering the Act. Most of its senior members, who later appointed themselves to the Court of Examiners, were not in medical practice. Indeed, it is

---

[39] Primary sources on the Association of Apothecaries and Surgeon–Apothecaries and the Apothecaries Act include the records of the Society of Apothecaries, London, Guildhall Library, especially MS 8211/1; *Transactions of the Associated Apothecaries and Surgeon–Apothecaries*, 1 (1823), i–cxxviii; *Medical and Physical Journal*, 29–31; *London Medical and Surgical Repository*, 1, (Jan.–June 1814); G. M. Burrows, *A Statement of Circumstances Connected with the Apothecaries Act and Its Administration*, (London, 1817); R. M. Kerrison, *An Inquiry into the Present State of the Medical Profession in England* (London, 1814). The most perceptive analysis of the Act of 1815 is S. W. F. Holloway, 'The Apothecaries Act 1815: a Reinterpretation', part 1, 'The Origins of the Act', *Medical History*, 10: 2 (1966), 107–29; part 2, 'The Consequences of the Act', *Medical History*, 10: 3 (1966), 221–36.

astonishing to find that when the Act was finally introduced in August 1815, many of them had only the haziest idea of the contents of the Act and the events which preceded it.

Because of the formidable opposition of the physicians, surgeons and pharmacists, the Apothecaries Act was an emasculated version of the original Bill drawn up by the Association. The licensing of midwives and druggists, the plans for a London College and 'fourth body', and the administration of an Act for the education and regulation of general practitioners by general practitioners – all these features were erased from the Bill. The Royal College of Physicians insisted on two additional clauses in the Act: first that they should still be allowed to search the premises of apothecaries (meaning general practitioners) to destroy unsatisfactory drugs; secondly that any new Act should be no more than an amendment to the original charter of the Society of Apothecaries. These were seen by general practitioners as deliberate slights. Licentiates of the Society of Apothecaries might call themselves general practitioners if they chose, but the College of Physicians wanted to label them as the same old subservient apothecaries, dressed up with a new name. Against this background the Act was introduced in an atmosphere of bitterness and disappointment, tempered only by the belief (mistaken as it happened) that subsequent legislation would be introduced to improve it.

Although the Society of Apothecaries administered the Act with efficiency, the Act itself can be criticized on a number of grounds. The examination for the LSA, with its emphasis on Latin and materia medica, was appropriate for the old style of apothecary whose main function was dispensing drugs, but not for the general practitioner who practised medicine, surgery and midwifery as well as pharmacy. The examination in surgery remained with the College of Surgeons (and was, of course, voluntary) and there was no examination in midwifery, the linchpin of general practice.

The licentiates of the Society, however, were delighted with one clause in the Act; this was the penal clause which empowered the Society to prosecute anyone 'practising as an apothecary' after 1 August 1815 without the licence of the Society. This should have provided the means for outlawing the irregulars; but in practice it had little effect.[40] There was, as Wakley pointed out in one of his forceful *Lancet* editorials, no

---

[40] 'Records of the Society of Apothecaries', London, Guildhall Library, MS 8212. This record provides the most comprehensive evidence of the difficulties surrounding the penal clause of the Act. See also the *Report of the Select Committee on Medical Education*, PP 1834, XIII, part III, Q. 270.

legal definition of 'acting as an apothecary'.[41] The prosecution of irregulars failed, however, chiefly because the Society had to bear the cost (estimated at £200) of every prosecution, and felt itself constitutionally unsuited for the role of public prosecutor. Many instances of illegal practice were reported by practitioners on which the Society took no action. In other instances the Society, with remarkable incompetence, prosecuted not the blatant irregulars, but well-qualified Edinburgh graduates who had excited the jealousy of their medical neighbours.[42] Technically a practitioner with an MD or LRCS from Edinburgh practised illegally unless he had also taken the LSA. No one had foreseen when it was introduced that the Act would be used in this spirit of spite and petty jealousy. The situation became so ridiculous that a writer was moved to remark 'the future historian will scarcely be able to believe that this was the state of medicine in the 1830s'.[43] The initial optimism of the general practitioners began to evaporate when they began to see the Act of which they had such high hopes as 'a very considerable failure'.

Intra-professional strife

The attempted rise of the general practitioners and the threat they posed to the physicians and surgeons was not the sole cause of instability in the medical profession of the early nineteenth century. Just as important was the apparent breakdown of the traditional divisions. The tripartite division of orthodox practitioners in the seventeenth century, and the subsequent appearance of the surgeon–apothecary is a commonplace. What, then, was the relation between the divisions of medical men during the period of medical reform? How did they perceive each other and how did those perceptions change? Was there a major revision of the tripartite system or merely a change in titles? For medical practitioners of all ranks these were burning questions, constantly discussed. Medical men were sensitive to a fault on questions of rank, status and medical qualifications which they saw, with reason, as the basis of professional power.

In the field of medical legislation, the power of the Royal College of Physicians was considerable and used almost exclusively in a negative

---

[41] Editorial, *Lancet*, 2 (1826–7), 514–17.

[42] *Report of the Select Committee on Medical Education*, PP 1834, XIII, part III, Q. 100.

[43] 'Repeal of the Apothecaries Act. Abuses in the Profession', *London Medical and Surgical Journal*, new series 3 (1833), 341–2.

fashion. Innovation was not the College's strong point. As one of their members expressed it:

Physician, surgeon and apothecary are the ancient, the true, the English arrangement. Interwoven with the very structure of English Society, the medical practice has been tripartite – physic, surgery, pharmacy, or surgery *united* with pharmacy. This adapted, this scientific, this ancient division of labour the medical reformer seeks to destroy.[44]

In the early nineteenth century, as in the eighteenth, the status of physicians rested on a liberal university education rather than a scientific training in medicine. As the gentlemen of the profession they studiously avoided manual activities and the dispensing of medicine. Social niceties were the basis of social superiority. Increasingly, however, the College was criticised for its snobbery and opposition to change. *The Lancet* attacked it unceasingly. *The London Medical and Surgical Journal* published a view of the College as 'a junta of time-serving, place-hunting intriguing men',[45] and the proletarian *Monthly Gazette of Health* openly mocked the College on numerous occasions, accusing its members of ignorance, arrogance and disgraceful habits such as colluding with druggists for the sake of profits.[46]

The Royal College of Surgeons was a more vigorous institution. The growth of the academic status of surgery and the growing influence of surgeons in the late eighteenth and early nineteenth century are well known. 'Times have changed', said Abernethy in 1812, 'and surgeons have changed too... and in consequence have got a kind of information which puts them on a par with others of the profession.'[47] The College protected its new position by creating a closed elite of London hospital surgeons. They, rather than the physicians tended to dominate the teaching hospitals and often commanded high fees and large incomes. But any surgeon who practised midwifery or pharmacy – in other words, a general practitioner – was excluded from office or privilege within the College.

Neither of the Royal Colleges was sympathetic to reform of the profession as a whole, fearing loss of privilege and power. Neither

---

[44] D. O. Edwards, 'Thoughts on the Real and Imaginary Grievances of the Profession', *Lancet*, 2 (1841–2), 510–14, 606–14, 742–7, 776–83.

[45] 'Repeal of the Apothecaries Act. Abuses in the Profession'.

[46] 'Knowledge of Diseases', *Monthly Gazette of Health*, 8 (1823), 571; and *ibid.*, 'Physician v. Apothecary', 4 (1819), 215–20, 'Of Living Biography', 6 (1821).

[47] Royal Society of Medicine, London, 'The Notebooks of John Greene Crosse of Norwich', MS 285.g.11. The quotation is from Crosse's notes as a student.

wanted to have anything to do with the general practitioner. Both, through connections with London society, had great influence with government, but it would be quite wrong to equate the general run of physicians or of surgeons with the leading members of their respective Colleges. In 1847 only half the London physicians and only 7 per cent of provincial physicians were licentiates or fellows of the College. Those who possessed an Oxford or Cambridge degree (and they alone were eligible for fellowship of the College) amounted to less than a quarter of the London physicians, and 6 per cent of those in the provinces. Most physicians held Scottish or continental degrees, the Edinburgh MD being by far the most common.[48] During this period, medicine (in the sense of physic, or 'internal medicine') owed most of its strength to Edinburgh graduates, many of whom were dissenters practising in the midlands or the north of England. The most important feature of medical practice in the period of medical reform, however, was the extent to which there was a large degree of overlap in everyday clinical practice, blurring the old tripartite distinctions between medical men. This meant that the period of medical reform was a transitional period in which the whole future of clinical practice was uncertain.

It was not until the second half of the nineteenth century that stability had returned. By that time physicians and surgeons had to a large degree become specialists, practising as consultants based on hospitals. General practitioners, excluded from major hospitals and the power associated with teaching, were firmly relegated to a subordinate status. Even though the separation was not complete until the twentieth century, by 1850 it was no longer the case, as it had been in 1827, that 'pure surgeons and consulting physicians are "rarae aves" certainly – to be met with only in very large towns; if we take another step down the ladder of professional distinctions we find everything jumbled, brayed and blended in the pretensions and pursuits of the general practitioner'.[49] Professional instability and intra-professional hostility was inevitable as long as there was 'the tendency ... to the union of medicine and surgery in practice, and to equalisation of rank; the inferior class pressing upwards to get on a level with the superior and the two classes in continual broils until that level [is] sustained'.[50] Even the 'pure' surgeons of London treated both medical and surgical cases. Where, in

[48] I. Loudon, 'Two Thousand Medical Men in 1847', *Bulletin of the Society for the Social History of Medicine*, 33 (1983), 4–8.
[49] Editorial, *London Medical Repository and Review*, new series 5 (1827), 188.
[50] Editorial, *British and Foreign Medical Review*, 14 (1842), 402–11.

the past, London surgeons had a virtual monopoly of major operations and patients were sent from great distances to the metropolis, the general practitioners had taken over. 'A considerable part of the practice of the Surgeons as well as the Physicians' said Sir James Clark in 1843, 'has thus fallen into the hands of the General Practitioners'.[51] As a result, the division of the profession into physician, surgeon and general practitioner was 'more ostensible than real' said one physician in 1834. Another physician believed that 'at present there are men of nearly equal distinction in all departments of the profession and the whole scheme of distinction is falling to pieces'.[52] What, they asked, was happening to the time-honoured divisions of medicine?

There had always been a tendency for surgeons to administer medical remedies to their patients when the occasion demanded; but they did so on a much larger scale in the early nineteenth century as surgery became more conservative and medical treatments often replaced operations. Physicians complained of this invasion of their territory. Not only were the old distinctions between practitioners disintegrating, but the divisions between physic and surgery were changing so much it was difficult to say where physic ended and surgery began. 'Distinctions between what belongs to the physician and what to the surgeon are indefinable', said the surgeon Sir Anthony Carlisle. 'Suppose a man has a disease of the lower intestine. If it is out of reach of the finger it belongs to the physician; but the moment it comes down and within reach of the finger, it belongs to the surgeon.'[53]

If the tendency, then, was to the fusion of physic and surgery, who could deny that this tendency was personified in the general practitioner who was by definition a practitioner of physic, surgery, midwifery and pharmacy? For:

It is only the general practitioner who, when called upon, does not stop to inquire if the patient is afflicted with a 'surgical' or a 'medical' disorder...and it is upon these grounds we take our stand. The title of general practitioner...is descriptive of what we are...and we want no other assumption to give us dignity.[54]

Specialization in medicine at this time was neither common nor admired. Indeed, it was often regarded as the refuge of the failed

---

[51] Sir James Clark, *Remarks on Medical Reform* (London, 1843).
[52] *Report of the Select Committee on Medical Education*, PP 1834, XIII, part I, Q.2121–31, 2467.
[53] *ibid.*, part II, Q.5981–3.
[54] Letter from 'Member of the Committee of the Metropolitan Society of General Practitioners', *Lancet*, 2 (1829–30), 653.

physician or surgeon; so it was logical to believe that 'no reform can have a chance of permanency unless...it adapts itself to those wants of the public which have been so unequivocally demonstrated; namely, by supplying an adequately qualified class of general practitioners'.[55] To the physicians and surgeons it seemed only too possible that the upwardly mobile general practitioner would take over the bulk of the practice of medicine.

The Countess of A or Mrs B the city millionaire's wife has a physician for one complaint, a surgeon for another, a physician accoucheur for a third, and an apothecary, probably, provides the medicines and attends the children and servants. But how is this possible for a person in ordinary circumstance?...It is therefore absolutely necessary that, to supply the wants of the middle and lower classes of the metropolis and of nearly all ranks in the provincial towns and villages, there should exist a branch of the profession, the members of which must be generally competent to undertake the management of all diseases. Whether this branch of the profession do or do not supply their patients with medicines is, in our opinion, quite immaterial.[56]

The struggles of the general practitioner

What happened to the general practitioners? Why did they fail in professional and public opinion to achieve the status of physicians and surgeons? One cannot attribute their failure solely to the inadequacies of the Apothecaries Act. For all its faults, the Act had made the middle classes more ambitious than ever to put their sons to a career in medicine. The dual qualification, the 'College and Hall', was at least a symbol of respectability and professional status. 'We know a few secrets in our profession, sir,' said Dr Jobling. 'Of course we do. We study for that; we pass the Hall and the College for that; and we take our station in society *by* that.'[57]

The popularity of general practice as a career was shown by the statistics. Between 1815 and 1850 some four to five hundred candidates a year obtained the LSA. At the same time, others returned from the Scottish medical schools to practise in England, and army and navy surgeons who had served in the Napoleonic wars resigned to enter

[55] Editorial, *British and Foreign Medical Review*, 19 (1840), 281–7.

[56] 'A Practitioner', *Is the Practice of Medicine a Degenerate Pursuit?* (London, 1850).

[57] Charles Dickens, *Martin Chuzzlewit* (London, no date, first published in monthly numbers between 1846 and 1848).

civilian practice. Medicine began to suffer seriously from the problems of overcrowding. By the 1840s the ratio of general practitioners to population was considerably higher than it has been at any time since, not only in London and the south of England but throughout Britain. Continual complaints of an overcrowded profession (commonly heard from all the professions at this period and therefore to be accepted with caution)[58] were justified. General practitioners, finding they were faced by even greater competition from their colleagues than their traditional enemy the irregular practitioner, were forced to lower their fees. Many went out of business or sank to the level of the dispensing druggist, selling articles of toilet as well as cheap medicines. Very few were able to abandon the practice of pharmacy with its degrading stigma of trade.

This was the reality when the very thing general practitioners were yearning for was professional respectability. They would, if they could, have seen themselves as 'physicians in ordinary'.[59] As the physician Neil Arnott said, most country practitioners would be content if they felt they belonged 'to an honourable body, as the curate who receives £80 to £90 a year belongs to an honourable body and is satisfied with being marked as a gentleman...much of the reward would be the station which the profession gave in society'.[60] Often no more than a hair's-breadth separated the physician and the general practitioner in actual practice and social spectrum of patients. But professional respectability eluded the general practitioner as long as he sold bottles of medicine for sixpence or less, and dug in his back pocket for the change of a shilling like a grocer. As he attempted to climb the ladder of professional distinction to catch the physician, there was the druggist, hard on his heels behind him. 'So long as the general practitioner vends medicine he is a mere poacher of the manor of the Physician, Surgeon and the Druggist.'[61]

---

[58] In the 1840s the ratio of general practitioners to population was 1:602 in London, 1:1,185 in England, 1:1,336 in Scotland and 1:1,691 in Wales. (1841 census, PP, 1844, XXVII, 31–44, 48–51). In the 1950s the ratio of general practitioners to population in the UK was approximately 1:2,500. The number of general practitioners relative to the population fell in the late nineteenth and early twentieth century reaching its lowest point just after the first world war. It then rose, but only slightly until the 1960s. Since then the ratio has increased. However, accurate estimates of secular trends in this ratio over the last 100–150 years are difficult because of changes in methods of recording statistics.

[59] The suggestion that the terms 'physician' and 'general practitioner' should be replaced by 'physician in ordinary' and 'consultant physician' was made in 'Medical Reform', *Medico-Chirurgical Review*, 20 (1834), 567–71.

[60] *Report of the Select Committee on Medical Education*, PP 1834, XIII, Q.2480.

[61] Letter from 'Ille ego qui Quondam', *Lancet*, 1 (1836–7), 647–8.

Faced with the difficulty of making a living at the start of his career, many general practitioners applied for posts as medical officers to the poor law, sick clubs and friendly societies, and factories, mills and mines. Almost all these posts were badly paid. It was a buyer's market which boards of guardians, committees of sick clubs, and industrialists exploited to the full. The post of poor law medical officer (or 'union surgeon') was so often so onerous and despised that it was either abandoned by the practitioner as soon as he had established a private practice, or it was retained solely to keep out 'interlopers'.[62]

A minority of general practitioners obtained posts as honorary surgeon to a hospital, while others accepted appointments at dispensaries, hoping for private practice from the introductions to the governors and subscribers.[63]

Competition, a low income derived largely from the practice of pharmacy, the need to accept poorly paid and degrading posts and the scorn of the upper ranks of the profession underlined the low status of the general practitioner. He became the victim of a series of scurrilous attacks on his status and competence, not only from the upper ranks but also from his peers. Self-denigration became an unattractive habit. The general practitioner was 'a mongrel kind of doctor, man-midwife, surgeon and druggist, a true jack-of-all-trades and master of none', looked upon by the public with 'a sort of good natured contempt'.[64] The general practitioner was, at the lowest level, 'the son of an ordinary trader' who practised in 'low pestiferous districts where he exercises his functions amongst the dirtiest and most ignorant'; above this came the general practitioner who was 'patronised by the shoe-maker and milkman...the huckster and greengrocer...he is in great force with domestic servants, and a great gun with the stable fraternity'.[65] He was even 'the scion of the chopper in love with amputations' who marries 'the red-headed daughter of the grocer' after a training spent in

---

[62] I. Loudon, "'I'd Rather Have Been a Parish Surgeon than a Union One'", *Bulletin of the Society for the Social History of Medicine*, 38 (1986), 68–73.

[63] 'Duties and Privations of Medical Practitioners', *London Medical Gazette*, new series 1 (1832), 633–5. The provident dispensaries, most of which were established after 1830, became an important source of income for general practitioners. At these, patients subscribed so much a week or month, and fees were given to medical officers in proportion to the number of patients who chose a particular doctor. The kind of income available to a medical officer at one of the largest dispensaries could be as much as £50 a year, or occasionally more.

[64] *Homeopathic Times*, 1 (1834), 34–6.

[65] George Allarton, MRCS LSA, *Mysteries of Medical Life* (London, 1856). Perhaps the author felt his position as a deputy coroner as well as a general practitioner entitled him to make such scathing comments about his colleagues.

'adultery, drinking, murder and what-not before the age of nineteen ... such as he is the immense majority of general practitioners'.[66] Such attacks, numerous and often brutal, were mostly the work of medical men and they showed how rapidly the optimism which infused the Association of Apothecaries and Surgeon–Apothecaries had turned sour.

Public attitudes, however, as revealed by novels and articles, were usually more sympathetic to the general practitioner than the physician. The typical London physician was portrayed as pompous, snobbish, rich and greedy. He was fond of scientific jargon but apt to prevaricate when it came to treatment or prognosis.[67] In contrast, the family doctor was portrayed as poor, often shabby, harried by overwork and constantly in demand night and day; but he was valued because he was a familiar figure, because he was discreet and because he was usually attentive to his patients. He had to be. In effect, he combined a pastoral and a clinical role in which it was on the whole an advantage if he was a bit old-fashioned in his ways and 'had no nonsensical ideas about new theories prescribing very much the same kinds of remedies which his late employer had been in the habit of prescribing'.[68] People never did quite trust the 'latest thing' in medicine.

An acid critic of the medical profession in Birmingham who must have made the doctors blush, made a special exception of the general practitioner: 'I know the family doctor is deservedly esteemed ... I know what consolation there is in his kindly assurance, what comfort in his smile.'[69] Notice the use of 'family doctor'. This was the practitioner who was a familiar figure of town or village; who 'had brought scores of matrons safely through their confinements, vaccinated hundreds of infants, drawn countless teeth, and physicked, cupped, bled, blistered

---

[66] *Dublin Medical Press*, 19 (1845), 205–6.

[67] One has only to think of Dr Omnicron Pie, Dr Fillgrave and Dr Mewdew in Anthony Trollope's novels, or Charles Dickens's insufferably pompous Dr Parker Peps in *Dombey and Son*. There is a fine specimen of the pompous physician in Amelia Edwards, *Barbara's History*, 2 vols. (London, 1864), I, p. 114. But it was the London physicians who were subjected to ridicule. The provincial practitioners of Victorian fiction include George Eliot's Dr Lydgate, and Anthony Trollope's Dr Thorne (best described as a physicianly general practitioner). Both are perceptive and sympathetic portraits.

[68] This was young Mr Mellidew, the general practitioner in Henry James Byron, 'Paid in Full', serialized in *Temple Bar Magazine*, 13 (1864–5), 246–7. As a characteristically poor and shabby GP, Mr Mellidew 'wore a cheap heavy hat which was brown from many showers. He enclosed his feet in clumsy half-wellingtons which were patched and mended until they lost all semblance of their original shape. There was generally a button or two missing from his waistcoat; and an obtrusive pin or two visible here and there about his garments.' For all the shabbiness the portrait is a kindly rather than a scornful one.

[69] 'Scrutator', *The Medical Charities of Birmingham* (Birmingham, 1863), p. 36.

and clystered generations upon generations'.[70] Even if Mr Hall in *Wives and Daughters* was old, going blind and a bit deaf 'he was still Mr Hall who could heal all their ailments'.[71] In short, the cult of the family doctor had arrived by the mid nineteenth century. Even physicians were sometimes excessive in their praise. [72] It can be argued that fiction is an unreliable source for historical conclusions; but fiction was not the only source of this rosy picture of the kind old family doctor. It can indeed be argued that the cult of the family doctor had more to do with the Victorian passion for sentimentality and nostalgia than professionalism or scientific competence. Nevertheless, as an ideal, the family doctor was established as the model for the development of general practice, and the so-called backbone of British medicine. As recently as 1967, Ann Cartwright described the concept of the family doctor as one of the sacred cows of general practice that no one except McKeown had dared to criticize.[73]

If the general practitioner had gained the affection of his patients, he had failed to achieve professional parity either in income or status. The average annual income of general practitioners in the first half of the nineteenth century was, at most, £150–£200. In Scotland it was lower. Even if the effects of inflation are discounted, this was significantly less than the income of the surgeon–apothecaries of the late eighteenth century.[74] General practitioners blamed their lack of political power and the absence of an institution to represent their views; it is significant that no one felt the Society of Apothecaries filled this role. Several general practitioner societies and associations were established for this purpose, notably the National Association of General Practitioners, created in 1845 for the purpose of founding a College of General Practitioners. After five years of setbacks and opposition from the physicians and surgeons, it very nearly succeeded. But an agreement that such a college should be established, already signed by the heads of all the medical corporations, was rejected at the last minute by Council of the Royal

[70] John Mills, *The Belle of the Village* (London, 1852).

[71] Elizabeth Gaskell, *Wives and Daughters* (first published 1862, paperback edn Penguin Books, 1969).

[72] W. A. Greenhill, an Oxford physician, wrote in his *Address to a Medical Student* (London, 1843), that 'the *perfect* specimen of a General Practitioner [with] his long and weary rides at all hours and in all weathers, and then his scanty payment [is] the noblest member of the whole medical profession...surely we may call him the *Missionary* of his profession.'

[73] Ann Cartwright, *Patients and their Doctors* (London, 1967).

[74] There was also the cost of medical training. In the mid to late eighteenth century the cost of training (apprenticeship and hospital) was equivalent to one year's income in mid-career, at most. By the mid nineteenth, the cost of medical training for a general practitioner was equal to about four years' income in mid-career.

College of Surgeons and ended the political activities of the general practitioners for many years to come.[75]

Eight years later the Medical Act was passed and the General Medical Council established. This was not a new initiative. The introduction of an Act to regulate the medical profession began in 1840 and ground through fifteen unsuccessful Bills before the sixteenth received the Royal assent in 1858.[76] By 1850, not only had the general practitioners failed to establish a college for themselves, but the profession and parliament had become weary of medical reform. As we hinted earlier, the Medical Act was a disappointment to the majority of practitioners. It provided only an external appearance of unity when the profession remained deeply divided. The power of the medical corporations was increased rather than diminished, and the plan for a 'single portal of entry' had failed. To this day British doctors possess such a wide variety of 'registerable qualifications' in the form of degrees, diplomas and licences that they mystify everyone except the members of the British medical profession. The outlawing of irregular practice (never a practical possibility, but nevertheless one of the major ambitions of the profession) did not take place. Many doctors were not properly trained, even by the standards of the mid nineteenth century. It was still possible to register as a qualified doctor on the basis of a single qualification in medicine or surgery until this and other features of the Medical Act of 1858 were changed by the passing of the Medical Act Amendment Act in 1886.

Conclusion

To describe the period of medical reform solely as a period dominated by self-interest and the attempt by the medical profession to create a monopoly of medical care would be as naive as to describe it as a glorious phase of uninterrupted progress. We have already stressed that the predominant feeling of the majority who practised medicine during the first half of the nineteenth century was frustration rather than exhilaration at the progress achieved. They were only too aware of the missed opportunities in the brief period of some thirty years from 1812 to the 1840s when radical change was still a possibility. For example, a rise in the status of the general practitioner *vis-à-vis* the surgeon and physician might have led to a system of medical education based on

---

[75] For an account of this attempt to establish a college of general practitioners see chapter 13 in Loudon, *Medical Care and the General Practitioner*.

[76] Charles Newman, *The Evolution of Medical Education in the Nineteenth Century* (London, 1957).

training in the community rather than hospitals, with a greater emphasis
on the common diseases and the problems of public health. The Poor
Law Amendment Act of 1834 provided the opportunity for a
comprehensive system of medical care for the poor when they
desperately needed it, but parsimony and prejudice against poverty
produced a miserable and inadequate system.[77] A low standard of
obstetric care, reflected in a persistently high maternal mortality rate,
was associated with the scorn of physicians and surgeons for this branch
of medicine. Elizabeth Garrett Anderson put the blame on the examiners,
and there is little doubt she was right.[78] All this makes the period of
medical reform a tempting subject for historically unprofitable
speculation on what might or might not have occurred had events taken
a different course.

With hindsight, however, no one can deny some progress was
achieved, chiefly in the education and regulation of the profession, and
most of all in the laying of foundations for future advances. Even if we
dispute the nature and extent of such progress, it is certain that the period
from the late eighteenth century to the mid nineteenth laid the
foundations of the medical profession as we know it today. Since the
1850s the only major structural change in the medical profession has been
the multiplication of specialities, and most of these were established
under the aegis of the Royal Colleges of Physicians and Surgeons.

There are many characteristics of modern British medicine that are
often taken for granted. For instance, the continuing control of the
medical colleges over specialist qualifications in spite of the growing
involvement of the universities in the process we have described as the
'academization' of medicine; the dominance of the teaching hospitals
and the high status of the consultant compared to the general practitioner,
associated with the centralization of clinical education on the hospitals
rather than the community; the growth of specialization; and the
peculiarly British principle of referral.[79] None of these features were the
preordained and inevitable consequences of the demands of society or
government, and only marginally were they determined by advances in

[77] M. W. Flinn, 'Medical Services Under the New Poor Law', in D. Fraser (ed.), *The New Poor Law in the Nineteenth Century* (London, 1984).
[78] E. G. Anderson, 'Deaths in Childbirth', *British Medical Journal*, 2 (1898), 839–40, 927.
[79] The principle of referral demands that consultants do not see patients directly but only those referred by general practitioners. It was a principle gradually introduced from the late nineteenth century at the insistence of general practitioners when a very large amount of primary care was being undertaken in hospital out-patient and casualty departments. Direct access of patients to consultants and to hospitals in Britain has, since the Second World War, been largely confined to accidents and a few special clinics.

medical care and medical science. They were to a much greater extent the products of intra-professional conflict during the period of medical reform, when high-minded determination to improve standards of medical education and medical care was inextricably mixed with personal ambition and aspirations towards professional, social, and financial success and respectability.

Public health, preventive medicine and professionalization: England and America in the nineteenth century

ELIZABETH FEE AND DOROTHY PORTER

Public health in both England and America began as a response to the social and health problems of rapid industrialization. Initially, the public health movement was created by social reformers including, but not led by, the medical profession. As public health became professionalized, physicians came to play a more dominant role. In England, the medical profession would eventually incorporate public health as 'preventive medicine'. In the United States, public health would retain a certain independence from medicine; as the medical profession remained wedded to fee-for-service practice and displayed little interest in salaried public health positions, public health evolved as a somewhat separate professional specialty, staffed by biologists, statisticians, engineers, and others with specialized training. In both England and America, however, the professionalization of public health involved a certain distancing from the original social reform impulses which had given it birth. Scientific methods tempered, when they did not replace, the initial commitment to improving the lives and living standards of the poor.

A great expansion of public health as social reform began in France and Germany in the mid nineteenth century. 1848 was the year of revolutions in Europe. Social, economic and political crises in France and Germany were matched by the physical and health crises of urbanism in the industrializing nations of the continent. Growing epidemic diseases from the late eighteenth century had brought the health of the community in ever-more densely populated mass societies into the arena of European politics. The year 1848 also saw, therefore, a high profile of political discussions regarding health and disease in France and Germany:

in England, the year was marked by the passing of the first Public Health Act.[1]

Panics generated by visitations into Europe of dramatic killer-diseases, such as Asiatic cholera in 1832, heightened the social disruptiveness of epidemic diseases but did not, in themselves, bring about substantial reforms.[2] The underlying conflicts of urbanization and urban health were better revealed in the indigenous, continuing problems of endemic fevers – smallpox, intermittent fever (malaria), typhus and typhoid – and chronic sicknesses which were reproduced by insanitary living conditions and nutritional deficiencies. Social movements developed across Europe during the 1830s and 1840s, concerned with the health of towns, the role of medicine as a political force, with health as a right of citizenship and with the relationship between sickness, poverty and death.[3]

The social historian of medicine, Richard Shryock, described the movements for sanitary reform in Europe in this period as led by individuals who were primarily interested in broad economic and social changes. Sanitarians, he suggested, viewed poverty and disease as forming a reciprocal cycle responsible for the dysfunctions of urban, industrial society.[4] Our reading of the lives and work of the central figures in the sanitary movements in Britain, France and Germany before 1850 supports this view.

After the end of the Napoleonic wars, the major educational reforms undertaken in France included the creation of a new medical academy in Paris with a department of hygiene under the direction of Jean Nöel Hallé. Hygienists studying at this department completed large-scale investigations into the disease consequences of population density and dirt in the urban centres of France.[5] A socio-political analysis emerged from this work, the essential arguments of which were articulated in the *Gazette Médicale* in 1848.[6] Here the term 'social medicine' was coined by Jules Guérin who outlined the political role of medicine in France as that of redressing the balance between industrial growth and the preservation

---

[1] See Richard H. Shryock, *The Development of Modern Medicine* (Madison, WI, 1979), pp. 211–47; and George Rosen, *A History of Public Health*, 3rd edn (New York, 1976), pp. 192–293.

[2] M. Pelling, *Cholera, Fever and English Medicine, 1825–1865* (London, 1978), pp. 1–33.

[3] George Rosen, *From Medical Police to Social Medicine* (New York, 1974). See also D. Porter and R. Porter, 'What Was Social Medicine? An Historiographical Essay', *The Journal of Historical Sociology*, 1 (1988), 90–106. [4] Shryock, *Development of Modern Medicine*, p. 221.

[5] E. H. Ackerknecht, 'Hygiene in France, 1815–1848', *Bulletin of the History of Medicine*, 22 (1948), 117–55.

[6] Iago Galdston, *Social and Historical Foundations of Modern Medicine* (New York, 1981), pp. 74–8.

of health.[7] The career of the leading French hygienist at this time, Louis René Villermé, illustrates these developments in medical politics.

Villermé and his contemporaries, from their economistic perspective, were pessimistic about solving the underlying problems of the social system. The sickness of civilization, they maintained, had no cure; in the view of the 'parti d'hygiène publique', medicine could at best rise to the challenge of *amelioration*. Epidemics could be addressed and their worst ravages reduced. Although the malfunctions of civilization lay deep in the structure of civil society, disease prevention and the reduction of mortality could be achieved through hygienic regulation of the environment and scientific investigation into the causes of disease.[8]

In Germany, members of the medical reform movement initially believed that the politics of health had a wider mandate. Salamon Neuman, Rudolf Virchow and their associates stated clearly in their broadsheet, *Die Medizinsche Reform* in 1848, that medicine *was* politics.[9] Virchow outlined a sociological explanation of the epidemiological patterns of disease in his essays on the outbreak of typhus in Upper Silesia.[10] Although he viewed communism as 'madness', Virchow was committed to a political ideal that the poor and the oppressed should not have to wait for heaven for their rewards; a healthful existence should be a right of citizenship in this life.[11] Throughout his career, the founder of cellular pathology rejected any monocausal aetiology, even after the bacteriological explanation of disease had been well established. He maintained his heterodox view of the multi-causality of disease and continued to assert that medicine should become part of a political process of change and transition to a fully democratic, welfare-based, society.[12] In this context the role of the physician should be as 'the natural attorney of the poor'.[13]

---

[7] René Sand, *Vers la médecine* (Paris and Brussels, 1948), pp. 573–4.

[8] William Coleman, *Death is a Social Disease. Public Health and Political Economy in Early Industrial France* (Madison, WI, 1982), pp. 277–306.

[9] Erwin Ackerknecht, *Rudolf Virchow: Doctor, Statesman, Anthropologist* (Madison, WI, 1953), pp. 130–46. [10] *Ibid.*, pp. 123–37.

[11] *Ibid.*, p. 166; H. G. Schlumberger, 'Rudolph Virchow – Revolutionist', *Annals of Medical History*, 3rd series, 4 (1942), 147–53.

[12] Ackerknecht, *Virchow*, pp. 105–18; David Pridan, 'Rudolph Virchow and Social Medicine in Historical Perspective', *Medical History*, 8 (1964), 275.

[13] Virchow as quoted by George Rosen in 'Disease and Social Criticism: A Contribution to a Theory of Medical History', *Bulletin of the History of Medicine*, 10 (1941), 15.

The origins of public health in England

In England, Edwin Chadwick, a civil servant and disciple of the political philosopher Jeremy Bentham, was the leader of the sanitary movement in the 1830s and 1840s.[14] As part of his work for the Poor Law Commission from 1834, Chadwick's view of the relationship between poverty and disease was similar to Virchow's. In contrast to Virchow, however, Chadwick believed that the science of engineering rather than medicine should play the greater role in the development of sanitary reform. According to Chadwick's 'sanitary idea', engineering should become the handmaiden to the political economy of felicific calculus in order to achieve the greatest happiness of the greatest number. This ideology, however, was not realized in the way Chadwick had envisaged it. From the outset, the public health service employed medical men.[15]

While Chadwick was secretary of the Poor Law Commission in 1838, it employed three medical practitioners as inspectors to inquire into the state of health and sickness in London. Neil Arnott, James Phillips Kay (later Kay-Shuttleworth) and Thomas Southwood Smith produced a report which revealed the desperate living conditions of the poor in London, and all three remained leading figures in the sanitary reform movement.[16] Smith, in particular, became Chadwick's close ally. He, like Chadwick, had served as a secretary to Jeremy Bentham. He helped to found the Metropolitan Health of Towns Association in 1844, which became a model for many more provincial Associations, acting as a major extra-parliamentary pressure group for public health reforms.[17]

In 1839, the Poor Law Commission was instructed to undertake inquiries into the health of the working classes throughout England and Wales, and later also in Scotland. The result, the largest social survey completed to that date, was published by Chadwick in 1842.[18] The thrust of the 1842 report was that epidemic diseases were caused by environmental filth and that the means of prevention were the provision of clean water supplies, effective sewerage and drainage, removal of nuisances such as refuse from all streets and roads, control of industrial

[14] S. E. Finer, *The Life and Times of Edwin Chadwick* (London, 1952), pp. 218–28.

[15] *Ibid.*, pp. 1–55. For further discussion of Chadwick see R. A. Lewis, *Edwin Chadwick and the Public Health Movement* (London, 1952).

[16] See discussion in John Simon, *English Sanitary Institutions* (London, 1890), pp. 178–87. See also W. M. Frazer, *The History of English Public Health, 1834–1839* (London, 1950), pp. 12–23.

[17] C. L. Lewes, *Dr Southwood Smith* (London and Edinburgh, 1898).

[18] E. Chadwick, *General Report on the Sanitary Conditions of the Labouring Classes of Great Britain, 1842*, edited and reprinted by M. W. Flinn (Edinburgh, 1965).

effluents, and the establishment of new standards of environmental and personal cleanliness. The report recommended that entirely new structures of administration be created, both in local and central government, for achieving these goals, including the appointment of 'district medical officers' constantly to inspect and report on local sanitary conditions.[19] As a result of the report, a Royal Commission was set up in 1843 to consider the health of towns; the substance of its proposals was eventually incorporated into the Public Health Act of 1848. The Act established a central government department to deal with public health, the General Board of Health, and local sanitary authorities to coordinate the municipal responsibilities for environmental regulation which had previously been chaotically distributed between myriad local commissions. A system for local inspection was created through the appointment of medical officers of health.[20] The power of the Act, however, was seriously undermined by being adoptive rather than compulsory, and it thus resulted in uneven standards of public health regulation throughout the kingdom.

Chadwick, supported by Thomas Southwood Smith's studies of fever, adopted the miasmatic theory of disease causation to legitimate an environmentalist programme of disease control.[21] This became the official orthodoxy of the General Board of Health and governed its policies.[22] The miasmatic theory offered an atmospheric explanation of disease causation wherein pollution in the air, which arose from decaying organic matter, provided the source of infection and epidemic spread. Erwin Ackerknecht has suggested that this 'anti-contagionist' theory dominated the thinking of sanitarians throughout Europe during the 1840s and 1850s.[23] It is not clear, however, that it was widely adopted among the medical profession in England. Margaret Pelling has demonstrated that the epidemiology of the sanitary era in England was characterized by a complex range of theories which incorporated both ideas of environmental pollution and explanations of disease transmission through contact.[24]

---

[19] *Ibid.* For contemporary discussion of the 1842 report see Simon, *English Sanitary Institutions*, pp. 187–202. See also Finer, *Chadwick*, pp. 209–29, 293–9.

[20] See Frazer, *English Public Health*, pp. 18–37; Finer, *Chadwick*, pp. 319–37. A model of local sanitary administration had already been established under a separate public health act for Liverpool in 1846 where the first medical officer of health, William Duncan, had been appointed. See W. M. Frazer, *Duncan of Liverpool* (London, 1947).

[21] See Thomas Southwood Smith, *Treatise on Fever* (London, 1830).

[22] See Pelling, *Cholera*.

[23] E. H. Ackerknecht, 'Anti Contagionism Between 1821–1867', *Bulletin of the History of Medicine*, 22 (1948), 568–93.   [24] Pelling, *Cholera*, pp. 70–9.

Despite variation in disease theories and policy tactics, sanitary science, both in England and on the continent during the 1840s, was ostensibly a political activity with social and economic change as its goal. Later, the sophistication of state medicine, at least as it emerged in England, began at mid century to shift the emphasis of reform from legislative change to administrative implementation. A new balance of aims altered the course of disease prevention up to the early years of the twentieth century.

Public health in the United States

The social crises generated by industrial development did not become obvious in the United States until the late nineteenth century. Until then, epidemic diseases were believed to pose only occasional threats to an otherwise healthy social order. By the last decades of the century, however, the burgeoning social problems of the industrial cities could no longer be ignored: the overwhelming influx of immigrants crowded into narrow alleys and tenement housing; the terrifying death and disease rates of working-class slums; the total inadequacy of water supplies and sewage systems for the rapidly growing population; the spread of endemic and epidemic diseases from the slums to the homes of the wealthy; and the escalating squalor and violence of the streets. Almost all families lost children to diphtheria, smallpox or other infectious diseases. Poverty and disease could no longer be treated simply as individual failings.

The early efforts of city health department officials to deal with health problems represented some attempt to mitigate the worst effects of unplanned and unregulated growth; a kind of rearguard action against the filth and congestion created by anarchic economic and urban development.[25] As cities grew in size, as the flow of immigrants continued, and as public health problems became ever more obvious, pressures mounted for more effective responses to the problems. New York, the largest city, and the one with some of the worst health conditions, produced some of the most active and progressive public

[25] John Blake, *Public Health in the Town of Boston, 1630–1822* (Cambridge, MA, 1959); Barbara Rosenkrantz, *Public Health and the State: Changing Views in Massachusetts, 1842–1936* (Cambridge, MA, 1972); John Duffy, *A History of Public Health in New York City, 1625–1866* (New York, 1968); John Duffy, *A History of Public Health in New York City, 1866–1966* (New York, 1974); Stuart Galishoff, *Safeguarding the Public Health: Newark, 1895–1918* (Westport, CT, 1975); Judith Walzer Leavitt, *The Healthiest City: Milwaukee and the Politics of Health Reform* (Princeton, NJ, 1982).

health leaders; Boston and Providence were also noted for their public health programmes; Baltimore and Philadelphia trailed far behind.[26]

Industrialization had meant new sources of affluence as well as of misery. America no longer fitted its self-image as a country of independent farmers and craftsmen; like the European countries, it displayed extremes of wealth and privilege, social misery and deprivation. Labour and social unrest pushed awareness of the need for social and health reforms. The great railroad strike of 1877, the assassination of President Garfield in 1881, the Haymarket bombing of 1886, the Homestead strike of 1892, and the Pullman strike of 1894 were just a few of the reminders that all was not well with the republic. The Noble Order of the Knights of Labor – dedicated to such measures as an income tax, an eight-hour day, social insurance, labour exchanges for the unemployed, the abolition of child labour, workmen's compensation and public ownership of railroads and utilities – grew from a membership of eleven to over 700,000 within a few years. Massive strikes for better wages and working conditions revealed deep class divisions and seemed to threaten social disorder. At the same time, the development of democratic machine politics challenged the dominance of the political and social elite, permitting some labour leaders to establish local bases of influence and power. The perceived social anarchy of the large industrial cities mocked the pretensions to social control of the traditional forces of church and state, and highlighted the need for more activist responses to the multiplicity of problems.

An increasing number of reform groups devoted themselves to social issues and improvements of every variety.[27] Health reformers, physicians and engineers urged improved sanitary conditions in the industrial cities. Medical men were prominent in reform organizations, but they were not alone.[28] Barbara Rosenkrantz contrasted public health in the late

[26] Charles-E. A. Winslow, *The Life of Hermann M. Biggs: Physician and Statesman of the Public Health* (Philadelphia, PA, 1929); E. O. Jordan, G. C. Whipple, C.-E. A. Winslow, *A Pioneer of Public Health: William Thompson Sedgwick* (New Haven, CT, 1924); James H. Cassedy, *Charles V. Chapin and the Public Health Movement* (Cambridge, MA, 1962); Rosenkrantz, *Public Health and the State*.

[27] Public health reform was a low priority for American social reformers generally. Slavery, for example, attracted much more attention a lot earlier. See Elizabeth Fee, *Disease and Discovery. A History of the Johns Hopkins School of Hygiene and Public Health 1916–1939* (Baltimore and London, 1987), pp. 1–30.

[28] Charles E. and Carroll S. Rosenberg, 'Pietism and the Origins of the American Public Health Movement', *Journal of the History of Medicine and Allied Sciences*, 23 (1968), 16–35; Richard H. Shryock, 'The Early American Public Health Movement', *American Journal of Public Health*, 27 (1937), 965–71.

nineteenth century with the internecine battles within general medicine: 'the field of public hygiene exemplified a happy marriage of engineers, physicians and public-spirited citizens providing a model of complementary comportment under the banner of sanitary science'.[29] The most formally organized and professional body, the American Public Health Association, included scientists, municipal officials, physicians, engineers, and the occasional architect and lawyer.[30]

Middle- and upper-class women, seizing an opportunity to escape from the narrow bounds of domestic responsibilities, joined in campaigns for improved housing, for the abolition of child labour, for maternal and child health, and for temperance; they were active in the settlement house movement (aiding the urban poor), trade union organizing, the suffrage movement, and municipal sanitary reform. The latter, as 'municipal housekeeping' was viewed as particularly suitable for women as a natural extension of women's training and experience as the housekeepers of the world.[31] These voluntary movements organized to support specific issues provided the organizational framework for many public health reforms. By the early years of the twentieth century, many such voluntary health organizations were established and active.[32]

The progressive reform groups in the public health movement advocated immediate change tempered by scientific knowledge and humanitarian concern. Sharing the revolutionaries' perception of the plight of the poor and the injustices of the system, they counselled less radical solutions.[33] They advocated public health reforms on political, economic, humanitarian and scientific grounds. Politically, public health reform offered a middle ground between the cutthroat principles of entrepreneurial capitalism and the revolutionary ideas of the socialists,

[29] Barbara Rosenkrantz, 'Cart Before Horse: Theory, Practice and Professional Image in American Public Health 1870–1920', *Journal of the History of Medicine and Allied Sciences*, 29 (1974), 57.

[30] Stephen Smith, 'The History of Public Health, 1871–1921', in Mazyck P. Ravenel (ed.), *A Half Century of Public Health* (New York, 1921), pp. 1–12; Mazyck P. Ravenel, 'The American Public Health Association: Past, Present, Future', in Ravenel, *Half Century*, pp. 13–55.

[31] See Mary P. Ryan, *Womanhood in America: From Colonial Times to the Present* (New York, 1975), pp. 225–34.

[32] The American Red Cross had been formed in 1882, the National Tuberculosis Association in 1904, the American Social Hygiene Association in 1905, the National Committee for Mental Hygiene in 1909, and the American Society for the Control of Cancer in 1919. See Wilson G. Smillie, *Public Health: Its Promise for the Future* (New York, 1955), pp. 450–8.

[33] Robert H. Wiebe, *The Search for Order, 1877–1920* (New York, 1967); Samuel P. Hays, 'The Politics of Reform in Municipal Government in the Progressive Era', in *American Political History as Social Analysis* (Knoxville, 1980), pp. 205–32; Samuel P. Hays, *Conservation and the Gospel of Efficiency: The Progressive Conservation Movement, 1890–1918* (Boston, 1968); Daniel T. Rogers, 'In Search of Progressivism', *Reviews in American History*, 10 (1982), 115–32.

anarchists and utopian visionaries. As William H. Welch expressed it to the Charity Organization Society, sanitary improvements offered the best way of improving the lot of the poor, short of the radical restructuring of society.[34]

An economic argument promoted by the progressive reformers was that public health should be viewed as a paying investment, giving higher returns than the stock market. In Germany, Max von Pettenkofer had first calculated the financial returns on public health 'investments' to prove the value of sanitary reform in reducing deaths from typhoid, and his argument would be repeated many times by American public health leaders.[35] As Welch explained:

merely from a mercenary and commercial point of view it is for the interest of the community to take care of the health of the poor. Philanthropy assumes a totally different aspect in the eyes of the world when it is able to demonstrate that it pays to keep people healthy.[36]

Whether progressives stressed the humanitarian need for reform or the business efficiency of improving public health, they emphasized the need for more scientific knowledge and training for those responsible for public health activities. They argued that public health should be a profession with appropriate training and income:

We hope that every local unit of government will have its health officer and that the iceman and the undertaker will not be considered suitable candidates, but that every health officer will be trained for his work. We hope that he will receive a reasonable reward for his services, and that the pay for saving a child's life with antitoxin will at least equal that received by a plumber for mending a leaky pipe; and that for managing a yellow fever outbreak a man may receive as much per week as a catcher on a baseball nine.[37]

The demand for centralized planning and business efficiency required scientific knowledge rather than the undisciplined enthusiasms of voluntary groups.[38] Public health decisions should be made by an

[34] William Henry Welch, 'Sanitation in Relation to the Poor'. An address to the Sanitation Organization Society of Baltimore, November 1892, in *Papers and Addresses by William Henry Welch*, vol. III (Baltimore, 1920), p. 598.

[35] For a classic statement of this argument, see Max von Pettenkofer, *The Value of Health to a City*. Translated with an introduction by Henry E. Sigerist (Baltimore, 1941), pp. 15–52.

[36] William Henry Welch, 'Sanitation in Relation to the Poor', p. 596.

[37] Charles Chapin, 'Pleasures and Hopes of the Health Officer', in *Papers of Charles V. Chapin, M.D.*, compiled by F. P. Gorham and C. L. Scamman (Oxford, 1934), p. 11; William Henry Welch, 'Sanitation in Relation to the Poor', p. 596.

[38] Thomas M. Rotch, 'The Position and Work of the American Pediatric Society Toward Public Questions', *Transactions of the American Pediatric Society*, 21 (1909), 12.

analysis of costs and benefits 'as an up-to-date manufacturer would count the cost of a new process'. The health officer, like the merchant, should learn 'which line of work yields the most for the sum expended'.[39]

Existing health departments were dominated more by patronage and political considerations than by economic or administrative efficiency. Progressives regretted 'the evil of politics' and wanted to increase the pay and minimum qualifications for health officers to attract personnel on the basis of skill rather than influence. The attempt to insulate boards of health from local political control was part of a broader movement to make all forms of public administration more 'rational' and 'efficient' by reducing the influence of political bosses and by promoting a new group of professional administrators.[40] The goal was for a well-trained professional elite to conduct social reform on scientific lines. It seemed only a matter of selecting the right people and giving them the best possible training for the job. As William Sedgwick argued:

If, as I believe, we are in fact moving irresistibly towards a bureaucracy, while clinging to the ideals of a democracy, we shall do well to pause and inquire what kind of bureaucracy we are building up about ourselves…scientists and technicians alike … must be employed and paid by the people, to rule over them as well as to guide and to guard them, to constitute a kind of official class, a kind of bureaucracy constituted for themselves by the people themselves…what kind of scientists and technicians shall we have in our public service?…I honestly believe that upon our ability to solve, and solve wisely, these fundamental problems of our American life will depend in large measure our comfort and success as a people in the 20th century.[41]

Public health was quickly becoming a national and even international issue. Although the United States congress was reluctant to enact federal health legislation, there were mounting pressures for United States attention to public health abroad. As American businessmen were seeking enlarged foreign markets, a vocal group of intellectuals and politicians argued for an assertive foreign policy. The United States began to challenge European dominance in the Far East and Latin America, seeking trade and political influence more than territory, but taking territory where it could. National defence goals included

[39] Charles Chapin, 'How Shall We Spend the Health Appropriation?', in *Papers of Charles V. Chapin, M.D.*, pp. 28–35.
[40] Martin J. Schiesl, *The Politics of Efficiency: Municipal Administration and Reform in America, 1880–1920* (Berkeley and London, 1980).
[41] William T. Sedgwick, 'Scientists and Technicians in the Public Service', as cited in E. O. Jordan, G. C. Whipple, C.-E. A. Winslow, *William Thompson Sedgwick*, pp. 133–4.

broadening control of trade routes, building a Central American canal, and establishing strategic bases in the Caribbean and western Pacific.

In 1898, the United States entered the Spanish–American War, expanded the army from 25,000 to 250,000 men, and sent troops to Cuba. That war showed that the United States could not afford military adventures overseas unless more attention was paid to sanitation and public health: 968 men died in battle, but 5,438 died of infectious diseases.[42] Nonetheless, the United States defeated Spain, and installed an army of occupation in Cuba. When yellow fever threatened the troops in 1900, the response was efficient and effective. An army commission under Walter Reed was sent to Cuba to study the disease and, in a dramatic series of human experiments, confirmed the hypothesis that it was spread by mosquitoes; Surgeon-Major William Gorgas then eliminated yellow fever from Havana.[43]

This experience confirmed the importance of public health for successful US efforts overseas. Earlier efforts to dig the Panama Canal had been attended by enormous mortality rates from disease.[44] But, in 1904, Gorgas, now promoted to General, took control of a campaign against malaria and yellow fever threatening canal operations. He was finally able to persuade the Canal Commission to institute an intensive campaign against mosquitoes; in one of the great triumphs of practical public health, yellow fever and malaria were brought under control and the canal successfully completed in 1914.

US industrialists brought some of the lessons of Cuba and the Panama Canal home to the southern United States. The south at that time resembled an underdeveloped country within the US, characterized by poor economic and social conditions. The northern industrialists were already investing heavily in southern education as well as in cotton mills and railroads; John D. Rockefeller had created the General Education Board to support 'the general organization of rural communities for economic, social and educational purposes'.[45] Charles Wardell Stiles managed to convince the secretary of the General Education Board that the real cause of misery and lack of productivity in the south was

---

[42] George M. Sternberg, 'Sanitary Lessons of the War', in *Sanitary Lessons of the War and Other Papers* (Washington, DC, 1912), p. 2; see also Graham A. Cosmas, *An Army for Empire: The United States Army in the Spanish-American War* (Columbia, MO, 1971).

[43] Howard A. Kelley, *Walter Reed and Yellow Fever* (Baltimore, 1906).

[44] George M. Sternberg, 'Sanitary Problems Connected with the Construction of the Isthmian Canal', in *Sanitary Lessons*, pp. 39–40.

[45] Raymond B. Fosdick, *Adventure in Giving: The Story of the General Education Board* (New York and Evanston, 1962), pp. 57–8.

hookworm, the 'germ of laziness'. In 1909, Rockefeller agreed to provide $1 million to create the Rockefeller Sanitary Commission for the Eradication of Hookworm Disease, with Wickliffe Rose as director.[46] This was to be the first instalment in Rockefeller's massive national and international investment in public health.

Rose went beyond the task of attempting to control a single disease and worked to establish an effective and permanent public health organization in the southern states.[47] At the end of five years of intensive effort, the campaign had failed to eradicate hookworm, but had greatly expanded the role of public health agencies. Many state health departments were greatly strengthened, and at the most local level, some rural areas began active health programmes. Between 1910 and 1914, total county appropriations for public health work increased from $240 to $110,000.[48] In 1914, the organizational experience gained in the southern states enabled the Rockefeller Foundation to extend the hookworm control programme to the Caribbean, Central America and Latin America.

Meanwhile, in Washington, the Committee of One Hundred on National Health, composed of such notables as Jane Addams, Andrew Carnegie, William H. Welch and Booker T. Washington, campaigned for the federal regulation of public health.[49] Its president, the economist Irving Fisher, argued that a public health service would be good policy and good economics, in conserving 'national vitality'.[50] In 1912, the federal government made its first real commitment to public health when it expanded the responsibilities of the Public Health Service, empowering it to investigate the causes and spread of diseases, and the pollution and sanitation of navigable streams and lakes.[51] By 1915, the Public Health Service, the US Army and the Rockefeller Foundation were the major agencies involved in public health activities, supplemented on a local level by a network of city and state health departments.

[46] For a detailed account of the Rockefeller Sanitary Commission, see John Ettling, *The Germ of Laziness: Rockefeller Philanthropy and Public Health in the New South* (Cambridge, MA, 1981).

[47] Wickliffe Rose, *First Annual Report of the Administrative Secretary of the Rockefeller Sanitary Commission* (1910), p. 4, as cited in Raymond B. Fosdick, *The Story of the Rockefeller Foundation* (New York, 1952), p. 33.   [48] Ettling, *Germ of Laziness*, pp. 220–1.

[49] George Rosen, 'The Committee of One Hundred on National Health and the Campaign for a National Health Department, 1906–1912', *American Journal of Public Health*, 62 (1972), 261–3; Alan I. Marcus, 'Disease Prevention in America: From a Local to a National Outlook, 1880–1910', *Bulletin of the History of Medicine*, 53 (1979), 184–203.

[50] Irving Fisher, *A Report on National Vitality, Its Wastes and Conservation*, Bulletin 30, Committee of One Hundred on National Health (Washington, DC, 1909).

[51] For a detailed history of the Public Health Service, see Ralph C. Williams, *The United States Public Health Service, 1798–1950* (Washington, DC, 1951).

State medicine and preventive medicine in England

Until the early years of the twentieth century, American public health reform had been directed largely by lay, non-professional personnel, a mixture of lawyers, philanthropists, engineers, evangelicals and some concerned doctors. In Europe, the medical profession dominated events from a much earlier date. Virchow in Germany and Villermé in France were leading scientists and physicians. And in England, the engineering and legalistic orthodoxies of the sanitary movement declined with the removal of Chadwick from the General Board of Health in 1854. The 'sanitary idea' was replaced by the rise of state medicine during the mid-Victorian period. The domination of medicine in the English context began with the appointment of John Simon to the General Board in 1854 and later at the Medical Department of the Privy Council in 1859.[52]

John Simon, a surgeon at St Thomas's Hospital, had taken an interest in public health since he had been a founding member of the Health of Towns Association in 1844. In 1848, the City of London Corporation appointed Simon local Medical Officer of Health. Chadwick's style of management at the General Board of Health had met with political resistance from the advocates of local government autonomy and had reached a critical point during 1854. When the Board was dissolved and reconstituted in 1855, Simon was appointed to the newly created post of Medical Officer of the Board.[53]

Before leaving the City of London, Simon published a collection of his reports to the authority. He took the opportunity 'to express...some thoughts on sanitary affairs in a fuller sense of the term'. He did not deal only with the City itself:

but speaking of the country in general, and pleading especially for the poorer masses of the population, I endeavoured to show how genuine and urgent a need there was, that the State should concern itself systematically and comprehensively with all chief interests of the public health. I submitted, as the state of the case, that except against wilful violence, the law was practically caring very little for the lives of the people.[54]

Simon admitted that in referring to the existing evils against which there was no legal protection, such as 'uncontrolled letting of houses unfit for human occupation; the unregulated industries of sorts endangering the health of persons employed in them; the unregulated nuisance-making

---

[52] Royston Lambert, *Sir John Simon 1816–1904 and English Social Administration* (London, 1963).
[53] *Ibid.*, pp. 221–32. [54] Simon, *English Sanitary Institutions*, p. 253.

business', he was dealing with social questions which 'I could not pretend to discuss'. Namely:

questions as to wages and poverty and pauperism; in relation to which I could only observe, as of medical common-sense, that, if given wages will not purchase such food and such lodgment as are necessary for health, the rate-payers who sooner or later have to doctor and perhaps bury the labourer, when starvation-disease or filth-disease has laid him low, are in effect paying the too late arrears of wages which might have hindered the suffering and sorrow.[55]

Simon argued that even if the law allowed wages to find their own level 'in the struggles of an unrestricted competition' then at least it should ensure that food standards be established to prevent starvation; that conditions of lodging be regulated consistent with decency and health; and that working conditions be inspected and regulated to reduce risk. Simon had a specific vision of how these goals could be achieved. They required:

comprehensive and scientific legislation, and generally in relation to sanitary government, I urged that the supervision of the public health, in the full sense indicated, ought to be the consolidated and sole charge of some one Minister: who...should be responsible, not only for the enforcement of existing laws...but likewise for their progress...as the growth of knowledge would make desirable.[56]

In 1858, a new Public Health Act moved Simon's medical department to the Privy Council, where its main function was to be 'Inquiry and Report'.[57] It had direct powers only with regard to the enactment of the vaccination acts and the Disease Prevention Act for control of epidemics. Apart from the special place that the administration of vaccination had in Simon's responsibilities, he perceived that the task of his department at the Privy Council was to:

develop a scientific basis for the progress of sanitary law and administration ... we had to aim at stamping on public hygiene a character of greater exactitude than it had hitherto had.[58]

Thus began a period of 'blue-books' wherein Simon and his inspectorate produced annual reports of investigations into disease prevalence in the country, 'measured and understood with precision ... in respect of their causes and modes of origin'. The investigations fell, said Simon, into two basic categories. The first studied the 'Excesses of

[55] Ibid., p. 254.   [56] Ibid., pp. 254-5.   [57] Ibid., p. 279.
[58] Ibid., p. 286.

Disease, epidemic or endemic, in particular districts or particular classes of the population'. The second focused on the 'distribution of the common *Necessaries of Health* among the population, and into the effect of deficiencies which were found existing'.

To realize his broad mandate Simon employed the leading medical and scientific experts of the day: Edward Seaton, John Burdon Sanderson, Henry Greenhow, William Thudichum, Robert Barnes, and John Syre Bristowe. Their reports, completed between 1858 and 1871, examined epidemic and endemic sicknesses: diphtheria, famine diseases, meningitis, yellow fever, cholera, cattle-plague, pulmonary diseases, mortality of infants and ague. Inquiries were also completed at the same time on 'standards which in great part were those of common social experience', such as the report on *Elementary Requisites for Popular Healthiness* which investigated the provision of food supply, house accommodation, physical surroundings, industrial circumstances and local precautions against the most notorious dangers in common life – 'local nuisances, and the contagions of disease from man and beast'. Further reports followed: *Dangerous Industries, Hospitals of the United Kingdom, Accidental and Criminal Poisoning, Dwellings of the Poorer Labouring Classes in Town and Country, Specialised Mortuary Statistics*, and the *Average Annual Proportions of Deaths*.[59]

During the first six years at the Privy Council, Simon and his inspectorate had amassed sufficient evidence to launch an appeal for a review of the law. This was achieved through a new Sanitary Act in 1866, which imposed a 'duty' upon local authorities to provide for proper inspection of their districts and the removal of nuisances. It gave local authorities new powers to intervene in the provision of clean water supplies, to regulate the tenement houses of the poor, and to impose penalties for those infected. Most importantly, the new 'grammar of common sanitary legislation' contained in the Act extended the power of the central government to coerce local authorities. The Act covered defaults of all kinds by local authorities and placed the power of determining faults, and ordering action into the hands of the Home Secretary. The Act was passed without the outrage and opposition earlier directed at Chadwick when he had attempted the same thing, largely because of the support of parliament's medical adviser.[60]

Simon had realized the ideals of a centrally administered state medical

[59] See Lambert, *Sir John Simon*, pp. 289–371; and Simon, *English Sanitary Institutions*, pp. 281–322.

[60] Lambert, *Sir John Simon*, pp. 377–91; Simon, *English Sanitary Institutions*, pp. 298–302.

policy as envisaged in 1856 by Henry Rumsey.[61] Between 1858 and 1871, Simon expanded his office from a single appointment to a state department with its own parliamentary secretary; the department occupied two buildings with a staff of over thirty. But state medicine, which arose at mid century, did not long survive. In 1867, the British Medical Association pressured parliament for an inquiry into the chaotic multiplicity of the public health laws, and the Royal Sanitary Commission was subsequently appointed in 1868. The end result of the inquiry was the great codifying legislation, the Public Health Act of 1875, and the establishment in 1871 of the Local Government Board to coordinate the administration of both the Poor Law and public health into one government department. Simon transferred to the Local Government Board but found the restriction of Poor Law administration upon his department made it impossible to function with the same breadth. He resigned the medical officership in 1876 and, as his excellent biographer, Royston Lambert, pointed out, his resignation signalled the eclipse of state medicine.[62]

The declining fortunes of state medicine in central government led to a shift in emphasis in public health matters. The subsequent development in disease control has been characterized as an era of 'preventive medicine'.[63] This was a much broader movement, outside the central corridors of power and beyond the elite provinces of the medical and scientific communities. It was not, however, a 'lay' movement, but was associated with the growth of prevention as a professional practice distinct from cure. It centred around doctors whose primary function was the provision of health in the community and who relinquished the treatment of illness.

The struggle for economic and social security by Medical Officers of Health in the 1890s helped them to develop an identity as practitioners of preventive medicine separate from the clinical profession as a whole.[64] There was also what might be called a 'community' of interests surrounding preventive medicine which was communicated through a journal literature and high-profile conferences, and was embodied in a variety of institutions set up for educational and research purposes. Together, the emerging preventive profession and preventive community constituted the social context in which preventive medicine

[61] Henry W. Rumsey, *Essays on State Medicine* (London, 1856).
[62] Lambert, *Sir John Simon*, pp. 347–77.   [63] Sand, *Vers la médecine*, p. 557.
[64] See Dorothy Porter, 'Stratification and Its Discontents: Professionalization and Conflict in the British Public Health Service 1848–1944', in Elizabeth Fee and Roy Acheson (eds.), *A History of Education in Public Health: Health that Mocks the Doctors' Rules* (Oxford, 1991), pp. 83–113.

developed as a practice and also as an ideal.[65] The ideological development of preventive medicine demonstrated how the economic and social values which underlay the environmentalist philosophy of sanitarianism were slowly replaced by technical neutrality.

In 1881, Chadwick addressed the Social Science Association on the relative merits of prevention and cure. He praised the achievements of preventive science and bemoaned its poor standing in the eyes of the medical profession, government, and public at large. He defined prevention in 'sanitary' terms and focused on the deaths avoided by the environmental regulation of water pollution, sewage disposal, street widening, and other civil engineering works.[66]

A decade later, the preventive community thought such views characterized an outdated era of disease control and a form of knowledge which, for future progress, must be unlearned.[67] The first professor of hygiene at the Army Medical School in Netley, Edmund Parkes, declared in *A Manual of Practical Hygiene* that prevention had, in the past, worked with generalized assumptions about the nature of disease causation and had used generalized methods, moving haphazardly in the dark. The scientific future of prevention, he said, lay in the discovery of the specific causes of individual diseases. Without the principle of specificity the science of hygiene was only 'working with shadows'.[68]

The impact of bacteriology

The historiography of medicine and science has rightly warned against assuming that what looks, with hindsight, to have been a revolution in knowledge, was perceived as such at the time.[69] The developments in bacteriology, which took place in the 1880s, were, however, embraced by the preventive community in England from the 1890s. And in the United States, the advent of bacteriology may have been even more important in helping to weld a new professional, scientific identity for public health.

[65] See D. E. Watkins, 'The English Revolution in Social Medicine' (University of London Ph.D. Thesis, 1984).

[66] Edwin Chadwick, 'Progress of Sanitation: Prevention as Compared with that of Curative Science', *Transactions of the National Association of Social Science* (1881), 625–49.

[67] See, for example, the presidential addresses of Joseph Ewart to the Epidemiological Society in 1891–2, *Transactions of the Epidemiological Society*, new series 10 (1890–1), 1–21, and 11 (1891–2), 1–26.

[68] Edmund Alexander Parkes, *A Manual of Practical Hygiene*, 4th edn (London, 1873), pp. 443–4.

[69] See, for example, the discussion in Roy Porter, 'The Scientific Revolution: A Spoke in the Wheel?', in Roy Porter and Mikulas Teich (eds.), *Revolution in History* (Cambridge, 1986), pp. 290–316.

ELIZABETH FEE AND DOROTHY PORTER

The 'sanitary idea' in England and the 'old public health' in America had attempted to procure the health of an undifferentiated 'public' with generalized methods of prevention. Towards the end of the nineteenth century, a shift in public health ideology began to categorize individuals into 'risk populations' based on what Edmund Parkes had termed 'the great principle of specificity'.[70] Bacteriology introduced the principle of specificity into understanding disease processes, and it also presented a powerful new way of differentiating scientific experts from mere social reformers. The response to the new science diverged, however, in America and England. New policy directives shared some common features in both national contexts, but other policy areas differed widely.

In the United States, in the period immediately following the brilliant experimental work of Pasteur, Koch and the German bacteriologists, the bacteriological laboratory became the primary symbol of a new, scientific public health. The clarity and simplicity of bacteriological methods and discoveries gave them tremendous cultural importance: the agents of particular diseases had been made visible under the microscope. The identification of specific bacteria had cut through the misty miasmas of disease and had defined the enemy in unmistakable terms. Bacteriology thus became an ideological marker, sharply differentiating the 'old' public health, the province of untrained amateurs, from the 'new' public health, which belonged to scientifically trained professionals.

Young Americans who had studied in Germany brought back the new knowledge of laboratory methods in bacteriology and started to teach others: William Henry Welch and T. Mitchell Prudden in New York, George Sternberg in Washington, and Alexander C. Abbott in Philadelphia were among the first to introduce the new bacteriology to the United States. These young scientists were convinced that other physicians spent too much time squabbling over medical ethics and politics, while they exemplified commitment to the purer values of laboratory research. The laboratory ideal rapidly influenced leading progressives in public health. By the 1880s, Charles Chapin had established a public health laboratory in Providence, Rhode Island; Victor C. Vaughan had created a state hygienic laboratory in Michigan; and William Sedgwick had used bacteriology to study water supplies and sewage disposal at the Lawrence Experiment Station in Massachusetts.[71]

[70] Parkes, *A Manual of Practical Hygiene*, pp. 443–4.
[71] For Sedgwick's rather lyrical view of bacteriology, see William T. Sedgwick, 'The Origin, Scope and Significance of Bacteriology', *Science*, 13 (1901), 121–8.

266

Sedgwick demonstrated the transmission of typhoid fever by polluted water supplies and developed quantitative methods for measuring the presence of bacteria in the air, water and milk. Describing the impact of bacteriological discoveries, he said: 'Before 1880 we knew nothing; after 1890 we knew it all; it was a glorious ten years.'[72]

The powerful new methods of identifying diseases through the microscope drew attention away from the larger and more diffuse problems of water supplies, street cleaning, housing reform and the living conditions of the poor. The approach of locating, identifying and isolating bacteria and their human hosts was a more elegant and efficient way of dealing with disease than worrying about environmental reform. The public health laboratory demonstrated the scientific and diagnostic power of the new public health. But by focusing on the diagnosis of infectious diseases, it narrowed the distance between medicine and public health, and brought public health into potential conflict with private medical practice. The use of bacteriological laboratory techniques also emphasized the importance of scientific training. Bacteriology thus narrowed the focus of public health, distinguished it from more general social and sanitary reform efforts, and reinforced the importance of scientific knowledge.

The new epidemiology, like the new bacteriology, was firmly oriented to the control of specific diseases. Charles Chapin, the superintendent of health of Providence, Rhode Island, was one of the leading proponents of the new epidemiology. Chapin had published a comprehensive text on municipal sanitation in 1901, but soon concluded that much of the effort devoted to cleaning up the cities was wasted; instead, public health officers should concentrate on controlling specific routes of infection.[73] In 1910, Chapin published a new text, *The Sources and Modes of Infection*, which became the gospel of infectious disease control.[74]

Hibbert Winslow Hill, director of the division of epidemiology of the Minnesota Board of Health, popularized Chapin's work in a lively series of articles first printed in 1,100 newspapers across the United States, and later published as a book, *The New Public Health*.[75] Hill likened the epidemiologist to a hunter trying to find a sheep-killing wolf. The old-fashioned amateur hunter covered the mountains with his assistants, and

---

[72] As cited in E. O. Jordan, G. C. Whipple, C.-E. A. Winslow, *Sedgwick*, p. 57.
[73] Charles V. Chapin, *Municipal Sanitation in the United States* (Providence, RI, 1901).
[74] Charles V. Chapin, *The Sources and Modes of Infection* (New York, 1910).
[75] Hibbert Winslow Hill, *The New Public Health* (New York, 1916).

told them to follow all wolf trails until they found the one that led to the slaughtered sheep. The new professional hunter, however, took a different approach:

Instead of finding in the mountains and following inward from them, say, 500 different wolf trails, 499 of which must necessarily be wrong, the experienced hunter goes directly to the slaughtered sheep, finding there and following outwards thence the only right trail... the one trail that is necessarily and inevitably the trail of the one actually guilty wolf.[76]

The new epidemiologist started with the 'slaughtered sheep' – the sick patient. From there, he traced back the single trail to the source of disease. All other unrelated environmental trails – decaying milk, flies in the market place, outdoor privies – were irrelevant.

Hill explained that modern scientific methods were more efficient than old-fashioned approaches to social reform. To control tuberculosis, for example, it was not necessary to improve the living conditions of the one hundred million people in the United States, only to prevent the 200,000 active tuberculosis cases from infecting others. He contrasted the expense and difficulty of trying to secure good food, decent housing and safe working conditions for the entire population with 'the expense of supervision of two hundred thousand people *merely to the extent of confining their infective discharges*... Need any more be said to indicate the superiority of the new principles, as practical business propositions, over the old?'[77] The vital statistician, Hill said, would be the future scientific and financial manager of public health:

Much abused, laughed at, neglected, he is, or will be, like the cost-of-production scientific manager of modern business, 'the most indispensable man on the staff'... a man who knows costs in each department in proportion to production, and where to cut cost, increase production, save time, unnecessary work, and waste in general.[78]

The dominance of the disease-oriented approach to public health was evident in the first handbook for practising public health officers, *A Manual for Health Officers*, published in 1915 by J. Scott MacNutt, and echoing the views of Chapin and Hill.[79] MacNutt devoted approximately half of his 600-page handbook to the contagious diseases, four pages to industrial hygiene, and gave only passing notice to housing, water supplies, public education and environmental health.

Although the bacteriological view was dominant, there were several

---

[76] *Ibid.*, p. 69.   [77] *Ibid.*, pp. 19–20.   [78] *Ibid.*, pp. 134–5.
[79] J. Scott MacNutt, *A Manual for Health Officers* (New York, 1915), p. 85.

other competing models for public health research and practice. Public health was not yet characterized by a single paradigm, but by a diversity of views and approaches. Compare, for example, Hill's narrow focus with the broad and expansive gaze of Charles-Edward A. Winslow, a public health spokesman who would become head of Yale's department of public health:

> Public health is the science and art of preventing disease, prolonging life, and promoting physical health and efficiency through organized community efforts for the sanitation of the environment, the control of community infections, the education of the individual in principles of personal hygiene, the organization of medical and nursing service for the early diagnosis and preventive treatment of disease, and the development of the social machinery which will ensure to every individual in the community a standard of living adequate for the maintenance of health.[80]

Winslow's was not the only alternative view. In the same year that Hill published his book on the new public health, Alice Hamilton in Illinois conducted a survey of industrial lead poisoning and established the fact that thousands of American workers were being slowly killed by white lead.[81] Hamilton's method was not that of following the single trail to the guilty wolf, but of following hundreds of trails to find the many guilty wolves in pottery glazing, bath-tub enamelling, cut-glass polishing, cigar wrapping, can sealing, and dozens of other industrial processes. Unaided by legislation, Hamilton argued, persuaded, shamed and flattered individual employers into improving working conditions. Almost single-handedly, she created the foundations of industrial hygiene in America.

Joseph Goldberger's epidemiological studies of pellagra for the Public Health Service offer an example of yet another approach to public health. In 1914, Goldberger announced that pellagra was due to dietary deficiencies and not to some unknown micro-organism; he and his colleagues had cured endemic pellagra in a Mississippi orphanage by feeding the children milk, eggs, beans and meat. He then teamed up with the economist, Edgar Sydenstricker, to survey the diets of southern wageworkers' families. They showed how the sharecropping system had impoverished tenant farmers, led to dietary deficiencies, and thus

---

[80] Charles-Edward A. Winslow, 'The Untilled Fields of Public Health', *Science*, 51 (1920), 23; see also C.-E. A. Winslow, *The Evolution and Significance of the Modern Public Health Campaign* (New Haven, CT, 1923).

[81] See Barbara Sicherman, *Alice Hamilton: A Life in Letters* (Cambridge and London, 1984), pp. 153–83.

produced endemic pellagra.[82] That guilty wolf – the economic system of cotton production and the pattern of land ownership – had swallowed much of the south.

Alice Hamilton, Joseph Goldberger and Edgar Sydenstricker were minority voices in America amid the growing majority focusing exclusively on bacteria. Only the minority continued to relate the problems of ill health and disease to the larger social environment. As most bacteriologists and epidemiologists concentrated on specific disease-causing organisms and the individuals who harboured them, the larger social environment became almost irrelevant.[83]

While the broader conceptions of public health required an understanding of economics and politics, the dominant model of public health knowledge was based almost exclusively on the biological sciences. In the United States, this latter definition of the problems of health and disease in bioscientific terms moved public health closer to medicine and reinforced the medical profession's claim to a dominant influence in the field – a claim that had already long been recognized in Britain, but which was still contested in the United States.

In England, knowledge of specific modes of transmission of different diseases encouraged new lines of preventive action. A new emphasis upon notification, isolation and disinfection had a high profile amongst medical officers of health in the 1890s. A list of the most common infections spread by social contact were made notifiable under an adoptive Act in 1889 and the law became compulsory in 1899.[84] Discussions of infectious disease control dominated the preventive journals up to 1900. All the preventive journals included bacteriological sections. Bacteriological diagnosis was made use of in incidents of notified infections and district public health officers increasingly demanded laboratory facilities from their sanitary authorities.[85]

One consequence of the new concern with notification was a growing awareness of the need for systematic and comprehensive planning of disease control amongst health officers in England. In the 1900s the

[82] Milton Terris (ed.), *Goldberger on Pellagra* (Baton Rouge, 1964). See especially Joseph Goldberger and Edgar Sydenstricker, 'Pellagra in the Mississippi Flood Area', pp. 271–91.

[83] For a detailed examination of this point in the case of tuberculosis, see Bonnie Kantor, 'The New Scientific Public Health Movement: A Case Study of Tuberculosis in Baltimore, Maryland, 1900–1910' (Sc.D. Dissertation, School of Hygiene and Public Health, The Johns Hopkins University, 1985).

[84] For discussion of the development of notification and the response of the public health service see Watkins, 'English Revolution in Social Medicine', pp. 214–38.

[85] See discussion of public health laboratories in D. S. Davies, 'Bacteriology in Public Health Work', *Public Health*, 11 (1898–9), 187–92.

Society of Medical Officers of Health discussed the desirability of adding tuberculosis to the list of notifiable diseases. Arthur Newsholme, when medical officer of health for Brighton, had established an efficient system in his district. He warned the Society, however, not to act hastily in demanding the notification of tuberculosis. He pointed out that a notification system could not work without the full cooperation of a sanitary authority in providing sufficient hospital and ambulance services for isolating sufferers. The need to plan health-care provision for a locality on the basis of its projected needs was drawn out sharply in Newsholme's discussion of the tuberculosis issue.[86]

Identification of specific diseases led preventive medicine in England to identify specific populations 'at risk'. The subsequent expansion of public health policy took its own particular form. This emerged from the debates around the popular concern with 'national fitness' and 'efficiency' in England before the First World War.

Public health and medicine

In Britain, after the defeats of the imperial army at the hands of South African farmers during the Boer War, concern over the physical fitness of the troops spilled over into a wider panic about physical deterioration in the nation as a whole. The Select Committee on Physical Deterioration was set up in the midst of a public and political alarm about 'national efficiency'. After the publication of the report in 1904, which highlighted acute health deficiencies amongst certain sections of the population, the Edwardian social and political consciousness became preoccupied with the degeneration of the imperial race by virtue of the Darwinian principle of natural selection.[87] By far the greatest response to the question of national efficiency, however, was the extension of the sociological classification of the health of the population.[88] A new focus emerged on the health of the schoolchild, antenatal care, infant welfare,

[86] Society of Medical Officers of Health, *Minutes of an Ordinary Meeting of the Society* (11 April 1890); see also *Public Health*, 3 (1890–1), 2–9.
[87] Geoffrey Searle, *The Quest for National Efficiency* (Oxford, 1971). For discussion of degeneration in the development of concepts of social hygiene in England during the Edwardian period see Greta Jones, *Social Hygiene in Twentieth Century Britain* (London, 1986). For discussion of the intellectual origins of degenerationism see J. E. Chamberlin and Sander Gilman, *Degeneration, The Dark Side of Progress* (New York, 1985); also Daniel Pick, *Faces of Degeneration, a European Disorder, c. 1848–c. 1918* (Cambridge, 1989).
[88] See discussion in Watkins, 'English Revolution in Social Medicine', pp. 291–322, and in David Armstrong, *The Political Anatomy of the Body: Medical Knowledge in Britain in the Twentieth Century* (Cambridge, 1983).

and the diseases of occupations.[89] The 1911 census provided the data for Thomas Stevenson to devise the first socio-economic classification of occupations for the Registrar General, thus extending the statistical tabulations of health risks.[90]

The sociological imagination enhanced the development of comprehensive planning for disease prevention and health preservation. Nowhere was this trend more pronounced than amongst medical officers of health. Closer allegiance grew up between them and the advocates of town planning, for example, in the search for integrated systems of municipal management which would ensure health efficiency.[91] But corporatism found its clearest expression in the increasingly strident demands amongst medical officers of health for a national system of health provision. Up to 1911, numerous articles and editorials in *Public Health* discussed proposals for the nationalization of health care, structured around the existing public health organization. Many envisaged a national system administered through the public health departments and coordinated by the new single government ministry to which all health authorities would be directly responsible. Influential medical officers of health argued for a national system of preventive health care in which they would play the crucial organizing role, no longer as local government officers, but as civil servants financed and salaried directly from the exchequer's purse.[92]

By the second decade of the twentieth century in the United States, non-medical public health officers were beginning to protest at the increasing dominance of public health by medical men. By this time, the sanitary engineers were the only professional group strong enough to challenge the physicians' assumption that the future of public health should be theirs. Civil and sanitary engineers had created clean city water supplies and adequate sewerage systems. The provision of uncontaminated water had been a major factor in declining death rates from infant diarrhoea and other infectious diseases. With the benefit of hindsight, we can say that the sanitary engineers, through their work in improving water supplies and sewerage systems, probably deserve much of the

---

[89] See Porter and Porter, 'What Was Social Medicine?'; A. Wohl, *Endangered Lives: Public Health in Victorian Britain* (London, 1984), pp. 329–41; Armstrong, *Political Anatomy*.

[90] Simon Szreter, 'The Importance of Social Intervention in Britain's Mortality Decline c. 1850–1914: A Reinterpretation of the Role of Public Health', *Social History of Medicine*, 1 (1988), 1–37.

[91] Dorothy Porter, '"Enemies of the Race": Biologism, Environmentalism and Public Health in Edwardian England', *Victorian Studies* (Winter 1991).

[92] Watkins, 'English Revolution and Social Medicine', pp. 214–38; Porter '"Enemies of the Race"'.

credit for the decline of infectious disease mortality and morbidity in the late nineteenth century.[93] The professional competition between sanitary engineers and physicians became intense in the early years of the twentieth century as physicians reinforced their dominance in public health departments, and as the sanitary engineers vociferously complained about the increasing 'medical monopoly' of public health.

By 1912, fifteen states required that all members of their boards of health be physicians, twenty-three states required that at least one member be a physician, and ten states had no professional requirement for eligibility.[94] The medical profession was well organized and making a strong claim for dominance in public health. The sanitary engineers' counter-claim was an uphill battle; the physicians were willing to concede their responsibility for public sanitation and water supplies, but little else.

The central task in creating a new profession of public health would be to weld unity of training, purpose and function from these diverse and often competing interests. Some resolution would have to be achieved between the different visions of public health, and some position taken with respect to the tensions between public health and medicine, between the biological and social views of public health, between the physicians and the sanitary engineers, and between the bacteriologists and those who sought a broader definition of the field. In order to create a more unified profession, decisions would have to be taken about the proper scope and content of public health, the kinds of knowledge and skills required of public health practitioners, the kinds of training to be provided and the kinds of credentials to be offered.

[93] It is difficult to be confident about mortality rates in the United States before 1900, when the death registration areas began regular reporting. The evidence seems, however, to suggest that mortality rates between 1850 and 1880 remained relatively constant, with wide annual variations depending on the presence of epidemics. In the 1880s the mortality rates began to decline, and continued this decline, with minor fluctuations, throughout the period from 1890 to 1915. The major component of the decline was in infant mortality, especially mortality rates from infectious diseases and infant diarrhoea. This pattern is consistent with the thesis that the extension of municipal water systems and the filtration of water supplies played a major role in the decline in mortality. The pasteurization of milk was probably also an important contributing factor. On the estimation of mortality rates for the period, see Edward Meeker, 'The Improving Health of the United States, 1850–1915', *Explorations in Economic History*, 9 (1972), 353–73; Michael R. Haines, 'The Use of Model Life Tables to Estimate Mortality for the United States in the Late Nineteenth Century', *Demography*, 16 (1979), 289–312; Frederick L. Hoffman, 'The General Death Rate of Large American Cities, 1871–1904', *Publications of the American Statistical Association*, 10 (1906–7), 1–75. For a general discussion of the social impact of infectious diseases, see John Duffy, 'Social Impact of Disease in the Late Nineteenth Century', *Bulletin of the New York Academy of Medicine*, 47 (1971), 797–811.

[94] Morris Knowles, 'Public Health Service not a Medical Monopoly', *American Journal of Public Health*, 3 (1913), 111–22.

In the United States, these questions would be worked out in the context of new schools of public health, largely founded and funded by the Rockefeller Foundation. These schools were open to physicians, but not limited to them. Indeed, when physicians displayed relatively little interest in public health training – given the much larger incomes to be made from private practice – the doors of public health were gradually opened wider to admit members of many other professions and those trained in a great variety of scientific disciplines. Some degree of professional unity was created among this diverse group through specialized public health training and the awarding of public health degrees. While physicians were usually preferred for public health administrative positions, non-physicians thus came to occupy important positions within public health departments, especially in specialized technical and research positions. In the United States, public health would continue to be partially independent of medicine, and the close but often strained relationship between the two fields would continue to structure the future development of public health as a profession.

Conclusion

A comparative analysis of the development of public health and preventive medicine in England and America has shown up both parallels and contrasts. The philosophy of public health in England was born in the 1830s and 1840s amidst a European-wide concern regarding the political dimensions of the role of medicine in ameliorating the ill health produced by urbanism, industrialism and the free-market economy. Public health in America also emerged as a social response to the disastrous health conditions of the industrial working class in the cities. Because industrial development occurred rather later in America than in Europe, however, public health also developed about fifty years later than in Britain.

In both America and England, the sanitary reform movements were initially dominated by non-medical personnel who pursued the prevention of disease within a broader framework for preventing poverty and social distress. From the mid-nineteenth century in England, however, medicine moved to centre stage through the establishment of a medical department and a senior civil service medical appointment. The career of John Simon made state medicine a reality. The transition from political philosophy to technocratic policy in public health was assisted by Simon's own strategy of replacing the need for legislative change with administrative planning to achieve his aims and goals. The rise of technocratic ideology, however, was assisted most by the rise of a new profession in the prevention of disease. This profession consolidated its identity with claims to legitimate authority in a new field of expertise, preventive medicine.

In the United States, public health remained somewhat separate from medicine. Public health as a profession only developed in the second decade of the twentieth century, at a time when reforms in medical education had already consolidated the professional identity and incomes of physicians. Relatively few were now interested in salaried public health positions. At least in part as a response to the relative disinterest of the medical profession, public health schools were open to non-physicians: to engineers, statisticians, biologists and others interested in specialized public health disciplines. Because public health was never assimilated to medicine, it tended to retain a rather broad definition of goals and interests, extending well beyond the boundaries of 'preventive medicine'. Relative to private medical practice, however, public health enjoyed less status and prestige than clinical medicine, and certainly less wealth. By retaining a separate identity from medicine, it also preserved some elements of the social reform impulse that marked its origins. As in Britain, public health became scientific, and its methods were moulded by the constraints of scientific and statistical methodology, but its relative independence from medicine represented an advantage as well as a constraint.

Madness and its institutions

ROY PORTER

In the eyes of some radical critics, mental illness should properly have no place in a book dealing with the history of sickness.[1] For, they would contend, there is no such disease (in the strict sense of the word) as insanity, 'psychiatric disorder' being nothing other than a stigma which the psychiatric profession, with the connivance of society at large, pins on those whose thoughts and actions are unacceptably 'deviant'. Society (it has been alleged) finds certain people 'disturbing' and, by a medicalizing sleight of hand, labels them 'disturbed', and therefore in need of treatment. Psychiatry is thus essentially a form of social control, a masked and medicalized mechanism of punishment.

This radical claim that 'mental illness' is itself a delusion commands only a small following even amongst critics of psychiatry. But it does highlight one feature which sets apart the social response to insanity from the handling of any of the other sorts of disease dealt with in this volume. This is the fact that, over the last two or three hundred years, those people suffering from serious mental disturbance have been subjected to compulsory and coercive medical treatment, usually under conditions of confinement and forfeiture of civil rights. Sick people in general (i.e. those suffering from somatic diseases such as measles or gout) have typically had the right to seek, or the right to refuse, medical treatment; have typically enjoyed their own choice of practitioner; and, insofar as they have been cared for in institutions such as hospitals, they have been legally free to come and go as they please.

[1] See for instance T. S. Szasz, *The Manufacture of Madness* (London, 1973); idem, *The Myth of Mental Illness* (London, 1972); idem, *The Myth of Psychotherapy* (New York, 1978); idem (ed.), *The Age of Madness. The History of Involuntary Mental Hospitalization Presented in Selected Texts* (Garden City, NY, 1973).

By contrast, the seriously mentally ill (that is, those generally in the past termed 'mad', 'maniacal', 'insane', or 'lunatic') have been subjected to a transformation in their legal status which has rendered their state more akin to that of criminals than that of the sick. Over the last few hundred years, the emergence of the madhouse (later termed the asylum or the mental hospital) spelt the coming of a 'total institution' which bore more likenesses to the prison than to the general infirmary.[2] The incarceration of mad people (and other comparable groups, such as the mentally handicapped) assumed gigantic proportions; by 1950, approximately half a million people were so confined in the USA and around 150,000 in Britain – perhaps some million all told in the Western world.[3] It has only been during the last generation, that the pattern of confinement has been reversed (in the movement variously called 'decarceration' or 'deinstitutionalization').[4] The aim of this chapter is neither to damn nor to defend the rise of the lunatic asylum as the archetypal site for treating mental illness. Rather it will seek to explain the social history of its emergence. It will not explore the history of the psychiatric profession or of psychiatry *per se*, viewed as the science of understanding and treating mental disorder, except in so far as the wider history of psychiatric medicine is inexorably associated with the emergence of the asylum.

There is very little evidence that mad people were confined in specialized institutions, designed exclusively for them, before the end of the Middle Ages.[5] That is, of course, not to say that lunatics were not singled out before modern times. Western medicine from Greek times

---

[2] Henri Vermorel and André Meylan, *Cent ans de psychiatrie: essai sur l'histoire des institutions psychiatriques en France de 1870 à nos jours* (Paris, 1969); Kathleen Jones, *A History of the Mental Health Services* (London, 1972); idem, *Mental Health and Social Policy 1845–1900* (London, 1960). For the history of opposition to asylums see D. A. Peterson (ed.), *A Mad People's History of Madness* (Pittsburgh, 1982).

[3] For a black interpretation of these developments see R. Castel, R. Castel and A. Lovell, *The Psychiatric Society* (Columbia, 1981).

[4] A. Scull, *Decarceration* (Englewood Cliffs, NJ, 1977; revised edn, Oxford, 1984).

[5] For broad introductions to the treatment of madness in Antiquity and the Middle Ages see Bennett Simon, *Mind and Madness in Ancient Greece* (Ithaca, 1978); Judith S. Neaman, *Suggestion of the Devil as the Origin of Madness* (New York, 1975); M. Screech, 'Good Madness in Christendom', in W. F. Bynum, Roy Porter and Michael Shepherd, *The Anatomy of Madness*, 3 vols. (London, 1985–8), I, pp. 25–39; Edith A. Wright, 'Medieval Attitudes Towards Mental Illness', *Bulletin of the History of Medicine*, 7 (1939), 352–6; Robert S. Kinsman, *The Darker Vision of the Renaissance. Beyond the Fields of Reason* (Berkeley, 1974); Basil Clarke, *Mental Disorder in Earlier Britain* (Cardiff, 1975); P. B. R. Doob, *Nebuchadnezzar's Children. Conventions of Madness in Middle English Literature* (New Haven and London, 1974); E. Welsford, *The Fool* (London, 1935); S. Billington, *The Social History of the Fool* (Brighton, 1984); R. Neugebauer, 'Treatment of the Mentally Ill in Medieval and Early Modern England' *Journal of the History of the Behavioral Sciences*, 14 (1978), 158–69.

onwards has offered its theories of the causes, diagnosis and prognosis of insanity, and two of the classic humours, yellow bile (choler) and black bile, were regarded as particularly responsible for mania and melancholia respectively. And from Antiquity onwards, legal systems routinely made special provision for the insane (with respect to making wills, holding property, signing contracts, etc.). But characteristically, it was the family which was held legally responsible for the deeds of its mad members, just as for children; and, not surprisingly, most of the shreds of evidence which have come down to us from classical and medieval times suggest that lunatics most commonly remained under family care (which may, of course, be a euphemism for family neglect).[6]

Detailed studies of English rural communities as late as the seventeenth and eighteenth centuries have demonstrated that families, aided by parish poor relief, were still typically expected to assume responsibility for their *non compos mentis* relatives, who might be kept at home, in a cellar, or hidden away in a barn, or sometimes under the care of a servant.[7] Such procedures may well have remained common in later centuries too, as the presence of the first Mrs Rochester, hidden away in the attic, in *Jane Eyre* may suggest. Insanity was commonly believed deeply shameful to a family, on account of its overtones either of diabolical possession or of hereditary taint. Home confinement was a way of maximizing secrecy. Almost by definition, it is quite impossible to say how many lunatics were looked after at home in previous centuries.

What is clear is that more formal segregative techniques for dealing with mad people also arose from early modern times. This departure probably registers a variety of quite different social and ideological currents. For one thing, piety seems to have encouraged the setting up of religious receptacles for the mad in certain countries. Some of the earliest known specialized lunatic asylums were established under religious auspices in fifteenth-century Spain, in Valencia, Zaragoza, Seville, Valladolid, Toledo and Barcelona (Islamic models may have

---

[6] J. Brydall, *Non Compos Mentis or the Law Relating to Natural fools, Mad Folkes and Lunatick Persons* (London, 1700); R. Neugebauer, 'Mental Illness and Government Policy in Sixteenth and Seventeenth Century England' (University of Columbia Ph.D. thesis, 1976).
[7] See Herbert Silvette, 'On Insanity in Seventeenth-Century England', *Bulletin of the History of Medicine*, 6 (1938), 22–33; George Rosen, 'The Mentally Ill and the Community in Western and Central Europe During the Late Middle Ages and the Renaissance', *Journal of the History of Medicine*, 19 (1964), 377–88; idem, 'Social Attitudes to Irrationality and Madness in 17th and 18th Century Europe', *Journal of the History of Medicine*, 18 (1963), 220–40; A. Fessler, 'The Management of Lunacy in 17th-Century England. An Investigation of Quarter-Sessions Records', *Proceedings of the Royal Society of Medicine*, 49 (1956), 901–7.

been influential).[8] In London the religious foundation of St Mary of Bethlehem (founded in 1247) was specializing in lunatics by the fifteenth century: it later became famous – or rather notorious – as Bethlem or 'Bedlam'.[9] By the same time, the Netherlandish town of Geel, which possessed the healing shrine of St Dymphna, was becoming celebrated as a healing shrine for the mentally disturbed.[10] And in Russia and various other parts of Europe, certain monasteries became known as sanctuaries for mad people, regarded as 'holy fools'.[11]

Piety continued to lie behind many philanthropic foundations even through the age of the Enlightenment. Appeals to religion were prominent in the founding of charitable asylums such as those set up in Liverpool, Manchester, Newcastle and York in eighteenth-century England. It is moreover extremely important not to underestimate the degree to which the custody and care of the insane lastingly remained in the hands of religious orders, in many parts of Europe right through into the present century. In Catholic nations such as France, Belgium, Poland, Spain and Portugal, most institutions for the insane in the eighteenth and nineteenth centuries were owned and controlled by brothers and sisters of charity, and funded by alms and pious donations. Elsewhere confessional strife led to rival religious asylums, resembling rival systems of schooling. As late as the last quarter of the nineteenth century, religiously exclusive Calvinist and Catholic lunatic asylums were being set up even in the 'modern' Netherlands – with the consequence that state psychiatry remained comparatively weak and the psychiatric profession divided.[12]

---

[8] A. S. Chamberlain, 'Early Mental Hospitals in Spain', *American Journal of Psychiatry*, 23 (1966), 143–9; Luis Garciá Ballester and Gerrardo Garciá-Gonzalez, 'Note sobre la asistencia a los locos...en la Cordoba medieval', *Asclepio*, 30 (1978/9), 199–207.

[9] R. R. Reed, *Bedlam on the Jacobean Stage* (Cambridge, MA, 1952). For corruption at Bethlem see P. Allderidge, 'Management and Mismanagement at Bedlam, 1547–1633', in Charles Webster (ed.), *Health, Medicine and Mortality in the Sixteenth Century* (Cambridge, 1979), pp. 141–64; M. Byrd, *Visits to Bedlam* (Columbia, SC, 1974); P. Allderidge, 'Bedlam: Fact or Fantasy?', in Bynum, Porter and Shepherd (eds.), *Anatomy of Madness*, II, pp. 17–23.

[10] For Gheel, including its later history, see J. Webster, *Notes on Belgian Lunatic Asylums, Including the Colony at Gheel* (London, 1857); W. L. Parry-Jones, 'The Model of the Gheel Lunatic Colony and its Influence on the Nineteenth Century Asylum System in Britain', in A. Scull (ed.), *Madhouses, Mad-doctors and Madmen* (London, 1981), pp. 207–17; J. A. Peeters, *Lettres médicales sur Gheel et le patronage familial* (Brussels, 1883); Eugeen Roosens, *Des fous dans la ville? (belgique) et sa thérapie séculaire* (Paris, 1977).

[11] K. S. Dix, 'Madness in Russia: 1775–1864, Official Attitudes and Institutions for the Insane' (University of California, Los Angeles, Ph.D. thesis, 1977).

[12] T. Bilikiewicz and M. Lyskanowski, 'Humanitarian Traditions of Treatment of the Mentally Ill Patients in Poland in the Sixteenth and Eighteenth Centuries', *International Congress of the History of Medicine 23rd. London, 1972. Proceedings*, I (1974), 427–9. On the Dutch case see H. Binneveld,

The emergence of the modern city state and nation state was also an important factor in the spread of confinement for the mad. The late Michel Foucault argued that the rise of absolutism – identified in particular with the accession of Louis XIV to the French throne in the mid seventeenth century – inaugurated a 'great confinement' (amounting to 'blind repression') throughout Europe.[13] In this, Foucault contended, all elements in society which stood for 'unreason' found themselves at risk of being shut away, constituting (as it was claimed they did) a scandal to law, order, and productive labour. Paupers, ne'er-do-wells, petty criminals, prostitutes, vagabonds and so forth formed the numerical majority of this abominable army of 'unreason'. But their symbolic leaders were the insane, the crazed and the idiotic. Already by the 1660s some 6,000 undesirables – including an unspecified number of mad people – had been locked away higgledy-piggledy in the Paris Hôpital Général. Similar hospitals were soon set up in the French provincial capitals.[14] And, Foucault argued, parallel institutions, such as the *Zuchthäuser* in the German principalities and assorted workhouses and bridewells in England, were soon burgeoning throughout Europe, shutting up the mad, together with other social nuisances and dangers, not as a therapeutic policy but as an act of state, essentially a police measure.[15]

Foucault argued that this 'great confinement' amounted to far more than a simple physical sequestration of the mad. For it also represented the utter degradation for the first time of the very existential condition of madness. Hitherto, by his strange peculiarity, the mad person had possessed a particular sort of fascination and power. In the figure of the holy fool, Christianity had permitted a 'good' religious madness. In the demoniac or the witch, there had also been a 'bad' religious madness which nevertheless bespoke power, albeit diabolical power.[16] Light-

'Lunacy Reform in the Netherlands. State Care and Private Initiative', in P. Spierenburg (ed.), *The Emergence of Carceral Institutions. Prisons, Galleys and Lunatic Asylums* (Rotterdam, 1984), pp. 165–86.

[13] M. Foucault, *Folie et déraison: histoire de la folie a l'âge classique. Civilisations d'hier et aujourd'hui* (Paris, 1961); this has been published in abridged translation as *Madness and Civilization: a History of Insanity in the Age of Reason*, trans. R. Howard (New York, 1965); see also George Rosen, 'Social Attitudes to Irrationality and Madness in Seventeenth and Eighteenth Century Europe', *Journal of the History of Medicine*, 18 (1963), 220–40.

[14] C. Jones, 'The Treatment of the Insane in Eighteenth- and Early Nineteenth-Century Montpellier', *Medical History*, 24 (1980), 371–90, p. 374.

[15] Compare A. Scull, 'A Convenient Place to Get Rid of Inconvenient People: The Victorian Lunatic Asylum', in A. D. King (ed.), *Buildings and Society* (London, 1980), pp. 37–60.

[16] See D. P. Walker, *Unclean Spirits: Possession and Exorcism in France and England in the Sixteenth and Seventeenth Centuries* (London, 1981).

headed zanies, acting as 'fools' and court jesters, had been permitted to utter their strange mad truths in riddles and snatches of song, and thus had enjoyed a license of free speech.[17] Through institutionalization, however, madness was robbed of all such positive features, its allure, its weird dignity. It was reduced to mere negation, the absence of all human characteristics. Small wonder, Foucault concluded, that lunatics in madhouses were often likened to, and treated like, wild beasts in a cage; for robbed of that essential human quality, reason, what were they but brutalized? In other words, the madman was not 'a sick man'; he was just an animal.

There is a certain core of truth in Foucault's characterization. The institutionalization of the insane undoubtedly accelerated, and (as he rightly stressed) this movement owed little to any tangible medical breakthroughs. But the interpretation needs much refinement.[18] For one thing, there is no reason to think that – France possibly excepted – the middle years of the seventeenth century constitute any dramatic watershed in the process of institutionalization. A fair amount of albeit scrappy evidence survives to show that civic authorities in Italy, in the Low Countries, in England and in the German-speaking lands had been occasionally providing facilities for locking up insane people at least from the sixteenth century. As custodial institutions such as houses of industry, workhouses, houses of improvement, and houses of correction emerged throughout urban Europe, offering putative solutions to the problems of urbanization, pauperization and proletarianization, so they necessarily caught some mad people in their nets.

But if institutionalization had been gradually emerging from long before, it certainly did not become the automatic blanket solution, across Europe, from the mid seventeenth century: in that sense, the term 'great confinement' is a misnomer. The type of action against the mad pursued by various states, and its level of intensity, differed quite fundamentally. Thus absolutist France centralized responses to the problem of the insane. From the time of Louis XIV through to the close of the *ancien régime*, it

[17] For some discussion see M. Macdonald, *Mystical Bedlam: Anxiety and Healing in Seventeenth-Century England* (Cambridge, 1981).

[18] For critiques of Foucault see H. C. E. Midelfort, 'Madness and Civilization in Early Modern Europe', in B. Malamont (ed.), *After the Reformation. Essays in Honor of J. H. Hexter* (Philadelphia, 1980), pp. 247–65; P. Sedgwick, *Psychopolitics* (London, 1981); Roy Porter, 'In the Eighteenth Century were Lunatic Asylums Total Institutions?', *Ego: Bulletin of the Department of Psychiatry, Guy's Hospital*, 4 (1983), 12–34. Most valuably see P. Spierenburg, 'The Sociogenesis of Confinement and its Development in Early Modern Europe', in Spierenburg (ed.), *Emergence of Carceral Institutions*, pp. 9–77.

became the responsibility of the civic authorities to provide institutional facilities for the mad poor (later, under the Napoleonic Code, prefects assumed these responsibilities). Families could have mad relatives legally confined upon obtaining a *lettre de cachet* from royal officials (such warrants effectively deprived the lunatic of all legal rights).[19] But the picture elsewhere in Europe remained very different.

In Russia, for example, state-organized receptacles for the insane hardly appeared before the second half of the nineteenth century. Before then, most confined mad people were kept in religious hands. In certain rural regions of Europe, few people seem to have undergone institutional confinement at all. Thus in Portugal, two lunatic asylums still sufficed for the entire nation at the close of the nineteenth century, holding no more than about 600 inmates.[20]

And England presents a case which does not easily square with the model of a 'great confinement'. It can hardly be denied that what Foucault called 'unreason' (i.e. the disturbing and dangerous classes) was at least as visible in England as in France. But state-activated confinement of the disturbed, disordered and distracted came very late. Not until 1808 was an Act of Parliament passed even permitting the use of public money for the establishment of voluntary county lunatic asylums; not until 1845 – almost two centuries after the beginning of Foucault's 'great confinement' – was the establishment of such asylums made compulsory. Figures on these matters are necessarily unreliable, but it appears that no more than perhaps 5,000 people were being held in specialized lunatic asylums in England around 1800, with perhaps as many mad people again housed in general workhouses, bridewells, jails and so forth. By that time, the aggregate national population was approaching 10 million. In other words, there is little evidence that the English ruling orders in the Georgian century felt that insanity or 'unreason' posed a terrible threat to the security of their regime.

Indeed, in England, and in other urbanized parts of Europe as well, the rise of the lunatic asylum is best seen less as a product of centralized acts

---

[19] See for example P. Sérieux, 'L'internement par "ordre de justice" des aliénés et des correctionnaires sous l'ancien régime, d'après des documents inédits', *Revue Historique du Droit Français et Etranger*, 77 (1932), 413–62; P. Sérieux and L. Libert, 'Le régime des aliénés en France au 18ème siècle d'après des documents inédits', *Annales Médico-psychologiques*, 10ème série, 6 (1914), 43–76, 196–219, 311–24, 470–97, 598–627; 7 (1914), 74–98; *idem*, 'Reglements de quelques maisons d'aliénés (documents pour servir à l'histoire de la psychiatrie en France)', *Bulletin de la Société de Médecine Mentale de Belgique*, 172 (1914), 209–50.

[20] J. J. Lopez Ibor, 'Spain and Portugal', in J. G. Howells (ed.), *World History of Psychiatry* (New York, 1968), pp. 90–118; Julian Espinosa, 'La assistencia psychiatrica en la Espana del siglo XIX', *Asclepio*, 21 (1969), 179–84.

of state than as an offshoot of the flourishing consumer society.[21] In England in 1800, most mad people in specialized institutions were secured in privately owned asylums, which operated for profit within the free market economy, as part of what contemporaries called the 'trade in lunacy'.[22] As late as the mid nineteenth century, more than half the confined lunatics in England were still housed in privately owned institutions. Because the private asylum was highly influential in the early development of psychiatry, but has been relatively neglected in recent historical accounts, it is worth dwelling for a moment on its emergence.

The early history of the private asylum is not, however, easy to trace. Such institutions presupposed a high level of discretion, not to say secrecy. A family which lodged a lunatic in a private asylum would clearly wish to avoid publicity (particularly if, as was alleged sometimes happened, the 'lunatic' in question was not truly insane but merely 'difficult' – an unruly son or daughter, or even a wife of whom her husband was tired). Not surprisingly, the keepers of such asylums did not admit visitors and rarely kept incriminating records. Moreover, not until 1774 were private lunatic asylums in England required even to be licensed in law.

Hence, our documentation on early private asylums is extremely scanty. It is clear, however, that such madhouses certainly existed in England before the middle of the seventeenth century. We know, for instance, that certain keepers of Bethlem Hospital also maintained their own private facilities for housing mad people. Likewise, when George Trosse of Exeter went mad in the 1650s, his friends carried him off (he was so violent they had to strap him to his horse) to a doctor in Glastonbury in Somerset who had a reputation for boarding and curing mad people.[23] And from about the same time, London newspapers begin to carry advertisements for private madhouses.

[21] See A. Scull, *Museums of Madness. The Social Organization of Insanity in Nineteenth Century England* (London, 1979). Note however that this comment does not apply to Ireland (where asylums were more centralized) or to Scotland, where voluntary, charitable asylums were typical. See M. Finnane, *Insanity and the Insane in Post-Famine Ireland* (London, 1981); Francis J. Rice, 'Madness and Industrial Society. A Study of the Origins and Early Growth of the Organisation of Insanity in Nineteenth Century Scotland c. 1830–1870' (University of Strathclyde Ph.D. thesis, 2 vols., 1981); Jane Feinmann, 'How a Lunatic Fared in 1781. (Transition of Montrose Lunatic Asylum to Sunnyside Royal Hospital)', *Medical News*, 13 (1981), 22–3; M. S. Thomson, 'The Mad, the Bad and the Sad: Psychiatric Care in the Royal Edinburgh Asylum (Morningside) 1813–1894' (Boston University Ph.D. thesis, 1984).

[22] William Parry-Jones, *The Trade in Lunacy. A Study of Private Madhouses in England in the Eighteenth and Nineteenth Centuries* (London, 1972).

[23] Roy Porter, *A Social History of Madness* (London, 1987), ch. 5.

By the close of the eighteenth century, the numbers of officially licensed private madhouses (licensed since the 1774 Act) had swollen in England to around fifty. This total perhaps should be regarded with some scepticism. There were probably more; some simply unlicensed, and some too small to require a license. We do not know, moreover, how many people made a living, or at least some surplus income, out of occasionally boarding one or two mad people. At the close of the eighteenth century, the water-colourist, J. R. Cozens, and the cartoonist, James Gillray, both went mad and were kept in private care; but no evidence survives about the sort of residence in which they were held. It is important to stress that the organized, inspected system of institutions for the mentally ill – the system which is presently being dismantled throughout Europe – is essentially a product of the nineteenth century. Before then, there was no system, but rather great diversity.[24]

Indeed, early asylums came in all shapes and sizes, big and small, good and bad.[25] Nowhere in Europe before the nineteenth century was there a legal requirement that asylums should be under the control of medically qualified personnel. In eighteenth-century England, some of the best asylums were indeed run by doctors. For example, Dr Thomas Arnold, who had been a pupil of Cullen at Edinburgh University, set up his own private asylum in Leicester in the 1760s. It quickly won a high reputation for its humane system of management. Arnold published extensively on the aetiology and classification of insanity. In his *Observations on the Nature, Kinds, Causes and Prevention of Insanity* (1782) he demonstrated that he was essentially an adherent of Locke's theory that insanity was primarily mental derangement dependent upon a deluded imagination.[26] But medical overlordship did not always secure good care. The medical dynasty of the Monro family at Bethlem – Dr James Monro was succeeded by his son John, who was succeeded by his

---

[24] See the discussion in Roy Porter, *Mind Forg'd Manacles. Madness in England from the Restoration to the Regency* (London, 1987), ch. 3.

[25] For a few examples of the range of asylums in England see A. D. Morris, *The Hoxton Madhouses* (March, Cambridgeshire, 1958); J. A. Bickford and M. E. Bickford, *The Private Lunatic Asylums of the East Riding* (Beverley, 1976); H. Temple Phillips, *The History of the Old Private Lunatic Asylum at Fishponds, Bristol, 1740–1859* (Bristol, 1973); Brenda Parry-Jones, *The Warneford Hospital Oxford, 1826–1976* (Oxford, 1976); idem, *The Warneford Hospital Oxford, 1826–1976. Guide to an Exhibition of Archives and Photographs to Celebrate the 150th Anniversary of the Hospital 10–14 July, 1976* (Oxford, 1976); R. Hunter and I. MacAlpine, *Psychiatry for the Poor. 1851 Colney Hatch Asylum, Friern Hospital 1973. A Medical and Social History* (London, 1974).

[26] T. Arnold, *Observations on the Nature, Kinds, Causes and Prevention of Insanity, Lunacy and Madness*, 2 vols. (Leicester, 1782–6). See also A. Walk, 'Some Aspects of the "Moral Management" of the Insane up to 1854', *Journal of Mental Sciences*, 100 (1954), 807–37.

son Thomas, who was succeeded by his son Edward – did not prevent that institution from becoming hidebound and corrupt.

It was perhaps not surprising, then, that one of the major reformist currents in asylum management should have been led by laymen. Around the turn of the nineteenth century, a series of scandals erupted at the York Asylum, a charitable institution under the control of local physicians, Dr Alexander Hunter and his successor Dr Charles Best. As a counter-measure, the local Quaker community, led by a York tea merchant, William Tuke, chose to establish their own asylum, opened in 1796 as the York Retreat. This was run by a lay superintendent, and possessed no resident physician.[27] In his *Description of the Retreat* (1813), William Tuke's grandson, Samuel, noted that medical therapies had been tried at the Retreat but with little success. Instead, they had largely abandoned 'medical' in favour of 'moral' means – an avoidance of force and restraint and the systematic deployment of kindness, reason and humanity, all within a family atmosphere – with excellent results.

The high repute of the Retreat was to prove something of a thorn in the flesh of attempts by the medical profession in the nineteenth century to secure monopolistic control for itself over the asylums. Nevertheless, a series of acts, passed from the 1820s onwards, was to require medical presence first in public and later in private asylums.

But early madhouses were differentiated by much more than the polarizing issue of medical *versus* lay control. For some were large, whereas others were tiny – a distinction which roughly corresponded to the social level of the clientele. In eighteenth- or early nineteenth-century England a large asylum (that is, one holding perhaps 60–100 inmates) catered mainly for lower-middle-class, or for pauper lunatics. These latter would be paid for by their parish of settlement at a rate of perhaps eight or ten shillings a week. But numerically speaking, the typical asylum remained much smaller.

Establishments such as Dr Nathaniel Cotton's asylum at St Albans (known as the Collegium Insanorum) housed no more than half a dozen lunatics. Rates were correspondingly higher. Cotton, for example, charged up to five guineas a week per client – a sum which was the equivalent of a year's wages for a maidservant. Obviously he catered for

---

[27] A. Digby, 'Changes in the Asylum: The Case of York, 1777–1815', *Economic History Review*, 36 (1983), 218–39; *idem, Madness, Morality and Medicine* (Cambridge, 1985); *idem*, 'The Changing Profile of a Nineteenth-Century Asylum: the York Retreat', *Psychological Medicine*, 14 (1984), 739–48.

a superior class of lunatic.[28] The same may be said for the very superior Ticehurst House, established in Sussex in the 1790s. There, patients were allowed to bring their own servants with them; a select few were lodged in individual houses in the grounds of the asylum; and the proprietors kept a pack of beagles so that gentlemen patients should not be deprived of their accustomed pleasures of the hunt. It must be added however that one patient's-eye view of Ticehurst, that of the prime minister's son, John Perceval, presents a rather jaundiced vision of conditions there.[29]

It is important to stress this broad class and cost spectrum of the asylum. For it gives the lie to one feature of Foucault's interpretation of the rise of the asylum – one endorsed by the German historian, Klaus Doerner.[30] Foucault and Doerner have claimed that confinement was essentially the sequestration of the mad poor; it was a reprisal conducted by advocates of the bourgeois imperative of labour against those who would not work. In Doerner's words, psychiatry was instituted 'specifically for the poor insane'. He contended that one of the key functions of the asylum lay in instructing the mad through work therapy. But the early history of the asylum offers little support to these hypotheses. Enterprising asylum proprietors naturally aimed to capture rich patients (and there seems to have been no shortage of these).[31] Moreover, there is little indication of organized labour in the early asylum (critics accused them in fact of being nests of idleness).[32]

All of this suggests that it would be simplistic to view the rise of institutional psychiatry in any crudely functional or conspiratorial terms, seeing it as a device to ensure the smoother running of the emergent capitalist economy, or as a tool for coping with the casualties of

---

[28] F. A. J. Harding, 'Dr Nathaniel Cotton of St Albans, Poet and Physician', *Herts. Countryside*, 23 (1969), 46–48.

[29] J. T. Perceval, *A Narrative of the Treatment Experienced by a Gentleman, during a state of Mental Derangement; Designed to Explain the Causes and the Nature of Insanity and to Expose the Injudicious Conduct Pursued Towards Many Unfortunate Sufferers Under that Calamity* (London, 1838); a modern abridged version is G. Bateson (ed.), *Perceval's Narrative* (Palo Alto, 1961); R. Hunter and I. MacAlpine, 'John Thomas Perceval (1803–1876) Patient and Reformer. (Review of "Perceval's Narrative"; a Patient's Account of his Psychosis, 1830–32)', *Medical History*, 6 (1962), 391–5. On Ticehurst see C. Mackenzie, 'Social Factors in the Admission, Discharge and Continuing Stay of Patients at Ticehurst Asylum, 1845–1917', in Bynum, Porter and Shepherd (eds.), *Anatomy of Madness*, II, pp. 147–74.

[30] Klaus Doerner, *Madmen and the Bourgeoisie: A Social History of Insanity and Psychiatry*, trans. Joachim Neugroschel and Jean Steinberg (Oxford, 1981).

[31] On mental disorder amongst the rich see the discussion in Roy Porter, 'The Rage of Party: a Glorious Revolution in English Psychiatry?', *Medical History*, 27 (1983), 35–50, and idem, *Mind Forg'd Manacles* ch. 2.

[32] Compare Michael Ignatieff, 'Total Institutions and Working Classes: a Review Essay', *History Workshop Journal*, 15 (1983), 167–73.

industrialization.[33] It is tempting to assume that the destabilizing effects of the market economy broke up old patterns of life, destroyed community and family ties, and created profound anxieties – in short, drove people crazy, while reducing the willingness or the ability of traditional support groups to cope with disturbed relatives.[34] But there is no certain evidence that proportionately more people became mentally unhinged during the era of industrialization. Contemporaries feared that this was happening, but they may simply have mistaken the greater visibility of madness (e.g. the attention focused upon the insane bouts of King George III) for its increasing incidence.[35] What is beyond dispute is that the supply of receptacles for the mad steadily increased through the eighteenth and into the nineteenth century – some private, some philanthropic, some official – and that the 'demand' for their facilities rose to meet the supply. Rather than seeing the emergence of the asylum in terms of manipulative social control, we should perhaps view it as the outcome of myriad small renegotiations of responsibilities, in an economy in which services were increasingly provided by cash payments.[36]

I have stressed the sheer diversity of the *ancien régime* lunatic asylum, in terms of size, level of medicalization, and its proprietorship. Not surprisingly, perhaps, they consequently differed widely in quality. Nineteenth-century reformers pictured early madhouses as utter abominations: riddled with neglect, cruelty, and corporal punishment – the use of the whip, of manacles, of beatings – masquerading as therapy. The published protestations of former inmates of such asylums give

[33] There has been some rather fruitless debate as to whether asylums were genuinely humanitarian or essentially instruments of social control. See K. Jones, 'Scull's Dilemma', *British Journal of Psychiatry*, 141 (1982), 221–6; for good discussion of social control see S. Cohen and A. Scull (eds.), *Social Control and the State* (Oxford, 1983); and A. Scull, 'Humanitarianism or Control? Some Observations on the Historiography of Anglo-American Psychiatry', *Rice University Studies*, 67 (1981), 35–7.

[34] See Peter L. Tyor and J. S. Zainoldin, 'Asylum and Society: An Approach to Industrial Change', *Journal of Social History*, 13 (1979), 23–48.

[35] For modern debate as to whether the increase of madness was 'real' see Edward Hare, 'Was Insanity on the Increase?', *British Journal of Psychiatry*, 142 (1983), 439–55; and A. Scull, 'Was Insanity Increasing? A Response to Edward Hare', *British Journal of Psychiatry*, 144 (1984), 432–6. See also W. S. Hallaran, *An Enquiry into the Causes Producing the Extraordinary Addition to the Number of Insane, Together with Extended Observations on the Cure of Insanity; with Hints as to the Better Management of Public Asylums for Insane Persons* (Cork, 1810); *idem*, *Practical Observations on the Causes and Cure of Insanity* (Cork, 1818).

[36] For excellent discussions see J. Walton, 'Casting out and Bringing Back in Victorian England', in Bynum, Porter and Shepherd (eds.), *Anatomy of Madness*, II, pp. 132–6; *idem*, 'Lunacy in the Industrial Revolution: a Study of Asylum Admissions in Lancashire, 1848–1850', *Journal of Social History*, 13 (1979/80), 1–22; *idem*, 'The Treatment of Pauper Lunatics in Victorian England: the Case of the Lancaster Asylum, 1834–1871', in Scull (ed.), *Madhouses*, pp. 166–200.

documentary backing to these denunciations. Yet the traditional asylum could be good as well as bad, even in the eyes of its patients. For example, the poet William Cowper, who went mad after several failed suicide attempts, spent eighteen months in Nathaniel Cotton's asylum at St Albans mentioned earlier. In his later autobiography he had nothing but praise for the care and attention he had received from the good doctor, 'ever watchful and apprehensive for my welfare'. So much did he approve of the attendants, that on his release, recovered, he persuaded Cotton to allow one of them to come with him as his personal servant.[37] The hundreds of pages of testimony given to the House of Commons committee on madhouses in 1815 gives abundant evidence of the positive qualities of certain madhouses – mainly private ones – while revealing the callousness and squalor of institutions such as Bethlem.[38]

Indeed, as I hinted earlier, the eighteenth-century private madhouse became a formative site for the development of psychiatry as an art and science. Asylums were not instituted for the practice of psychiatry; rather psychiatry was the practice which developed once the problem of managing asylum inmates arose. In other words, theories of insanity had been quite rudimentary before doctors and other proprietors had gained extensive experience of treating the mad in sizable numbers at close quarters. It had been widely assumed that the mad were little better than wild beasts, requiring stern discipline while hoping that nature might perhaps work a cure; and a range of antique therapies and drugs had been used time out of mind: bloodlettings, purgings, vomits, cold-water shock treatments. But practical psychiatry was transformed during the course of the eighteenth century through asylum experience, buoyed up also by the optimism generated by the new institution.

For one thing, it was widely claimed that the well-designed, well-managed asylum would in fact restore to mental health a high percentage of the insane. In mid-eighteenth-century England, William Battie, physician to the newly founded St Luke's Asylum in London,[39] admitted that a certain proportion of the insane did indeed suffer from 'original insanity' which – rather like original sin – was essentially incurable; yet he contended that far more common was 'consequential insanity' – i.e. insanity brought about as a result of some accident – for

[37] W. Cowper, *Memoir of the Early Life of William Cowper* (London, 1816), p. 99. See also Porter, *Social History of Madness*, ch. 5.
[38] See *First Report. Minutes of Evidence Taken Before the Select Committee Appointed to Consider of Provisions Being Made for the Better Regulation of Madhouses in England* (Ordered, by the House of Commons, to be Printed, 25 May 1815).
[39] C. N. French, *The Story of St Lukes* (London, 1951).

which the prognosis was good. To maximize cures, argued Battie and his many followers, what was required was early diagnosis, early confinement (before the madness grew confirmed), and then a regime tailored to the needs of the individual case. Routine and general therapeutics (such as the annual spring bloodletting deployed at Bethlem) were useless. Indeed, Battie argued, medical, surgical and mechanical techniques would in general avail little: medicine would accomplish far less than management, by which he meant close person-to-person encounters designed to understand and overcome the particular delusions or moral perversions of the individual sufferer.[40]

Throughout Europe, the last decades of the eighteenth century and the early ones of the nineteenth saw a blossoming of faith in the prospect of cures accomplished in the sheltered environment of the asylum ('far from the madding crowd') by the astute therapist. In England, such doctors as Thomas Arnold, William Pargeter,[41] Joseph Mason Cox (who stressed the value of 'gentleness') and Francis Willis – the man called in to treat King George III when he became deranged in 1788[42] – followed in the footsteps of William Battie with his watchword that 'management did more than medicine'. They devised the techniques of 'moral management', through which the expert and astute mind of the therapist would outmanoeuvre the deluded consciousness of his charge. Shortly afterwards, the Tukes at the York Retreat developed their philosophy of 'moral therapy' with its systematic emphasis upon creating a family atmosphere of humanity, as an environment for reconditioning the behaviour of the lunatic.[43]

Comparable developments occurred elsewhere. In late-eighteenth-century Tuscany, fired by Enlightenment ideals, Dr Vicenzo Chiarugi repudiated the old carceral regime, with its emphasis upon mere custody, traditional medication, and restraint, and proclaimed the superiority of

[40] See discussion in R. Hunter and I. MacAlpine, introduction to *A Treatise on Madness by William Battie and Remarks on Dr Battie's Treatise on Madness by John Monro* (London, 1962). See also M. Hay, 'Understanding Madness. Some Approaches to Mental Illness, 1650–1800' (University of York Ph.D. thesis, 1979); and for more general discussion of therapeutic innovation, W. L. Jones, *Ministering to Minds Diseased. A History of Psychiatric Treatment* (London, 1983).

[41] See W. Pargeter, *Observations on Maniacal Disorders* (Reading, 1792).

[42] See I. MacAlpine and R. Hunter, *George III and the Mad-business* (London, 1969).

[43] S. Tuke, *Description of the Retreat, an Institution near York for Insane Persons of the Society of Friends*, facsimile edition ed. R. Hunter and I. MacAlpine (London, 1964, first edition 1813); A. Digby, 'Moral Treatment at the York Retreat', in Bynum, Porter and Shepherd (eds.), *Anatomy of Madness*, II, pp. 52–72. For a critical evaluation see A. Scull, 'Moral Treatment Reconsidered: Some Sociological Comments on an Episode in the History of British Psychiatry', in Scull (ed.), *Madhouses*, pp. 105–18, and Roy Porter, 'Was there a Moral Therapy in 18th Century Psychiatry?', *Lychnos* (1981/2), 12–26.

therapies which treated the madman as a human being.[44] A more
specifically Christian reformist programme was advocated in the
German-speaking world by Dr Reil. He stressed how madness was a
sickness of the soul, and regarded the asylum doctor as somewhat akin
to a latter-day exorcist. For Reil, the environment of the asylum should
ideally provide a stage whose many distinct scenarios – of terror,
punishment, fear and hope, doom and forgiveness – would provide
traumatic and purgative moral and spiritual experiences – a kind of
pilgrim's progress eventually leading the sufferer back to sanity.[45]

Most spectacular of all, perhaps, was the psychiatric reform initiated
in Paris by Dr Philippe Pinel. Specifically inspired by the ideals of
liberty, equality, and fraternity disseminated by the French Revolution,
Pinel literally and figuratively removed the chains from the mad patients
at the Salpetrière and Bicêtre Hospitals in 1793. It was a fine symbolic
gesture. But Pinel's act also embodied the best constructive and
progressive thinking about curative therapies. If insanity was a mental
disorder, a set of mental shackles imprisoning the patient, it had to be
cured through mental approaches. Physical restraint was at best an
irrelevance, at worst an irritant for the patient and a lazy alternative to
real treatment. For Pinel and all the other psychiatric reformers just
mentioned, madness was tantamount to a failure of internal, rational
discipline on the part of the sufferer. His moral faculties needed to be
reawakened and rekindled so that inner self-discipline and self-control
could come to replace external coercion. In other words, psychiatry's
task was to re-animate the rational consciousness or conscience (though
modern sceptics would say that Pinel's revolution merely exchanged one
set of chains for another).[46]

[44] George Mora, 'The 1774 Ordinance for the Hospitalization of the Mentally Ill in Tuscany:
a Reassessment', *Journal for the History of the Behavioral Sciences*, 11 (1975), 246–56; *idem*, 'Bi-
centenary of the Birth of Vincenzo Chiarugi (1749–1820): a Pioneer of the Modern Mental
Hospital', *American Journal of Psychiatry*, 116 (1959), 267–71; *idem*, 'Pietro Pisani (1760–1837): a
Precursor of Modern Mental Hospital Treatment', *American Journal of Psychiatry*, 117 (1960), 79–81;
Luigi Stropplana, 'La riforma degli ospedali psichiatrici di chiarugi nel quadro del riformiso',
Rivista di Storia Medica, 20 (1976) 168–79.
[45] M. Schrenk, *Über den Umgang mit Geisterskranken: Die Entwicklung der Psychiatrischen Therapie
vom 'Moralischen Regime' in England und Frankreich zu den 'Psychischen Curmethoden' in Deutschland*
(New York and Heidelberg, 1973). For Reil see ch. 12–13 of E. Harms, *Origins of Modern Psychiatry*
(Springfield, Il., 1967); and Sir A. Lewis, 'J. C. Reil, Innovator and Battler', *Journal of the History
of the Behavioral Sciences*, 1 (1965), 178–90.
[46] C. Jones, 'The "New Treatment" of the Insane in Paris', *History Today* (October 1980), 5–10.
J. Postel, 'Les premières expériences psychiatriques de Philippe Pinel à la maison de Santé
Belhomme', *Canadian Journal of Psychiatry*, 28 (1983), 571–5; K. Grange, 'Pinel and Eighteenth
Century Psychiatry', *Bulletin of the History of Medicine*, 35 (1961), 442–53.

The 'new psychiatries', the reformist ideals just discussed, were children of their time, and they harmonized well with the socio-political optimism abroad at the beginning of the nineteenth century. In many European nations, liberals and reformers wished to do away with all the last vestiges of the corrupt and benighted *ancien régime* of madhouses. Insofar as traditional institutions such as London's Bethlem were reminders of mere repression, mindless coercion, and hopeless confinement, reformers urged they be thoroughly purged and transformed. Insofar as private asylums had allowed wicked families improperly to lock up their parents, wives, daughters, or even had been exploited for political purposes, they needed to be hedged around with protective legal safeguards. Insofar as the madhouse had been a secret space, hidden from public scrutiny, it now needed to be opened up to proper public inspection and control. Exposés such as John Mitford's *The Crimes and Horrors in the Interior of Warburton's Private Madhouses at Hoxton and Bethnal Green* (1825) made a great stir.

Hence, in many parts of Europe, the generation following the French Revolution proved immensely influential in transforming the institutionalization of the mad from an *ad hoc* expedient, which had 'just growed', into an idealistic system with a formal place within the protocols of a paternalistic state. (To put this another way, criticism led not to the abolition of the asylum, but to its refurbishing in a reformed guise.) In France, for example, the reforms of Pinel and the new legal requirements of the Napoleonic Code were further codified in the extremely important statute of 1838. This formally required each *département* for the first time either to establish its own network of public asylums for the mad, or at least to ensure the provision of adequate facilities for them. It furthermore aimed to provide against improper confinement by establishing rules for the certification of confined lunatics by medical officers (though for pauper lunatics the signature of the prefect remained sufficient warrant for confinement).[47] Prefects were given powers to inspect asylums. Very similar legislation was passed in Belgium in 1850.[48]

A comparable programme of reform was put through in England, in the teeth of opposition from vested interests within the medical

---

[47] R. G. Hillman, 'The Imprisonment of Mentally Ill Patients in Early Nineteenth-Century Provincial France: Legal Proceedings', *23rd International Congress of the History of Medicine* (London, 1972), *Proceedings*, 1 (1974), 416–21.

[48] R. Pierott, 'Belgium', in J. G. Howells (ed.), *World History of Psychiatry* (New York, 1968), 136–49.

profession, who feared that the independence and profitability of the private asylum would be undermined. Scandals revealing the widespread practice of the improper confinement of the sane in private asylums had already led to one important legislative safeguard in the eighteenth century. The Madhouses Act of 1774 had set up a rudimentary system of licensing and certification. Under its provisions, all private madhouses had to be licensed annually by magistrates. A maximum size for each asylum was established. The renewal of licenses would depend upon satisfactory maintainance of admissions registers.[49] Magistrates were empowered to carry out visitations (in London the inspecting body was a committee of the Royal College of Physicians). Most importantly, a system of medical certification was for the first time instituted. Henceforth, although paupers could continue to be confined at the nod of magistrates, the written statement of a regular medical practitioner would be required before confinement was lawful.

Further reforms followed in the nineteenth century. A combination of further scandalous revelations and reformist zeal led to parliamentary committees in 1807 and 1815 which assembled an unparalleled quantity of evidence on the provision and condition of madhouses throughout the nation. Evidence of gross mismanagement at Bethlem (where it was said that the recently deceased surgeon, Bryan Crowther, had himself been so mad as to require being kept in a straitjacket) led to the dismissal of the medical staff.[50] The ineffectiveness of the 1774 Act led to its strengthening in a series of Acts passed from the 1820s, above all establishing the Commissioners in Lunacy, first merely for the metropolitan area and then for the whole of England.[51] The Lunacy Commissioners constituted a permanent body of inspectors (some members were doctors, others lawyers) charged to report on the state of asylums. They had powers to prosecute illegal practices and to refuse renewals of licenses. They also possessed a remit to standardize and improve conditions of care and treatment. It is possible that the Lunacy Commissioners helped introduce a stultifying uniformity; they un-

[49] See R. A. Hunter, I. MacAlpine and L. M. Payne, 'The County Register of Houses for the Reception of Lunatics, 1798–1812', *Journal of Mental Science*, 102 (1963), 856–63.

[50] A. Scull, 'The Social History of Psychiatry in the Victorian Era', in Scull (ed.), *Madhouses*, pp. 5–34; Peter McCandless, 'Insanity and Society: A Study of the English Lunacy Reform Movement, 1815–1870' (University of Wisconsin Ph.D. thesis, 1974); E. G. O'Donoghue, *The Story of Bethlehem Hospital, from its Foundation in 1247* (London, 1914).

[51] N. Hervey, 'A Slavish Bowing Down', in Bynum, Porter and Shepherd (eds.), *Anatomy of Madness*, II, pp. 98–131; Sir Allan Powell, *The Metropolitan Asylums Board and its Work, 1867–1930* (London, 1930); D. J. Mellett, 'Bureaucracy and Mental Illness: the Commissioners in Lunacy 1845–90', *Medical History*, 25 (1981), 221–50.

doubtedly also ensured the eradication of the worst abuses in the madhouse system (e.g. by insisting on the formal keeping of patient records and by requiring that all cases of the use of coercion should be recorded on paper).

Safeguards against the dangers of the improper confinement of the sane in lunatic asylums were further tightened.[52] Under the influential consolidating act of 1890, two medical certificates were required for the first time for the confinement of all patients. In the long run, this liberal and legalistic concern lest asylums be used as carceral institutions may have proved counter-productive. For by insisting that only formally certified lunatics be lodged in asylums, it delayed the possibility of the asylum turning into an 'open' institution, easy of access and easy of exit. Rather the asylum was confirmed as the institution of last resort; certification thus all too readily became associated with protracted detention. The result was a failure to provide institutional care appropriate for bouts of insanity merely of short duration, or indeed for those who were only moderately psychiatrically disturbed.[53]

Throughout Europe, it was the nineteenth century which witnessed the most rapid rise in the number of mental hospitals and the aggregate of patients confined therein. In England, patient numbers rose from perhaps 10,000 (in all types of institution) in 1800 to some 100,000 in 1900. The rise was especially rapid in the new nation states. In Italy, for example, some 18,000 had been confined in 1881; by 1907 the number had soared to 40,000. Such increases are not hard to explain. The bureaucratic and utilitarian mentalities of the nineteenth century entertained an immense faith in the powers of institutional solutions, indeed quite literally in bricks and mortar. Schools, reformatories, prisons, hospitals, asylums – all these would solve the superabundant social problems of an age of rapid population rise, urbanization and

[52] T. Butler, *Mental Health, Social Policy and the Law* (London, 1985). See also for contemporary fears James Parkinson, *Mad-houses. Observations on the Act for Regulation of Mad-Houses, and a Correction of the Statements of the Case of Benjamin Elliott, convicted of Illegally Confining Mary Daintree: With Remarks Addressed to the Friends of Insane Persons* (London, 1811).

[53] A further contemporary development, which cannot be explored here, was the interface between law and psychiatry. See for Britain D. J. West and A. Walk, *Daniel McNaughton: His Trial and Aftermath* (Ashford, 1977); Richard Moran, *Knowing Right from Wrong. The Insanity Defense of Daniel McNaughton* (New York, 1983); Roger Smith, 'The Boundary Between Insanity and Criminal Responsibility in Nineteenth Century England', in Scull (ed.), *Madhouses*, pp. 363–83; P. H. Allderidge, 'Criminal Insanity: Bethlem to Broadmoor', *Proceedings of the Royal Society of Medicine*, 67 (1974), 897–904; N. Walker, *Crime and Insanity in England*, 1 (Edinburgh, 1968); J. Eigen, 'Intentionality and Insanity: What the 18th-Century Juror Heard', in Bynum, Porter and Shepherd (eds.), *Anatomy of Madness*, 11, pp. 34–51; Kathleen Jones, *Lunacy, Law, and Conscience, 1744–1845. The Social History of the Care of the Insane* (London, 1955).

industrialization. The spirit of reform helped to convince the public and legislatures alike that the new asylums would not be mere dungeons of repressive inhumanity. The new psychiatries of Pinel, Chiarugi, the Tukes etc. specifically promised that the properly managed asylum would not merely secure the mad but cure them as well.[54]

The first two thirds of the nineteenth century thus constituted a period of intense (and intensely optimistic) thought and action focusing on the asylum as the site for treating insanity. Many important innovations were pioneered. In England the new philosophy of 'non-restraint' was selectively introduced from the 1830s onwards, above all thanks to the efforts of Robert Gardiner Hill at the Lincoln Asylum, and John Conolly[55] at the large public asylum at Hanwell on the western outskirts of London.[56] Extending the aims of moral therapy, Hill and Conolly programmatically abolished all forms of mechanical coercion what-soever. They argued that not just manacles and shackles but even straitjackets could advantageously be dispensed with. Their functions could be taken over by the surveillance of vigilant attendants within a total asylum regime of disciplined, organized work and activity which would stimulate the mind and inculcate self-control. Hill claimed non-restraint was a great success. In 1834 647 incidents occurred at the Lincoln Asylum requiring manual restraint; by 1838 there were none; and this had been achieved without any deaths or suicides.

[54] For a characteristic text see William Alexander Francis Browne, *What Asylums Were, Are and Ought to Be: Being the Substance of Five Lectures Delivered Before the Managers of the Montrose Royal Lunatic Asylum* (Edinburgh, 1837). See also M. Fears, 'Therapeutic Optimism and the Treatment of the Insane', in R. Dingwall (ed.), *Health Care and Health Knowledge* (London, 1977), pp. 66–81; *idem*, 'The "Moral Treatment" of Insanity: A Study in the Social Construction of Human Nature' (University of Edinburgh Ph.D. Thesis, 1978); J. M. Leniaud, 'La cité utopie ou l'asile dans la première moitié du XIXe siècle', in Lyons, Université Claude Bernard, Institut d'Histoire de la Médecine, *Conférences d'Histoire de la Médecine*, 82 (1983), 129–44.

[55] See A. Scull, 'John Conolly: a Victorian Psychiatric Reformer', in Bynum, Porter and Shepherd (eds.), *Anatomy of Madness*, pp. 103–50; J. Conolly, *Treatment of the Insane without Mechanical Restraints* (London, 1973, reprint of 1856 edn); *idem*, *The Construction of Government of Lunatic Asylums and Hospitals for the Insane* (London, 1968, reprint of 1847 edn).

[56] See A. Walk, 'Some Aspects of the Moral Treatment of the Insane up to 1854', *Journal of Mental Science*, 100 (1954), 807–37; Robert Gardiner Hill, *A Concise History of the Entire Abolition of Mechanical Restraint in the Treatment of the Insane and of the Introduction, success and final triumphs of the Non-Restraint System together with a Reprint of a Lecture delivered on the Subject in the Year 1838* (London, 1857); J. A. Frank, 'Non-restraint and Robert Gardiner Hill', *Bulletin of the History of Medicine*, 41 (1967), 140–60; A. Walk, 'Lincoln and Non-restraint', *British Journal of Psychiatry*, 117 (1970), 481–95. For the fate of non-restraint elsewhere see C. Geduldig, *Die Behandlung der Geisteskranken Ohne Psysischen Zwang. Die Rezeption des Non-Restraint im Deutschen Sprachgebiet* (Zurich, 1975); N. Raskin, 'Non-restraint (Introduction of the Principle into Russia, by S. S. Korsakov in 1881)', *American Journal of Psychiatry*, 115 (1958), 471; M. Lyskanowski, 'Recognition of the English "No-Restraint System" in the Warsaw Medical Milieu of the Nineteenth Century', *23rd International Congress of the History of Medicine* (London, 1972), *Proceedings*, 1 (1974), 759–61.

Despite Pinel's freeing of the mad from their chains, *total* non-restraint was seen by continental reformers as a peculiarly English *idée fixe*, an example of doctrinaire liberalism, and was little imitated. But reformers in France, Germany and Italy made similarly inventive use of the asylum environment. Work therapy was widely favoured. Sited in the countryside, the nineteenth-century asylum typically became a self-sufficient colony, running its own farms, laundries and workshops, partly for reasons of economy, partly implementing an ideology of cure through labour. In France the systematic use of balneological treatments became a key feature of 'asylum science', or what was known as *police intérieure*.[57] In Germany, C. F. W. Roller's *Die Irrenanstalt nach ihren Beziehung* (1831) influentially spelt out detailed desiderata in such matters as patient dress, diet and exercise.[58] There the asylum was often closely linked to the university medical faculty, with the aim of providing clinical instruction for students.[59]

Everywhere, the care and cure of the mad came to be closely associated with a new 'science': asylum management. Asylum keepers grouped together to form the nucleus of the psychiatric profession, and professional journals such as the *Asylum Journal* and the *Annales Médico-psychologiques* were established.[60] Professional congresses and publications

[57] Gerard Bleandonu and Guy Le Gaufey, 'Naissance des asiles d'alienée (Auxerre–Paris)', *Annales, Economies, Sociétés, Civilisations*, 30 (1975), 93–121; English translation in R. Forster and O. Ranum, *Deviants and the Abandoned in French Society (Selections from the Annales Economies Sociétés, Civilizations)*, IV (Baltimore and London, 1978), pp. 180–212; C. Jones, 'The Treatment of the Insane in Eighteenth and Early Nineteenth-Century Montpellier', *Medical History*, 29 (1980), 371–90; *idem, Charity and Bienfaisance* (Cambridge, 1983), pp. 176f.; for Charenton's early history, see C. F. S. Giraudy, *Mémoire sur la maison nationale de Charenton* (Paris, Year 12); and J. Esquirol, *Mémoire historique et statistique sur la maison royale de Charenton* (Paris, 1824); see also C. Quétel, 'Garder les fous dans un asile de province au XIXe siècle. Le Bon-Sauveur de Caen', *Annales Normandie*, 29 (1979), 193–224.

[58] O. M. Marx, 'Diet in European Psychiatric Hospitals, Jails, and General Hospitals in the First Half of the 19th-Century according to Travellers' Reports', *Journal of the History of Medicine*, 23 (1968), 217–47. Compare J. Hawkes, *On the General Management of Public Lunatic Asylums in England and Wales. An Essay* (London, 1871).

[59] E. Kraepelin, *One Hundred Years of Psychiatry* (London, 1962). For German mental institutions see H. Kranz and K. Heinrich, *Bilanz und Ausblick der Anstaltpsychiatrie. 100 Jahre Rheinisches Landeskrankenhaus-Psychiatrische Klinik der Universität Düsseldorf, 1876–1976* (Stuttgart, 1977); and H. Schadewaldt, 'Geschichtlicher Überblick über die Entwicklung des Rheinischen Landeskranken-hauses-Psychiatrische Klinik der Universität Düsseldorf 1876 bis 1976', in Kranz and Heinrich, *Bilanz und Ausblick der Anstaltpsychiatrie*, pp. 7–15; D. Blasius, 'The Asylum in Germany before 1860', in Spierenburg (ed.), *Emergence of Carceral Institutions*, pp. 148–64.

[60] A. Scull, 'From Madness to Mental Illness. Medical Men as Moral Entrepreneurs', *European Journal of Sociology*, 16 (1975), 219–61; *idem*, 'Mad-Doctors and Magistrates: English Psychiatry's Struggle for Professional Autonomy in the Nineteenth Century', *European Journal of Sociology*, 17 (1976), 279–305; W. F. Bynum, 'The Nervous Patient in Eighteenth and Nineteenth Century England: The Psychiatric Origins of British Neurology', in Bynum, Porter and Shepherd (eds.), *Anatomy of Madness*, I, pp. 89–102.

were preoccupied above all not with the theory of insanity but with the practical issues of managing the well-run asylum.[61]

Questions of architecture were of cardinal importance.[62] Asylum design had to ensure maximum security, ample ventilation, efficient drainage, optimal visibility (Bentham's target of panopticism, i.e. total surveillance, though few asylums were actually built following his precise blueprint for the panopticon prison), and, not least, efficient classification of the different grades of lunatics. Men had to be separated from women, incurables from curables, the violent from the peaceable, the clean from the dirty, and a ladder of progress established so that improving lunatics could see themselves moving onwards from ward to ward, getting ever nearer to the final door of discharge. Meticulous classification of the inmates became the first commandment of asylum managers and of the English lunacy commissioners. And all these aims had to be achieved in ways compatible with order, economy, efficiency and discipline. The art of management had to combine the highest goals of statecraft (the asylum as a form of Utopia, better organized even than sane society) together with expertise in such matters as non-slip, fireproof floor materials and self-locking door fittings.

Asylums had never been without their critics.[63] Institutions such as Bedlam early became a byword for man's inhumanity to man. An extensive literature of patient protest grew up from the eighteenth century onwards complaining of brutality and neglect.[64] And a radical undercurrent within the medical profession itself had always insisted

[61] Otto M. Marx, 'Descriptions of Psychiatric Care in Some Hospitals During the First Half of the 19th-Century', *Bulletin of the History of Medicine*, 41 (1967), 208–14.

[62] See Michael Ignatiaff, *A Just Measure of Pain* (London, 1978); M. Donnelly, *Managing the Mind* (London, 1983); Robin Evans, *The Fabrication of Virtue. English Prison Architecture, 1750–1840* (Cambridge, 1982); T. Markus (ed.), *Order in Space and Society* (Edinburgh, 1982), especially T. Markus, 'Buildings for the Bad and the Mad in Urban Scotland', pp. 25–114; Sir H. C. Burdett, *Hospitals and Asylums of the World: Their Origin, History, Construction, Administration, Management and Legislation ... the Portfolio of Plans of ... British, Colonial American and Foreign Hospitals ... in Addition to Plans of all the Hospitals of London*, 4 vols. (London, 1983); D. Jetter, *Geschichte des Hospitals* (Wiesbaden, 1966/1971); J. D. Thompson and G. Goldin, *The Hospital: A Social and Architectural History* (New Haven, 1975). See also Peter McCandless, 'Build! Build! The Controversy over the Care of the Chronically Insane in England, 1855–1870', *Bulletin of the History of Medicine*, 53 (1979), 553–74.

[63] This is well brought out in D. M. Mellett, *The Prerogative of Asylumdom* (New York, 1982).

[64] For the confined protesting their sanity in such cases see Samuel Bruckshaw, *The Case, Petition and Address of Samuel Bruckshaw, who Suffered a Most Severe Imprisonment, for Very Near a Whole Year, Loaded with Irons, without Being Heard in his Defence, Nay even without Being Accused, and at last Denied an Appeal to a Jury, Humbly Offered to the Perusal and Consideration of the Public* (London, 1774); and Alexander Cruden, *The London Citizen Exceedingly injured: or a British Inquisition Display'd in Account of the Unparallel'd Case of a Citizen of London, Bookseller to the late Queen, Who Was Sent to a Private Madhouse* (London, 1739). For later instances see N. Hervey, 'Advocacy or Folly: The Alleged

that, with the best will in the world, the asylum must necessarily prove counter-productive. For (argued critics such as Andrew Harper and George Nesse Hill)[65] mad people herded together would inevitably reduce each other to the lowest common denominator; in this sense, madhouses were bound to be 'manufactories of madness'. What the insane needed (critics claimed) was the mental and moral stimulus of the sane not the inevitable stigma of seclusion. But up to perhaps the mid-nineteenth-century advocates had outnumbered critics, and the asylum movement had been buoyed up on a wave of optimism.

This changed. A new pessimism becomes conspicuous in the second half of the nineteenth century. Asylum discharge figures left no one in any doubt that the expectations that the asylum would become an engine of almost universal cure-power were proving grossly over-optimistic. Recent studies have demonstrated that, despite a popular stereotype, it was by no means true that admission to the late-nineteenth-century asylum was effectively a death-certificate; that people left only in hearses.[66] All the same, success rates (though largely statistically meaningless) even in the best asylums, such as the York Retreat, dipped during the course of the century, and public asylums above all silted up with large complements of long-stay patients (the older they became, the greater the likelihood that they would stay for life).

To some extent, asylum psychiatrists had proved the victims of their own ideology. In developing categories such as 'monomania', 'klep-tomania', 'dipsomania', 'moral insanity' etc., they had argued that many of the kinds of aberrant conduct traditionally labelled vice, sin, and crime were true mental disorders which should be treated in the asylum.[67] As a result, magistrates and prison authorities had been encouraged to divert difficult and recidivist cases from the workhouse or the jail to the asylum, where superintendents discovered to their cost that regeneration posed more problems than anticipated. Furthermore, the senile and the demented, along with epileptics, paralytics, sufferers from

Lunatics' Friend Society, 1845–63', *Medical History*, 30 (1986), 245–75; R. Paternoster, *The Madhouse System* (London, 1841); Louisa Lowe, *The Bastilles of England, or the Lunacy Laws* (London, 1883).

[65] See A. Harper, *A Treatise on the Real Cause and Cure of Insanity in Which the Nature and Distinction of this Disease are Fully Explained, and the Treatment Established on New Principles* (London, 1789); and for Hill, Roy Porter, 'Brunonian Psychiatry: The Case of George Nesse Hill', *Medical History Supplement*, 8 (London, 1988), 89–99.

[66] R. Russell, 'Mental Physicians and their Patients: Psychological Medicine in the English Pauper Lunatic Asylums of the Later Nineteenth-Century' (Sheffield University Ph.D. thesis, 1983), especially pp. 154f.

[67] V. Skultans, *Madness and Morals: Ideas on Insanity in the Nineteenth Century* (London, 1975), part III, 'Psychiatric Darwinism'.

tertiary syphilis, ataxias and neurological sensory-motor disorders increasingly found their way into the asylum warehouse. For all such conditions, the prognosis was gloomy. In time, the asylum became a dustbin for hopeless cases.

In the second half of the nineteenth century, psychiatry necessarily adjusted itself to cope with this newly bleak prognosis. If 'moral therapy' did not work, that seemed to indicate that much insanity was actually organic disease, indeed was ingrained and constitutional, probably a hereditary taint.[68] Researches seemed to show that madness was passed on from generation to generation, that alcoholics and syphilitics produced subnormal offspring, indeed that society harboured a vast 'iceberg' of atavistic degenerates and defectives. Confronted with these intractible problems, 'degenerationist' psychiatrists such as Henry Maudsley in England, Morel and Moreau de la Tours in France,[69] Griesinger, Friedrich and Jacobi in Germany[70] and Lombroso in Italy[71]

---

[68] J. C. Prichard, *A Treatise on Insanity and Other Disorders Affecting the Mind* (London, 1835). See also for England W. F. Bynum, 'Theory and Practice in British Psychiatry from J. C. Prichard (1786–1848) to Henry Maudsley (1835–1918)', in T. Ogawa (ed.), *History of Psychiatry* (Osaka, 1982), pp. 196–216, and more generally, E. T. Carlson and N. Dain, 'The Meaning of Moral Insanity', *Bulletin of the History of Medicine*, 36 (1962), 130–40.

[69] For France see Ian Dowbiggin, 'Degeneration in French Psychiatry', in Bynum, Porter and Shepherd (eds.), *Anatomy of Madness*, I, pp. 188–232; Ruth Harris, 'Murder under Hypnosis', in Bynum, Porter and Shepherd (eds.), *Anatomy of Madness*, II, pp. 197–241; R. Nye, *Crime, Madness and Policies in Modern France* (Princeton, NJ, 1984); R. Friedlander, *Benedict-Augustin Morel and the Development of the Theory of Degenerescence (the Introduction of Anthropology into Psychiatry)* (Ann Arbor, MI, 1973); J. Goldstein, '"Moral Contagion": A Professional Ideology of Medicine and Psychiatry in Eighteenth and Nineteenth Century France', in G. E. Geison (ed.), *Professions and the French State 1700–1900* (Philadelphia, 1984), pp. 181–223; M. D. Alexander, 'The Administration of Madness and Attitudes Toward the Insane in Nineteenth-Century Paris' (Johns Hopkins University Ph.D. thesis, 1976). For important contemporary texts see Prosper Lucas, *Traité philosophique et physiologique de l'heredité naturelle dans les états de santé et de maladie du système nerveux*, 2 vols. (Paris, 1847–50); J. Déjérine, *L'hérédité dans les maladies du système nerveux* (Paris, 1886); B. A. Morel, *Traité de dégénérescences physiques, intellectuelles, et morales de l'espèce humaine* (Paris, 1857); Antoine Ritti, *Histoire des travaux de la société médico-psychologique et eloges de ses membres*, 2 vols. (Paris, 1913–14).

[70] W. Griesinger, *Mental Pathology and Therapeutics*, trans. C. Lockhart Robertson and James Rutherford (New York, reprint of 1867 London translation of German 2nd edn, 1965); A. Mette, *Wilhelm Griesinger: der Begrunder der Wissenschaftlichen Psychiatrie in Deutschland* (Leipzig, 1976); O. Marx, 'Wilhelm Griesinger and the History of Psychiatry: a Reassessment', *Bulletin of the History of Medicine*, 46 (1972), 519–44.

[71] For Italy see A. Tagliavini, 'Aspects of the History of Psychiatry in Italy in the Second Half of the 19th Century', in Bynum, Porter and Shepherd (eds.), *Anatomy of Madness*, II, pp. 175–96; V. P. Babini, M. Cott, F. Minuz, A. Tagliavini, *Tra sapere e potere* (Milan, 1982); R. Canosa, *Storia del manicomio in Italia dall' unita ad oggi* (Milano, 1979); for a history of asylums in Milan, see A. de Bernardi, F. Peri, L. Panzeri, *Tempo e catene. Manicomio, psichiatria e classi subalterne* (Milano, 1980). For key contemporary texts see C. Lombroso, *L'uomo delinquente studiato in rapporto alla antropologia, alla medicina legale e alle discipline carcerarie* (Milan, 1876); A. Verga, 'Se come si possa definire la pazzia', *Archivio Italiano per le Malattie Nervose* (1874), 3–22, 73–83; E. Morselli, 'Psichiatria e neuropatologia', *Revista Sperimentale di Freniatria* (1905), 15–43.

believed there was little that could be done beyond placing such threats in the asylum where they would at least be prevented from breeding future generations of inbeciles and perverts. The Irish inspectors of lunacy had expressed the new pessimism as early as 1851, announcing that 'the uniform tendency of all asylums is to degenerate from their original object, that of being hospitals for the treatment of insanity, into domiciles for incurable lunatics'.

In this atmosphere, the large public asylum became larger (the average public asylum in England housed 116 patients in 1827, 802 patients in 1890) and degenerated into a centre of routine work, formal drills and financial stringency. Greater recourse was had to drug treatments designed essentially to sedate and stupefy. Therapeutic innovation was to focus chiefly upon experimental organic treatments such as the use in the present century of insulin coma therapy and of electro-convulsive therapy. The high ideals of the asylum gradually disappeared into thin air. In the USA – where developments initially followed an almost parallel course to those in England, moving from the optimism of moral therapy to an increasing preoccupation with safety and sedation – Nancy Tomes has traced a falling off of standards of care during the course of the nineteenth century.

Institutions such as the Pennsylvania Asylum, set up in the first half of the nineteenth century, initially showed high levels of community and family involvement, underpinning a curative ideology. By the last decades of the century, a more organic psychiatry had become dominant, which at its worst could serve as a cover-up for the indiscriminate use of sedatives (bromides, chloral) and a decline in personal therapy.[72]

It is open to real dispute how far the science of psychiatry as a whole is 'objective knowledge', or how far it rather constitutes an objectification of social values. Notions of the hierarchical structure of the mind (such as Plato's vision of reason governing the appetites in the mind, rather as the philosopher–kings should rule the people in the state, latterly translated into the Freudian super-ego, ego and id) seem suspiciously to mirror traditional concepts of the social hierarchy, indeed to exemplify the old microcosm/macrocosm analogy, linking individual to cosmos. And more generally, it is easy to claim that every society gets the kinds of 'psychiatric disorders' it deserves. Thus modern Western

[72] Nancy Tomes, *A Generous Confidence* (Cambridge, 1984). See also A. Scull, 'The Discovery of the Asylum Revisited', in Scull (ed.), *Madhouses*, pp. 144–65, for an assessment of scholarship on the early history of the asylum in America. For an excellent up-to-date survey of American developments in tandem to British ones, see Tomes's 'The Great Restraint Controversy', in Bynum, Porter and Shepherd (eds.), *Anatomy of Madness*, III.

societies have legitimated the concept of mild mental illness under the heading of 'neurosis'. Because we feel we have a right to happiness, we have a corresponding right to express our unhappiness in medical terms and to seek therapy. Such a resort would be unthinkable in today's China. There comparable symptoms (depression, lethargy, 'functional' disorders) are not 'psychiatrized' but rather 'somatized'. For in the Communist East, with its highly collective values, 'mental disorder' is a mark of socio-political deviation, whereas the presentation of organic disturbance commands a real claim on attention, sympathy and excuse. Thus sickness and its labels, and the sick role, are both culture-bound.[73]

It is a matter of debate how far we should see our very notion of mental illness as socially and culturally determined. What is beyond dispute, however, is that the strategy of institutionalizing the mad in lunatic asylums quite expressly puts into practice many of the key values of Western society since the Renaissance.[74] It represents a fusion of the imperatives of the rationalist state wedded to the expedients of a market economy. Its therapeutic optimism, developing since the late eighteenth century, displays enlightened optimism (carrying however a sting in the tail, the idea that certain groups in society have the right and duty to improve others). And not least it reflects the long-term secularizing culture-shift from religion to an ethos of science. Before the Renaissance and the Scientific Revolution, the crucial divide within the key values of the culture of Christendom lay between the godly and the ungodly. In that, the distinction between the sane and the crazy counted for relatively little. Increasingly, that has changed, and the salient polarity, since what we may call the 'age of reason', has become the division between the rational and the rest.[75] The institution of the asylum set up a *cordon sanitaire*, protecting the 'normal' from the 'mad', served to underline the Otherhood of the insane, and provided a managerial milieu in which that alienness could be confirmed. How far today's policies of returning the mentally ill to the community will reverse that process remains to be seen.

[73] A. Kleinman, *Social Origins of Distress and Disease* (New Haven and London, 1986).

[74] Bill Luckin, 'Towards a Social History of Institutionalization', *Social History*, 8 (1983), 87–94.

[75] Important discussions of this are contained in M. MacDonald, 'Religion, Social Change and Psychological Healing in England 1600–1800', in W. Shiels (ed.), *The Church and Healing* (Oxford, 1982), pp. 101–26; *idem*, 'Popular Belief about Mental Disorder in Early Modern England', in W. Eckart and J. Geyer-Kordesch (eds.), *Heilberufe und Kranke in 17 und 18 Jahrhundert* (Munster, 1982), pp. 148–73; *idem*, 'Insanity and the Realities of History in Early Modern England', *Psychological Medicine*, 11 (1981), 11–25.

From infectious to chronic diseases: changing patterns of sickness in the nineteenth and twentieth centuries

PAUL WEINDLING

The relationship between the rise of modern medicine and the incidence of disease is controversial. It might be expected that the greater a society's investment in medical research and health care, the less disease there would occur. But while it is possible to target certain problems for solution, a multiplicity of factors produce overall improvements in health, and it must be appreciated that medicine, disease and society are not constant and uniform categories. The history of medicine shows that relations between medical practitioners, medical institutions, patients' expectations and diseases have been constantly changing. Calculating the costs of medical services, and the extent of sickness in past societies are immensely complex tasks. Another way of perceiving the relationship between the advent of modern scientific medical services and disease is to see not so much a diminishing quantity of disease, but a change in the quality – i.e. in the types and virulence – of diseases. Demographers often refer to an 'epidemiological transition' from pre-industrial patterns of epidemic infectious diseases to a modern pattern of deaths from chronic degenerative diseases.[1] This raises the question whether morbidity and mortality patterns have fundamentally differed before and after industrialization, or whether only changes in perceptions and managing diseases have taken place.

Coupled with the rapid and substantial decline in infant mortality, the increased registered incidence of heart disease and cancers (the ills of middle and old age) has been an outstanding feature of industrial societies

[1] For a succinct analysis of these problems see R. Spree, *Health and Social Class in Imperial Germany* (Oxford, 1988). For the epidemiological transition see A. Omran, 'The Epidemiologic Transition. A Theory of the Epidemiology of Population Change', *Milbank Memorial Fund Quarterly*, 49 (1971), part 1.

during the twentieth century. The reasons for these supposed changes and for the consequent increase of life expectancy are far from clear. Various explanations for the changing spectrum of diseases have been advanced ranging from new therapies to improvements in diet and housing, and the limitation of family size. A major concern of nineteenth-century medicine was the combatting of epidemic infectious diseases. Most striking were the waves of cholera epidemics.[2] Less sensational but also a high risk to life were the diseases of poor sanitation such as typhoid, and of overcrowding such as typhus. There was attention to the diagnosis and contagious nature of these diseases, and to improving the environment in order to prevent the generation of 'miasmas' – or foul vapours – to which the origins of infections were attributed. Whether diseases were blamed on environmental causes, on microscopic germs or on a combination of environmentalist and contagionist theories, improvements in sanitation were required.[3] During the 1840s medical reformers mounted a vociferous crusade for public health reforms in European cities, which resulted in professional appointments for municipal and state medical officers, and specialized departments of public health. By the 1890s when epidemic infectious diseases were on the wane, interest increased in chronic degenerative diseases. Some, like tuberculosis and sexually transmitted diseases, were infections that weakened the sufferer over many years. Other illnesses, like alcoholism, heart disease and cancer, were stigmatized as 'diseases of civilization' or 'racial poisons'. Accordingly, medical thinking and practice was reoriented to problems of chronic ill health. This chapter seeks to examine the shift from infectious diseases to the modern mortality pattern of chronic degenerative diseases in industrial societies.

The impact on diseases of investment in medical training, and of large-scale institutions for medical education, research, care and treatments is far from clear. Germany is the classic case of high investment in medical education and research during the rapid industrialization after 1870 when science-based industries were an important factor in economic growth.[4] Medical services were financed by insurance and provided by scientifically trained doctors; rapid growth of hospitals and sanatoria occurred; and manufacture of pharmaceutical products also took off. In

[2] R. H. Shryock, *The Development of Modern Medicine* (Madison, WI, 1979); R. J. Evans, *Death in Hamburg* (Oxford, 1987).

[3] M. Pelling, *Cholera, Fever and English Public Medicine* (Oxford, 1976).

[4] P. J. Weindling, 'Medicine and Modernisation: the Social History of German Health and Medicine', *History of Science*, 24 (1986), 277–301; H-H. Eulner, *Die Entwicklung der medizinischen Spezialfächer an den Universitäten des deutschen Sprachgebietes* (Stuttgart, 1970).

this context of the emergence of a model system of modern medicine, serum therapy for diphtheria marked the advent of a new era of laboratory-based immunization and 'chemotherapies'. Until the advent of serum therapy in the 1890s there were only a few specific therapies for disease, such as quinine for malaria. Yet serum therapy coincided with intensified measures to improve housing and environmental conditions on the basis of concepts of 'natural immunity' – that of improving the body's resistance to infections. The complex interaction between medical innovation and social change make the impact of even major scientific breakthroughs difficult to evaluate. The origins of antiseptic surgery during the 1860s and of bacteriology during the 1870s coincided with more general attempts to clean up the urban environment, and with improvements in diet, housing and income. It has been pointed out that improved nutrition was a factor in increasing the rise in the number of successful operations.[5] It is thus difficult to disentangle what improvements in health were due to medical research and what to economic factors.

One indisputable consequence of modern systems of scientific medicine has been a rise in the professional status of doctors, and the establishment of widespread networks of primary care and of hospital referral systems.[6] While there has been improved diagnosis there have not always been improved therapies. Indeed, there was a venerable tradition of non-interventionism in nineteenth-century medicine. At the Vienna Medical School, brilliant clinical diagnosis was often accompanied by scepticism of drugs and interventive treatments.[7] The more medical facilities that have been provided, the greater the professional and public awareness of disease has become. A submerged mass of already existing aches, pains, carbuncles and infections has thus been rendered visible. As the hospital has replaced the home as the fit and proper place for serious diseases to be treated, so professional and public awareness of sickness – and of its costs – has risen.

The changing pattern of diseases

This shift from infectious to chronic degenerative diseases as an 'epidemiological transition' is presumed to be the counterpart of the 'demographic transition' of the early twentieth century from large

[5] D. Hamilton, 'The Nineteenth-century Surgical Revolution – Antisepsis or Better Nutrition', *Bulletin of the History of Medicine*, 56 (1982), 39–40.

[6] S. Webb and B. Webb. *The State and the Doctor* (London, 1910).

[7] E. Lesky, *The Vienna Medical School of the 19th Century* (Baltimore and London, 1976).

families suffering high mortality rates to small families with a low infant
and child mortality. The concept of linking demographic to morbidity
changes has a number of advantages. Thus modern methods of
contraception can be regarded as one of the most effective means of self-
help in improving personal health.[8] Relating population movements to
health offers the possibility of linking demographic and morbidity shifts
with social processes such as industrialization and urbanization.
However, a disadvantage of this way of looking at health in the context
of industrialization is that it might be assumed that chronic degenerative
diseases were not important in earlier periods: for they might simply
have been underdiagnosed, or masked by the onset of rapid and
spectacular infections. Thus tuberculosis, cancers and heart disease might
have been widespread in the past, but imperfectly diagnosed. The large
category of deaths from 'old age' in pre-twentieth-century mortality
tables should be noted. This category might well have concealed strokes
and cancers. It should also be noted that organisms vary in their
virulence, as well as the body's capacity of resistance to infections. Some
diseases such as 'chlorosis' have disappeared and others like hayfever
have become commonplace.[9] It is difficult to decide what was meant by
such outmoded concepts, for example whether chlorosis frequently
diagnosed in adolescent girls was anorexia nervosa, anaemia, exhaustion
due to poverty and overwork, or a product of the repressive social
attitudes. Thus it is puzzling whether the disappearance of such diseases
was due to changes in medical approaches, or to real differences due to
the transformation of diet, culture and life style in modern mass
industrial societies. As medical sociologists have pointed out, scientific
analysis of disease narrows the framework of reference and so excludes
relevant social factors.[10] Given the lack of understanding of the
interaction between working patterns and economic standing with
health, the social causes of diseases have been neglected. For these
reasons, the term 'epidemiological transition' is an oversimplification.

An analysis of medical approaches in terms of fashions or paradigms
rather than in terms of advances in medical science has much in its
favour. The procedures and rationales of science have in themselves
exercised power to shape the institutions and professional standards of
modern medicine. There have been numerous shifts between social and

[8] F. Ronsin, La grève de ventres (Paris, 1978).
[9] I. S. L. Loudon, 'The Diseases called Chlorosis', Psychological Medicine, 14 (1984), 27–36.
[10] D. Milles, 'From Workmen's Diseases to Occupational Diseases', in P. J. Weindling, The Social History of Occupation Health (London, 1985), pp. 55–77.

biological approaches to diseases. Between 1840 and 1890 there was an emphasis on 'cellular pathology'. It has often been said that cell theory was a distinctive German achievement, although it should be noted that many pioneers such as Purkyne or Remak emphasized their non-German identities and French research such as Henri Milne Edwards's work on the theory of physiological division of labour or Dujardin's sarcode theory was fundamental. Following the discovery by Matthias Schleiden and Theodor Schwann in 1838 that cells were common structural units of plant and animal life, Johannes Müller, the professor of physiology in Berlin, exemplified an influential approach to the organism and its functioning in terms of the study of its cellular constituents. An approach to tumours and infections was developed in terms of cellular pathology. Virchow, a political liberal, argued against humoral theories of disease.[11] The cell provided a unit of empirical observation and explanation for disease which could be explained in terms of cellular malfunctioning. Virchow and Remak emphasized the growth of cells from pre-existing cells by a process of continuous division, so replacing the Schleiden–Schwann theory of the crystallization of cells from the blastema (a structureless ground substance). The Bonn anatomist, Max Schultze, in the early 1860s redefined the cell as 'a clump of protoplasm surrounding a nucleus', so breaking with the Schleiden–Schwann emphasis on the cell as a membrane containing fluids of virtually no importance. Human anatomy thus became concerned with problems of cellular structure, growth and function. It should be appreciated that there were many variants of cell theory in the nineteenth century partly arising from discoveries about constituents of the cell, and partly from varieties of theoretical interpretation ranging from vitalism to mechanistic reductionism. This meant that ideas about the causes of tumour formation and diseases varied because of different views about cell division and the role of the nucleus, as well as about the responsiveness of cells to change in the organism and environment. Such division of opinion can be seen in debates on the origins of cancerous tumours. Virchow abandoned the blastema theory of tumours arising from a structureless ground substance and argued that tumours arose by cell division as a result of external stimuli on undifferentiated cells. Such a view combined physiological, histological and social factors.[12]

---

[11] R. Virchow, *Cellular pathology as Based upon Physiology and Pathological Histology* (repr. New York, 1971).
[12] L. J. Rather, *The Genesis of Cancer* (Baltimore and London, 1978); P. J. Weindling, *Darwinism and Social Darwinism in Imperial Germany* (Stuttgart, 1991).

During the nineteenth century there was a virtually utopian belief in the value of the transfer of discoveries in biology and physiology to clinical medicine. Despite persistent criticisms that the vivisection experiments on laboratory animals could not correspond to human physiology or diseases, and of the need to take environmental and psychological facts into account, confidence grew in the potential powers of medical science.[13] In France, the physiological experimentalism was enshrined in a great Parisian tradition stretching from Bichat at the beginning of the nineteenth century to the mid-century hegemony of Magendie and culminated in the supremely powerful Bernard. This was contested by the Montpellier school in which notably Barthes insisted on the essential unity of living beings and on the vital properties of varied organs and parts of the body. In Germany there was a greater degree of criticism of physiological experimentalism, and a search for the vital qualities and distinctive organizational structures of biological organisms. While the *Naturphilosophen* were renowned for abstract theorizing on the unity of man and nature, Johannes Müller symbolized the distinctive German biological concerns which found expression in rapid advances in cell biology and embryology. Müller, despite an early death in 1858, came to be regarded as a central figure in German biology and medicine as he unified philosophical and experimental modes of analysis so providing a stimulus to embryology, histology and cell biology, on which were based the achievements of German experimental medicine later in the century. Research was frequently histological and concentrated on reconstruction of morbid processes as a preliminary to providing causal explanation. The ultimate aims were prevention and therapy of disease on the basis of a thorough scientific understanding of the animal and human organism.

The hegemony of cellular pathology was challenged when Emil Behring, a bacteriologist working under Koch, claimed firstly that Virchow's prescription of social reform as an antidote to disease was impotent, and secondly that diseases were the result of parasite infections attacking the humoral constitution of the body. Behring was in the forefront of the development of a bacteriologically based serum therapy.[14] There was a shift from classification of diseases on the basis of signs and symptoms observed at a patient's bedside to laboratory-based diagnosis of causal organisms. Despite the enormous impact of

---

[13] N. A. Rupke (ed.), *Vivisection in Historical Perspective* (London, 1987).
[14] H. Zeiss and R. Bieling, *Behring, Gestalt und Werk* (Berlin, 1940).

bacteriology on medical thinking, the influence and effects of the introduction of effective bacteriologically based methods of prevention, whether by disinfection or by immunization, and of therapy remain controversial owing to a lack of systematic historical study of the biology and bacteriology of this crucial period. Leading figures in British public health thus continued to emphasize holistic and sanitarian approaches in preference to bacteriology until the mid twentieth century.[15] During the early twentieth century there was renewed emphasis on an inherited constitution to explain illness. The importance of the emergence of perceptions of chronic degenerative diseases can be seen with the rise of eugenics from the 1890s. Doctors took a lead in the eugenics movements in several European countries and North America. Eugenicists were among the first medical commentators on the prevalence of chronic degenerative diseases such as tuberculosis, alcoholism and venereal disease, although they warned against treatment as perpetuating genetically poor population groups. Their draconian emphasis on the breeding out of diseases, and preventive medicine can be seen in their concern with, for example, syphilis. Eugenicists also sought to eradicate the supposed germs of mental diseases such as schizophrenia by isolation and detention. During the 1920s and 30s constitutional medicine as an explanation for susceptibility to disease was in vogue, boosted by discoveries in genetics, endocrinology and nutrition. Although early attempts to apply genetics to medicine in the form of eugenics were ill-fated, the more cautious and more rigorously scientific approaches of human geneticists have had some success since the 1940s.[16] While high hopes are today pinned on genetic engineering and on molecular biology as providing keys to the problem of cancer, these have been preceded by an earlier generation of hereditary theories.

New therapies and theories

In considering the shift in diagnostic fashion from social to biological diseases, a more detailed examination of the advent of bacteriology is helpful. In the mid nineteenth century, cellular pathology was the counterpart of a chemical approach by Pasteur and Pettenkofer.[17] Both

---

[15] L. G. Stevenson, 'Science Down the Drain. On the Hostility of Certain Sanitarians to Animal Experimentation, Bacteriology and Immunology', *Bulletin of the History of Medicine*, 29 (1955), 1–26.
[16] D. J. Kevles, *In the Name of Eugenics. Genetics and the Uses of Human Heredity* (New York, 1985).   [17] C. Salomon Bayet (ed.), *Pasteur et la révolution pastorienne* (Paris, 1986).

Pasteur and Pettenkofer were convinced that industrial advance would lead to overall improvements in health. Their researches had economic implications as with Pasteur's efforts to eradicate chicken cholera and vine diseases, and with Pettenkofer's developing of a meat extract in association with Liebig.[18] This confidence in the benefits of medicine as providing the cure for the social ills resulting from industrialization during the 1860s was reversed by public health experts during the 1890s, who condemned unrestricted economic liberalism as damaging to health because it gave rise to slums, pollution and mass poverty.

Modern immunology arose from a synthesis between two schools of research: that of Koch's bacteriology and Pasteurian microbiology. Between 1873 and 1900 the causal organisms of almost all bacterial diseases were isolated. A turning point came with the simultaneous discovery of the anthrax bacillus by Koch and Pasteur in 1876. Koch argued that it was necessary to isolate a bacillus by staining; it was necessary to obtain pure cultures, and then to inject the cultures into an animal organisms so as to recreate the disease under experimental conditions. Known as 'Koch's postulates' these established the methodological basis for tackling the causes of infectious diseases.[19] Advances in experimental biology – with high-powered microscopes and aniline dyestuffs – were applied to medicine. During the nineteenth century efforts intensified to promote systematic monitoring of environmental and housing conditions. In the 1880s research and production of disinfectants gathered momentum. A search for disinfectants for homes and such public institutions as schools, offices and of course hospitals, led to research into what were referred to as internal disinfectants. This paved the way for the discovery of the immunizing properties of infected blood sera in the cases of tetanus and diphtheria. This was also of relevance to tropical medicine, as with international commissions against plague and cholera and sleeping sickness in 1890s. Large-scale research institutes were founded such as the Institut Pasteur in Paris in 1888 and Koch's Institut für Infectionskrankheiten in Berlin in 1891.[20] Virtually every European metropolis possessed a central institute for medical research, and the Rockefeller Institute for Medical Research was founded in New York in 1901. The British (from 1897 'Jenner' and

[18] H. Breyer, *Max von Pettenkofer* (Leipzig, 1980).
[19] The classic history of bacteriology remains W. Bulloch, *The History of Bacteriology* (London, 1938).
[20] A. Delaunay, *L'Institut Pasteur des origines à aujourd'hui* (Paris, 1962); B. Möllers, *Robert Koch* (Hannover, 1950).

from 1903 'Lister') Institute of Preventive Medicine derived from amalgamation with the College of State Medicine in 1893, but clinical research did not develop on any substantial scale in Britain until the founding of the Medical Research Council.[21]

Tuberculosis provides an illuminating case study of the impact of bacteriology. The discovery of the tuberculosis bacillus by Koch in 1882 was an international sensation, even though localist critics like Virchow argued that the discovery did not explain why tuberculosis took so many distinct clinical forms. The principle of the infectiousness of the disease was helpful in instigating preventive measures such as isolation and disinfection, although in practice these were pursued in too random a way to be effective. Even if the principle of the infectiousness of tuberculosis was accepted, there was no therapy. Koch's attempts to introduce 'tuberculin' therapy during the 1890s created a sensation as hopeful patients flocked to Berlin, but after widespread use its efficacy was challenged. After some modifications, tuberculin was recognized by Clemens von Pirquet in Vienna in 1907 as of diagnostic rather than therapeutic value. Yet the decline in tuberculosis mortality was occurring before an effective therapy was introduced. The disease had reached a low level by the time antibiotics became generally available in the late 1940s. Tuberculosis is thus an example of a chronic infectious disease exacerbated by poor social conditions of housing and diet.

The control of diphtheria marked a turning point in the rise of modern medicine as an effective means of preventing infection was developed. Although the bacillus was observed by Edwin Klebs in Zürich in 1882, it was a pupil of Koch, Friedrich Loeffler, who succeeded in culturing the bacillus in 1884. Loeffler took scientific research one step further by separating the poison from the bacillus. Behring was much influenced by Loeffler's concept of the disease process as an enzyme and by the demand for disinfectants. In 1890 Behring discovered that the broth used in culturing the bacillus had poisonous qualities. Kitasato, Behring's Japanese co-worker, noticed this for tetanus culture medium. Experiments showed that animals to whom large doses of diphtheria serum were administered acquired immunity when subsequently exposed to the diphtheria bacilli. In 1890 Behring injected the poison or 'toxin' of diphtheria into healthy animals and ensured their immunity to infection. Behring and Kitasato described this as the formation of an antibody to a toxin, which they referred to as an 'antitoxin'. The

[21] R. J. Godlee, *Lord Lister* (London, 1917).

conceptual foundations for immunization and immunology were thereby established.[22]

Diphtheria exemplifies the difficulties in making the transition from laboratory research to clinical practice. It was pointed out at the time that a disease which could be controlled in guinea pigs might not be cured in the very different human organism. Here important refinements were made by Emile Roux and Paul Ehrlich. Roux suggested that horses could produce substantial quantities of serum. Ehrlich was persuaded to take on serum testing after pioneering work in the quantification of dosages.[23] The ensuing immunization campaigns against diphtheria helped to establish the scientific credentials of pediatrics as a legitimate medical discipline. It is important to keep in mind that many leading public health experts remained sceptical of the effects of interventive therapies, and preferred to see diseases as the outcome of the interaction of climatic and social conditions.[24]

After centuries of neglect because of their moral stigma, venereal diseases became recognized as a major hazard, damaging overall levels of health. The discovery of the bacterial cause of gonorrhoea provoked a change of heart. During the 1890s, concern with the declining birth rate prompted the fear of sterility. Gonorrhoea was widely prevalent among the population. However, the search for a serum proved a disappointment in the 1890s. Alfred Fournier's study of syphilis and marriage had a great public impact, and his demand for effective medical controls was popularized by the drama *Damaged Goods* (*Les Avariés*) by Eugène Brieux. The doctor assumed the important role of adjudicating when someone who had contracted syphilis might marry. Doctors pointed out that early marriage would be helpful in preventing the spread of venereal disease. Therapeutic developments did not occur until the early twentieth century. A breakthrough in sero-diagnosis was achieved by Wassermann. Ehrlich's development of salvarsan, an arsenic compound, resulted in an effective although difficult cure to administer. VD prevention by condoms, as a barrier to infection, was increasingly appreciated from the 1890s. Public associations to prevent VD were founded throughout the Western world on the model of that in Germany established by Neisser and Blaschko in 1902 and by Fournier in France in 1901. These mounted a mass publicity campaign with plays and

[22] H. J. Parish, *A History of Immunization* (Edinburgh and London, 1965); Parish, *Victory with Vaccines* (London, 1968).

[23] P. Bäumler, *Paul Ehrlich. Scientist for Life* (New York and London, 1984).

[24] G. Newsholme, *Epidemic Diphtheria* (Oxford, 1900).

pamphlets, and were a basis for health education and emphasis on earlier marriage. Most controversial was the issue of whether condoms could be recommended as prophylactics. Some hygienists objected that this would facilitate public immorality and further weaken population reserves as birth rates were in decline. Yet contraception can be regarded as one of the most important means of improving women's health on the basis of self-help rather than medical intervention. Parallels with issues surrounding AIDS are striking.

Reasons for the changing pattern of diseases could also lie in changing living conditions, in particular housing and diet. McKeown's theories highlighting the role of improved nutrition in promoting improved health merit historical investigation.[25] Here recent historical research into the decline of infant mortality and tuberculosis provides valuable evidence on the role of public associations, sanatoria and dispensary clinics in reducing mortality.[26] The questions of infant welfare and tuberculosis came together when it was suggested that purer milk from tuberculin-tested cattle could do much to reduce mortality rates. While the quality of the milk supply may well have been a factor, broader issues such as domestic hygiene, consumption patterns and economic levels of prosperity should not be overlooked in their effects on health. Whatever the effect on actual health, it should be noted that infant welfare and anti-tuberculosis measures greatly extended professional opportunities in medicine and nursing, as well as providing an issue for promoting public understanding of domestic hygiene. Successful chemotherapy with the introduction of antibiotics came only at the tail end of the disease in Western Europe. It should be further noted that the anti-tuberculosis services were remodelled and redeployed against heart and circulatory diseases from the 1950s and 60s, so maintaining the extensive services and accumulated expertise. Thus the National Association for the Prevention of Tuberculosis altered its constitution in 1956 so as to embrace non-tuberculous diseases, and it metamorphosed into the Chest, Heart and Stroke Association.

Yet at the time that the concept of specific serum therapies for infectious diseases was introduced in the 1890s, doctors also developed concepts of natural immunity. Critics of Koch like the public health experts Gottstein and the bacteriologist Hueppe argued for the importance of studying resistance to diseases. They emphasized the

[25] T. McKeown, *The Role of Medicine. Dream, Mirage or Nemesis?* (London, 1976).
[26] L. Bryder, *Below the Magic Mountain. A Social History of Tuberculosis in Twentieth-Century Britain* (Oxford, 1988); F. B. Smith, *The Retreat of Tuberculosis* (London, 1988).

importance of strengthening the body's natural resistance to disease rather than promoting 'artificial immunity' through mass immunization with injections of sera. Gottstein pioneered open air schools for tubercular children as part of model schemes for child welfare in pre-1914 Berlin. Hueppe became interested in how heredity, race and constitutional powers promoted resistance to infections. Laboratory researchers such as Hans Buchner pointed out that the blood leucocytes had the bactericidal powers to resist and to destroy infections. Awareness of how exposure to air, sun and light killed bacteria provided a medical rationale for natural therapies, as deployed in sanatoria. It also was a rationale for environmental and social reforms. Improved diet, housing and exercise thus could improve natural resistance. Laboratory research thus assisted environmental and social reforms. This can be seen in a later generation of researchers interested in the connections between vitamin deficiencies and disease.[27]

The corollary of the shift in causes of deaths and diseases was changes in medical services. Hospitals largely changed from being isolation and detention centres to being curative institutions. The medical profession added many new specialisms. Medical techniques were extended on the basis of discoveries in biology, and its offshoot bacteriology, and with chemical discoveries enabling disinfection and the use of chemical drugs. Doctors certainly acquired a new scientific armoury of drugs, diagnostic techniques and preventive ideas. There was also a shift in priorities from the health of adult males to mothers and children. By the first decade of the twentieth century there was a pronounced down-turn in infant mortality rates, which until then were the group suffering the highest mortality. Clinics and welfare services for mothers and babies became a priority.[28] Provision of medical care also reflected this shift. Sickness insurance systems were originally provided only for the sick adult worker. Such widespread diseases as sexually transmitted diseases were omitted, as they were considered the moral responsibility of the insured. French schemes for 'maternity insurance' during the 1890s and initiatives by progressive German sickness insurances in the first decade of the twentieth century influenced Lloyd George's National Insurance Act of 1911. The spread of sickness insurance meant that ever increasing proportions of the population were brought into contact with scientifically based medical practice.

[27] P. J. Weindling, *Health, Race and German Politics Between National Unification and Nazism* (Cambridge, 1989).

[28] D. Dwork, *War is Good for Babies and Other Young Children* (London and New York, 1987).

David Armstrong's view that the hospital was a type of utilitarian panopticon for detention and surveillance can be supported by the evidence of the 'epidemiological transition'.[29] For armies of home visitors and public health officials used the prevalence of submerged reservoirs of chronic degenerative diseases to intervene in the domestic sphere. The TB dispensary, pioneered in France from 1899, was then extended to infant-care clinics, alcoholism, VD and cancer throughout Europe and North America. Their implications for preventive medicine and public health are examined in this volume in the chapter by Fee and Porter. As sickness insurance was extended to a worker's dependants, the result was a broadening of the scope and public demand for scientific medicine. The extension of the market for medical care enabled the financing of professional medical attention and hospital treatment.[30] A further repercussion was the improvement of standards in hospitals, and their emergence as the mainstays of modern medical services.

Conclusions

The integration of health services has seen the involvement of individual practitioners, municipalities, state authorities, insurances and voluntary agencies. Modern concepts of the welfare state conceal the reality of a broad-ranging diversity of services. These have been difficult to integrate into a single, adequate and uniform system of medical care to which all population groups have equal access. That modern medicine has ultimately emerged as scientific and hospital based should not obscure how such medical institutions as hospitals and sanatoria developed to provide an ideal type of domestic environment, and as antidotes to mass urban poverty and slum life arising from industrialization. In terms of bacteriologically based therapies and preventive measures, successful therapies such as serum therapy or the improved toxoid immunization against diphtheria, or the BCG vaccination against tuberculosis were deployed on a restricted scale during the 1920s and 1930s. In evaluating the impact of scientifically based preventive and curative methods, it is necessary to consider not only the intrinsic qualities of the innovation, but also to compare national, regional and local trends, and to evaluate factors in population groups affected such as differences of age, gender, class, income, and occupation. McKeown's theory of disease as declining

[29] D. Armstrong, *Political Anatomy of the Body. Medical Knowledge in Britain in the Twentieth Century* (Cambridge, 1983).
[30] C. Huerkamp, *Der Aufstieg der Ärzte* (Göttingen, 1985).

due to improved nutrition rather than to medical advance confronts historians with a stark dichotomy between 'medical' and 'social' factors. This dichotomy does not reflect the way doctors saw environmental, reproductive, economic and nutritional factors as promoting health. The concept of 'natural immunity' led to the social involvement of medical science, and public health officials. There is, however, a lack of research into the financial, institutional and professional implications of the twentieth-century growth of scientific medicine. Yet it should be observed that health care cannot be simply measured in terms of mortality rates and the proliferation of medical services. Perhaps one of the most profound repercussions of medical advance has been the life-style changing function of medicine. Further insight will be gained from an approach to the social history of health based on the changing social environment of population groups and consumer patterns.

Providers, 'consumers', the state and the delivery of health-care services in twentieth-century Britain

JANE LEWIS*

Introduction

Debates about twentieth-century medicine have been characterized above all by an increased preoccupation with the delivery of health-care services. Underlying this preoccupation has been the fundamental assumption that personal health care delivered by a doctor to a patient, whether in the home or in a hospital, is a worthy endeavour that should be widely available. The belief in the progressive power of scientific medicine to cure has been largely shared by policy makers and consumers, as well as by the medical profession itself. In turn, this belief has sustained the view first, that doctors are the best people to determine the content of medical services and second, that developments in medical care should be made available to as many people as possible. The latter view has necessarily involved greater collective effort and a larger role for the state. It is only very recently that faith in the capacity of the medical profession and state medical services has begun to falter. During the 1980s, support for the medical profession in its task of making us healthier and for an increasing role for the state in making medical services more widely available has been questioned.

While the twentieth century has thus been marked by an overarching consensus as to the value of scientific medicine, below this there has nevertheless been considerable room for conflict. The interests of the three major groups of protagonists – the medical profession, 'consumers' and the state – have often differed, and these conflicts have become of

* I would like to thank Charles Webster for his help and encouragement in the preparation of this chapter.

317

paramount importance when faith in the medical profession and in the role of the state in providing medical care are called into question. While doctors are imbued with 'an absolutist ethic of treatment',[1] the concern of policy makers has been distinctly utilitarian and state provision has been accompanied by a belief in the ability of medical care to work for the collective and not merely the individual good. Thus public expenditure on health care has often been justified in terms of improving the national health and hence national efficiency. The views of recipients of health care are much harder to distinguish. But there is evidence to suggest that a majority continue to approve of collective provision through the National Health Service (NHS) because it enables them to obtain the kind of care they are told is best; even though, as individuals, they may remain sceptical or even fatalistic about the treatment they receive.[2] Of course none of these three major groups is monolithic. Particularly important have been the conflicts within the medical profession, between general practitioners (GPs), hospital doctors and public health doctors. Indeed, it is impossible to see debates over twentieth-century medicine and medical care in terms of either simple consensus or conflict. Rather there are layers of consensus and conflict to be unpacked. This chapter can only sketch some of the blunter alliances and divisions, but it is important to remember that during the twentieth century divisions between providers of health have become increasingly complicated by sex and skill.

The first part of this chapter examines the growing emphasis within medicine on the importance of personal health care and the growing role of the state in providing such services before the First World War. While both phenomena were common to all Western industrial nations the form that collective provision took varied considerably. By the end of the nineteenth century, Britain had an extensive poor law medical service which provided both domiciliary medical relief on application to the relieving officer, and hospital beds. Indeed, the hospital service, both voluntary and poor law, constituted the dominant part of the early twentieth-century health-care system. However, from a political point of view, the decision to expand the role of the state in 1911 by introducing a National Health Insurance scheme was to prove crucial because of the way in which it shaped the pattern of relationships within the health-care system. Britain followed Germany in adopting an

---

[1] The phrase is R. Kelin's *The Politics of the NHS* (London, 1983).

[2] See for example Mildred Blaxter and Elizabeth Paterson with the assistance of Sheila Murray, *Mothers and Daughters: a three generation study of health attitudes and behaviour* (London, 1982).

insurance model, but the United States did not follow this path despite the fact that the Progressives' rhetoric regarding the relationship between health and national efficiency was remarkably similar to the dominant strain in the British debate. The reasons for the introduction of National Health Insurance (NHI) are beyond the scope of this chapter, the major concern here being the subsequent significance of the policy. For, as the second part of the chapter shows, the nature of the debate between the medical profession and the state and between different groups of doctors over medical care has been in large part determined by the structural framework.

The battle for control between providers and policy makers has revolved around the question of money – costs, financing and payment – and has remained a constant, both influencing and being influenced by subsequent shifts in the structure of provision. Until recently the medical profession has succeeded in wielding most power and its success is intimately related to the privacy of the patient–doctor relationship and the control over resources that it gives to the doctor, as well as to our belief that we should obey doctors' prescriptions for fear of what will happen if we do not. Indeed, collective provision served to enhance the power of the profession based on the individual patient–doctor relationship. Argument in the interwar years centred on the best way of extending personal health-care provision, with doctors favouring an extension of insurance and government, fearing the cost of such a policy, preferring to extend provision piecemeal through the public health service.

Excluded from the mainstream debate until recently has been the question of the relationship between health status and medical care. This was raised particularly during the 1930s and 1940s, the impetus coming largely from people and groups outside the medical profession (including social scientists, women's organizations and political lobby groups), although with the efforts of social medicine in the 1940s to study health and disease in relation to structural determinants, an effort was made to redirect the whole emphasis of medical training and health-care services. However, the power of the hospital within medicine and of the existing structures erected to deliver medical care proved too strong. Nor has the consumer's voice been heard. Increased access to medical care appears to have resulted in decreasing control by the consumer, which may explain his/her often mixed views about health-care services.

In fact these apparent paradoxes – that medical services may have little to do with health and that consumers of medical care may have better access to, but less control over services – are fundamental to the current debate over health services which appears to mark a significant departure from previous developments. For in the 1980s, the power of scientific medicine and the beneficial consequences of making it available for all became a contested rather than a shared concept and, as a result, the conflicts between providers, consumers and the state have been thrown into sharper relief. Government has taken on board the idea that scientific medicine may not be able substantially to improve health status. Nevertheless the debate between providers and policy makers has been, and continues to be, contained within narrow confines. Policy makers have responded to social scientists' and health economists' questions as to scientific medicine's ability to deliver health, first by seeking to exert greater control over decision making (and hence over doctors) and thereby to shift resources away from the expensive acute-care sector and towards community care; and second by managing health services more efficiently, which has entailed the exploration of alternatives to the state's involvement in delivering services. In pursuing these new strategies government has sought an alliance with the patient or 'consumer', who should, it argues, be allowed greater choice in health care. Despite the apparent willingness of policy makers to address the issue of the content of medical care and the position of the consumer for the first time, the policy response has been dictated primarily by concerns over costs; government has raised the question as to whether the drain on national resources resulting from the vast National Health Services might not constitute on balance a diswelfare.

The importance of personal health-care services and the increasing involvement of the state, 1900–18

By the early twentieth century much more regard was being attached to the medical profession and to personal medical care. The reasons for this are complicated. Traditionally it has been thought that the rise in the status and power of the medical profession was intrinsically related to its increased ability to cure the patient, with the rise of germ theory playing a particularly important part. However, M. Jeanne Peterson has argued that Victorians did not judge occupational status by efficiency and that increasing secularization and more concern about physical health, human life and productivity provided a social environment in which knowledge of the human body, even in the absence of effective treatment, began to be significant.[3] Such an environment permitted the independent authority of the physician to grow. Paul Starr has identified a complicated conjuncture for the USA, including the growth of the market for medical care as incomes rose; the standardization and expansion of medical education providing additional legitimacy for the profession; and the rise of new structures of dependency, such as national insurance, replacing the doctor's reliance on lay patronage thereby tipping the balance of power and authority in favour of the profession rather than the layperson.[4] Undoubtedly the increased interest in medical care was a product of much more than suppliers creating their own demand or professionalization internal to the profession. Changing attitudes to health and disease, the high premium attached to health, and changing market conditions, as well as changes in the training and organization of the medical profession (legitimated by scientific advances) all played a part.[5]

The increasing importance attached to personal health-care services is clearly apparent in the growth of the poor law and public health medical services provided by the state. In theory the poor law provided both hospital treatment and GP services (outdoor medical relief) to the destitute, but in the 1870s one third of those entering poor law hospitals were not paupers at the time of admission and, in recognition of this, from 1885 those using the poor law hospitals were no longer deprived of their right to vote. In 1911, more than twice as many hospital beds were to be found in poor law hospitals as in voluntary hospitals.[6] There was therefore both a greater demand for medical relief and an eagerness on the part of doctors to take on the office of medical officer. While fees increased considerably in the 1880s, 25 per cent of doctors still earned less than £195 in 1913–14[7]; late-nineteenth-century medical men were growing in status and authority, but could still be described as 'marginal men' in terms of their income.

However, standard accounts of nineteenth-century health policy concentrated on the heroic battles for sewerage and clean water and against infectious disease, led by pioneers of public health such as Edwin Chadwick, William Farr and Sir John Simon. Industrialization and rapid urbanization made more extensive and more formal protection of the

---

[3] M. Jeanne Peterson, *The Medical Profession in Mid-Victorian London* (Berkeley, 1978).

[4] Paul Starr, *The Social Transformation of American Medicine* (New York, 1982).

[5] Ivan Waddington, *The Medical Profession in the Industrial Revolution* (London, 1984).

[6] Frank Honigsbaum, *The Division in British Medicine* (London, 1980); and Brian Abel-Smith, *The Hospitals, 1800–1948* (London, 1964).   [7] Peterson, *Medical Profession*, p. 194.

community's health a major concern of government. 'Slum' and 'fever den' were terms used interchangeably in the nineteenth century.[8] Both they and their inhabitants were feared as agents of infection before it was understood how this occurred. Indeed state intervention went furthest in matters of health policy, largely because of the threat diseases such as cholera and smallpox posed to the whole community; vaccination against smallpox was the only measure that central government made the obligatory responsibility of local authorities.[9]

The focus of nineteenth-century health policy was preeminently environmental: all dirt was considered dangerous.[10] By the end of the century, social investigators were convinced that physical well-being was a necessary prerequisite for further social progress. The nineteenth-century vision of health policy was convincingly broad. In particular, the Public Health Acts were permitted to serve as a filter for more general social reform. Typically, major Public Health Acts were also Housing Acts. As Sutcliffe has perceptively argued, the 'urban variable' acted as a spur to state intervention because a large number of social questions concerned with poverty and housing as well as health were packed into the fear of urban degeneration and physical deterioration.[11] The urban environment was feared to be producing a race of degenerates, physically stunted and morally inferior. The slippage between social and moral categories, so characteristic of Victorian social science, only served to intensify fear of contamination. Fear, together with religious zeal and civic pride (albeit often moderated by ratepayer parsimony) combined to produce the sanitary reform associated with nineteenth-century health reform.

The images of early-twentieth-century debates about health and ideas for reform are rather different and are indicative of the growing emphasis on personal health care that was legitimated by scientific advances, particularly in bacteriology. Increasingly emphasis was placed on what the individual should do to ensure personal hygiene. The campaign to reduce infant mortality provides an especially clear example of this approach. The campaign to 'glorify, dignify and purify' motherhood began in earnest after the Boer War. In the late 1900s, epidemiological studies of the problem conducted by medical officers of

[8] Anthony Wohl, *Endangered Lives: Public Health in Victorian Britain* (Cambridge, MA, 1983), p. 45. [9] R. Lambert, 'A Victorian NHS', *Historical Journal*, 5 (1962), 1–18.
[10] Starr, *Social Transformation of American Medicine*, p. 189.
[11] A. Sutcliffe, 'In Search of the Urban Variable', in D. Fraser and H. Sutcliffe (eds.), *The Pursuit of Urban History* (London, 1983).

health employed by local authority public health departments revealed the death rate to be highest in poor inner city slums, yet government officials and public health doctors tended to view maternal and child welfare in terms of a series of discrete personal health problems, to be solved by the provision of health visitors, infant welfare centres and better maternity services. Before World War I, the bulk of their attention was focused on health education, encouraging mothers to breast feed and strive for higher standards of domestic hygiene. Clinic work was seen as 'applied physiology', a new kind of personal preventive clinical medicine.[12] Thus, once it was realized that dirt per se did not cause infectious disease, the broad mandate of public health to deal with all aspects of environmental sanitation and housing as the means of promoting cleanliness disappeared. In Starr's words, the concept of dirt 'narrowed', thereby also proving considerably cheaper to clean up.[13] Germ theory deflected attention from the primary cause of disease in the environment and from the individual's relationship to that environment, thus making a direct appeal from mortality figures to social reform much more difficult.[14]

The shift to personal health-care services must also be related to the movement for national efficiency and the debate about the relationship between poverty and sickness. Sidney and Beatrice Webb, who as leading Fabian socialists expended considerable effort advocating new approaches to the problem of poor law administration, stressed that any diminution in the prevalence of disease among the working class could be classed as an economy measure. They rightly pointed out that both public health reform and medical treatment under the nineteenth-century poor law shared the hope that better health would save the nation money.[15] Edwin Chadwick, after all, had been inspired to action on health reform by the idea that disease brought large numbers on to the poor law. In their work for the 1909 Royal Commission on the Poor Laws, the Webbs argued strongly for a system of health care that ensured the poor adopted hygienic habits. This early appeal to 'healthy life styles' was broadly shared by social investigators, policy makers and public health doctors in the early twentieth century. Only thorough-going eugenicists (referred to as the better-dead school by contemporaries) remained convinced that personal habits were a matter of

---

[12] For further discussion of this concept, see J. Lewis, *What Price Community Medicine?* (Brighton, 1986), ch. 1.   [13] Starr, *Social Transformation of American Medicine*, p. 189.
[14] J. Eyler, *Victorian Social Medicine* (Baltimore, 1979).
[15] Sidney and Beatrice Webb, *The State and the Doctor* (London, 1910).

heredity rather than environment and therefore held out against the idea that some further effort should be made to improve the health status of a population whose low level of physical fitness had been exposed in the course of recruitment for the Boer War and investigated at length by the 1904 Interdepartmental Committee on Physical Deterioration.

Public health legislation provided the major vehicle for social reform and the Public Health Acts of the nineteenth century isolated infectious people and began the work of clearing the slums that were the product of poverty. Health issues were defined in such a way that a wide range of social problems fell within its compass, however no attempt was made to tackle the issue of poverty directly or to build houses. The Edwardian years saw the introduction of a wide range of legislation in the field of social policy, the centrepiece being national insurance for periods of sickness and unemployment. Health legislation was thus more formally separated from welfare and at the same time the mandate of public health was thereby narrowed.

Both the growing demand for personal health-care services and the conviction that the inculcation of proper habits of personal hygiene could improve national health and efficiency prompted a change in the role of the state in the delivery of health-care services. Linda Bryder has argued that it was as much the movement for national efficiency as the discovery of germ theory that led to the provision of state assistance for tuberculosis sufferers under the 1911 National Health Insurance Act.[16] Certainly it was the threat infant mortality posed to the quantity and quality of population that fuelled the Edwardian campaign to reduce the mortality rate. It was recognized that unfit soldiers may well have been sickly infants and children, and during World War I the campaign to stop the wastage of infant life became stronger as it was realized that had the infant mortality rate been reduced to the 1917 levels for the previous fifty years, an extra half a million men would have been available for the armed forces.[17]

However there was no consensus as to what form of state intervention was most appropriate. Health-care services at the beginning of the century consisted of a confusing patchwork of provision. Public health provided little by way of personal health care at the turn of the century, although individual medical officers of health supported the various

[16] Linda Bryder, 'The Problems of TB in England and Wales, 1900–1950' (unpublished D. Phil. thesis, Oxford, 1985).
[17] Carnegie UK Trust, *Report on the Physical Welfare of Mothers and Children*, vol. I (London, 1917).

voluntary organizations providing infant welfare clinics. The ordinary sick person could seek private medical attention from a GP if he or she could afford to pay; the minimum official fee for a surgery consultation for the poorest class (classified as those paying rents from £10–25 a year) was two shillings and sixpence, although in practice this dropped as low as a shilling. For the worker earning round about a pound a week and for his wife struggling to balance the family budget, such a sum was often impossible to find and they would rely on the services of a charitable dispensary, the out-patients department of a voluntary hospital, or in the final event on the poor law medical officer. The poor law doctor was in particularly heavy demand for childbirth. Large numbers of poor women found themselves unable to find the ten shillings (twelve and sixpence in London) asked by midwives for first births. The regularly employed were likely to be members of friendly societies or trade unions and to be able to call on the 'club' doctors they employed for attention. Beveridge calculated that about 4.75 million were members of registered societies offering medical benefits in 1910.[18] In his recent study of club practice, D. G. Green suggests that as many again were members of unregistered societies and that 9 of the 12 million originally included in the NHI scheme introduced in 1911 were thus already members of societies offering medical care.[19]

One of the two major models for reform was promoted by the Webbs who felt that a choice had to be made between the two existing forms of state provision – the poor law medical service and the public health service – and who argued strongly against the former. They viewed any reform of the poor law medical services to be impossible. Any increase in efficiency or humanity, or in preventive services would merely tempt more people to pauperize themselves in order to obtain medical relief. They therefore believed the only viable form of state medicine to be that based on the local authority public health departments which served to create 'in the recipient an increased feeling of personal obligation and even a new sense of social responsibility ... the very aim of the sanitarians is to train the people to better habits of life'.[20] The new state service proposed by the Webbs would set charges in order not to pauperize recipients. Ill health, like sweated wages and unemployment, was to the Webbs a barrier to national efficiency. Their solutions to all three problems were essentially administrative, imposing a national minimum

[18] William Beveridge, *Voluntary Action* (London, 1948), p. 76.
[19] David G. Green, *Working Class Patients and the Medical Establishment* (Aldershot, 1985), p. 85.
[20] S. and B. Webb, *State and the Doctor*, p. 206.

standard of provision with no quarter given to those who refused to cooperate. Workers who were too 'inefficient' (often by reason of poor health) to earn the minimum rates they proposed for certain sweated trades would necessarily suffer unemployment; those who did not find work through labour exchanges would be incarcerated in labour camps. Similarly, hygienic habits were to be imposed from above with the explicit intention of improving not merely the health but also the 'character of the race'.[21] They regarded the educational work of health visitors and local authority infant welfare centres as models for the future.

Starting from a similar concern with national efficiency, the Liberal government of the period enacted a rather different model of health reform based on state insurance. The National Health Insurance Act of 1911 provided both sickness benefits and access to a 'panel' doctor for insured workers. Lloyd George who was primarily responsible for the Act was clearly worried about the level of physical fitness, remarking that a C3 population would not do for an A1 empire.[22] However, the focus of government attention was not the determination to abolish the poor law as it was the Webb's, but rather the relationship between poverty and disease. Like Chadwick, Lloyd George believed that sickness caused poverty. Insurance offered a two-pronged attack on this problem. First and foremost it offered a means of income maintenance for wage earners during periods of sickness and, second, access to medical care that would restore their wage-earning capacity. (This is not to deny that Lloyd George was undoubtedly concerned to provide directly for tuberculosis sufferers in particular: access to sanatorium beds was provided under the Act.[23]) Thus while the focus of attention was very much on the physical efficiency of (mainly male) wage earners, the primary concern was not so much with the nature of health care being offered as with the intention to treat pauperism due to sickness.

The Webbs argued against the idea of a compulsory state insurance scheme. They felt that an insurance system which allowed for free choice of doctor and which remunerated doctors according to the number of patients allocated to them would only 'intensify the popular superstition as to the value of medicine [i.e. medication] and the popular reluctance to adopt hygienic methods of life'.[24] They felt that such a system would

---

[21] Ibid., p. 259.
[22] B. B. Gilbert, British Social Policy, 1914–39 (London, 1970), p. 15.
[23] Honigsbaum, Division in British Medicine, part I.
[24] S. and B. Webb, State and the Doctor, p. 259.

end up not being genuinely preventive or curative medicine, but rather a form of medical relief akin to the poor law, with the additional disadvantage that it would be unconditional. The Webbs have been credited with rethinking the whole concept of health and with focusing on preventive rather than curative medicine. In fact this is rather misleading. The Webbs shared the belief of public health doctors that 'health springs from the domestic, social and personal life of the people'[25] and their conviction that health education was all important. They believed that the inevitably deterrent nature of the poor law authority which acted only to relieve the destitute prevented early diagnosis and the giving of medical advice, and felt that an insurance scheme merely increased reliance on bottles of medicine and permitted malingering rather than encouraging hygienic habits. What they do not seem to have realized was that in practice the personal preventive medicine adopted by the public health doctor was derived from clinical medicine and was hard to distinguish from that of the ordinary GP. The work of the infant welfare clinics, for example, amounted in large measure to diagnosis with a minimal amount of treatment. Even this aroused the hostility of GPs and led them to mount a strong campaign against the clinics as a threat to private practice in the 1920s. The Webbs thought honestly about prevention, but their model for health-care delivery was, like health insurance, only capable of ensuring greater access to medical care.

Neither an insurance nor a local-authority-based scheme gave much consideration to consumer preference. The Webbs would have wanted doctors to impose proper habits of personal hygiene on their patients. The NHI Act removed the lay control of doctors exercised through the friendly societies (which were mutual aid organizations serving some six million members of the better-off working classes at the turn of the century) and thereby increased the power of the medical profession which had not been Lloyd George's intention. In making friendly societies the approved societies administering the Act, he had sought to build on and extend the principle of working-class voluntary mutual aid. However the Act removed the power of the Approved societies to set rates of contribution and doctors' fees, as well as giving registered doctors a monopoly over practice at the expense of 'alternative' practitioners such as homeopaths. As a result, doctors made significant advances in terms of pay under the state insurance system.

---

[25] G. Newman, *The Foundation of National Health* (London, 1928), the Charles Hastings Lecture.

The treatment of working-class consumers, and in particular the shift in the balance of power between doctor and consumer in favour of the former, has recently been the focus of considerable attention from right and left-wing commentators.[26] Older interpretations insisted that friendly societies protected their own funds first and their members health and welfare second.[27] But more detailed investigation has revealed the extensive rules governing the clubs' contracts with the doctors they employed and the power of lay committees to enforce them. Recent evidence that the state insurance scheme enacted in 1911 neither greatly improved access to medical care – women and children were the largest group left unprovided for – nor the quality of care is impressive. The findings are not wholly surprising given that the measure was inspired more by the desire to do something about poverty due to sickness than about health status.

The disregard for the consumer's view is particularly glaring in the case of women and children. Infant welfare had become a major focus of local-authority public health work and of public debate after the Boer War because of concern about physical efficiency of the population. The 32,000 strong Women's Cooperative Guild campaigned actively for improvements in the maternal and child-welfare services and for the maternity benefit that was included in the 1911 NHI Act, which in 1913 they succeeded in getting paid to women. However the Women's Industrial Council and the Fabian Women's Group were correct in their assessment that national insurance offered little to married women, merely intensifying 'the regrettable tendency to consider the work of the wife and mother in her home of no money value'.[28] One of the major reasons for excluding women from national insurance was of course the cost of including them, especially when it was widely believed that women were more vulnerable to sickness than men. Club doctors had also usually refused to take women members for the same reason prior to 1911.[29] Women were very active in the campaign for a Ministry of Health which they hoped would result in more attention being given to women's health needs. Representatives of women's organizations, led by Lady Rhondda, an active feminist, forced the first Minister of Health,

[26] Green, *Working Class Patients*, and S. Yeo, 'Working class associations, private capital and the state in the late nineteenth and early twentieth centuries', in Noel Parry, Michael Rustin and Carole Satyamati (eds.), *Social Work, Welfare and the State* (London, 1979), pp. 48–71.
[27] E.g. R. Klein, *Complaints against Doctors* (London, 1973), and B. B. Gilbert, *The Evolution of National Insurance in Great Britain. The Origins of the Welfare State* (London, 1966).
[28] Women's Industrial Council, Memo on the National Insurance Bill as it Affects Women (TS, 1911, BLPES). [29] Green, *Working Class Patients*, pp. 104–6.

Addison, to set up a Consultative Council for patients on which women
were given the majority of seats, but Lady Rhondda herself soon
resigned out of frustration at the lack of attention paid to the Council's
views. Most women's groups favoured a fully fledged state system of
medical care as their best hope of improving their access to health
services. Both the collection of 'maternity letters' put together by the
Women's Cooperative Guild in 1915 and the survey carried out by the
Women's Health Inquiry at the end of the 1930s[30] indicated the extent
to which high levels of morbidity prevailed among women. There is no
doubt but that full state provision in the form of the National Health
Service did enable large numbers of women to seek medical attention
regularly for the first time, but women's other major concern, to make
health-care services responsive to their demands, continued to be
ignored.

National insurance was accepted in Britain with little debate. Yet in
the United States, where the progressives argued for health insurance on
very similar grounds, no legislation was introduced.[31] The underlying
consensus as to the value of personal health care and the importance of
promoting national efficiency existed in both countries, but the way in
which state subsidy of health services was increased differed profoundly.
The US showed a marked reluctance to engage in social spending, but
nevertheless promoted the growth of the health industry through
indirect and direct subsidy to medical education, hospitals, research, and
eventually to vulnerable groups in the population via Medicare and
Medicaid.[32] The most influential recent explanation of these different
developments has focused particularly on the differences in the phasing
and relationship between electoral politics and the building of
bureaucracies in the two countries. These are argued to be more
important than economic variables, differences in values, or working-
class strength.[33] In respect to health care, it certainly seems that the
origins of the conviction that improving health-care provision was
important were very similar, and in neither country was it due to
working-class pressure. Economic considerations, such as the differences

[30] M. Llewellyn Davies, *Maternity: Letters from Working Women* (London, 1915) and M. Spring
Rice, *Working Class Wives* (Harmondsworth, 1939).
[31] Paul Starr, 'Transformation in Defeat: the Changing Objectives of National Health Insurance,
1915–1980', in Ronald C. Numbers (ed.), (Westport, CT, 1982).
[32] Dan Fox, 'History and Health Policy', *Journal of Social History*, 18 (1985), 349–64.
[33] Ann Skola Orloff and Theda Skocpol, 'Why Not Equal Provision? Explaining the Politics of
Public Social Spending in Britain, 1900–1911 and the United States, 1880s–1920', *American
Sociological Review*, 49 (1980), 726–50.

in phasing of industrialization and urbanization and the differences in the pressures exerted upon the workforces in various countries, warrant much more close research. In Canada, for example, the rapid urbanization of the first two decades of the twentieth century ushered in a heroic period of public health measures in respect to environmental sanitation and vaccination similar to that of nineteenth-century Britain, and these paralleled the development of personal health care. Nevertheless, it certainly appears, as Paul Johnson has observed, that the pattern of expansion of welfare provision generally in most countries was for expert administrators to establish a monopoly of information which they then used to further welfare expansion.[34] Given this, the relative lack of an established independent bureaucracy in the US assumes greater importance in any explanatory model. Also, it becomes important to understand the larger framework within which administrative experts were thinking about health and health policy. In the US, the larger goals of the progressives were to attack monopoly and corruption, in Britain social policy issues in the early twentieth century not only assumed a more independent existence, but were always related to, the central pillar of Victorian provision, the poor law. Both the Webbs' ideas for increasing the state's role in health service provision, and the prospects for health insurance were linked to the issue of poor law reform. While the Webbs planned to abolish the poor law, national insurance planned to circumvent it by removing the regularly employed male worker from its auspices.

The adoption of state insurance in Britain not only substantially increased state involvement in health care, but also tipped the balance of power firmly in the direction of the medical profession. The GP was the direct beneficiary of the introduction of insurance, but, more important still, the consensus as to the importance of personal health care legitimated the dominant position occupied by clinical medicine, where developments were dominated by the voluntary hospital. Between 1911 and 1948 Britain had essentially a tripartite system of health service delivery (via GPs, public health departments and hospitals) and the conflicts that are often described as characteristic of the period after the setting up of the NHS were as much a part of the health insurance years.

[34] Paul Johnson, *The Historical Dimensions of the Welfare State Crisis* (London, 1985).

Doctors versus doctors and doctors versus the state, 1918–48

During the interwar years, the fundamental assumption regarding the value of making personal health-care services widely available persisted, but opinion differed over the speed with which the state should expand provision and whether insurance cover should be expanded or public health provision increased.

National insurance created a structure which ensured doctors a large measure of professional autonomy and control. The major concern of the majority was to ensure that any extension of state provision did not call this into question. Thus GPs were suspicious of the expansion of local-authority services largely because public health doctors were salaried and they regarded salaried practice as a fundamental threat to their professional autonomy. Voluntary hospitals also fought hard to retain their independent status. For its part government extended provision piecemeal, using local authority public health departments (particularly for services designed to increase national efficiency), and strove to keep costs in check. The latter involved conflict with providers, over the issue of payments to panel doctors, for example. It may be argued that neither the majority of doctors nor government paid much attention to issues respecting the meaning and measurement of health or the nature of health-care services. Such criticism was made during the period, but it tended to come from outside the framework of medical services, particularly from women's groups and independent social investigators.

In 1919 the new Minister of Health asked his Consultative Council on Medical and Allied Services to prepare a report on a scheme for the provision of medical services. The resulting Dawson Report,[35] published less than twelve months later, is popularly remembered on the one hand for its advocacy of health centres and its stress on the importance of positive health and 'physical culture', and on the other for its reluctance to face the crucial issues of payment for services by patients and terms and conditions for doctors. The Report argued that the changes it recommended were necessary because medicine was poorly organized and because it failed to bring new medical knowledge 'within the reach of the people'.[36] The real significance of the report in terms of medical organization was the way in which it made the GP the key figure in the scheme for the delivery of medical services. The health centre was

[35] PP., Report of the Consultative Council on Medical and Allied Services, Cmd 693, 1920, XVII, 1001.   [36] Ibid., para 3.

intended to end the GP's intellectual isolation and provide him with access to laboratory and radiology services, operating rooms and a dispensary. In effect the Report advocated passing the personal preventive health services developed by local authorities in the fields of infant welfare, VD and tuberculosis control to GPs. The chairman, Lord Dawson, was himself vehemently opposed to a state medical service and firmly committed to promoting the cause of the independent GP.

The Dawson Report advocated a particular direction for increasing the availability of health care that left the precise role of the state unspecified in respect to patient charges and doctors' conditions of service, but which was clearly intended to crush the most immediate threat of control by the state in the form of an expanded public health service. The Ministry of Health however took little notice of the Report, in part because it left so many controversial issues open, particularly in respect to finance, in part because the Ministry experienced severe financial constraints soon after the publication of the Report, and in part because it did not share Lord Dawson's antipathy to the local-authority medical service. Between 1918 and 1939, some twenty pieces of legislation effectively expanding the local-authority health services were passed and local authorities were given additional responsibility for maternal and child-welfare services, tuberculosis and VD schemes, a school medical service, health centres, cancer treatment and, by the Local Government Act of 1929, the administration of what had been the poor law hospitals. Local-authority public health departments provided a convenient administrative framework for this incremental increase in the scope of state provision of particular services and throughout the interwar years they continued to claim that 'public health work is mainly clinical medicine, but clinical medicine of a special kind',[37] even though public health doctors were preoccupied with the administration of municipal hospitals after 1929.

The British Medical Association (BMA) continued to fight the issue of what was referred to as 'encroachment' by local authority clinics into the territory of the independent practitioner. The Final Report of the BMA's Committee on 'encroachment' stated firmly that medical practice with individuals, whether sick or requiring knowledge on how best to maintain their health, 'naturally belongs to, because is best provided by private practitioners'.[38] The BMA's proposals for a general

---

[37] Editorial, 'The Public Health Service', *Medical Officer*, 34 (1925), 99.

[38] 'Report on Encroachments in the Sphere of Private Practice', *British Medical Journal*, 1 (1929), 130.

medical service, first published in 1930, proposed a scheme in which, like the recommendations of the Dawson Report, the GP would become the lynchpin.[39] Unlike the Dawson Report, the BMA came down firmly in favour of increasing GP, specialist, laboratory, nursing and dental services within a national contributory insurance scheme. National insurance was now seen as the safest way of broadening service provision without threatening the autonomy and control of the medical profession. Public health doctors found themselves in a minority in advocating the establishment of a full salaried state medical service. However, because of their expanding sphere of responsibility, they remained confident both that the government was moving towards the establishment of a state service and that their role within it would be central. However, the combined weight of the BMA and the voluntary hospitals was to prove sufficient to thwart their minority vision of the way in which the health service should be expanded.

Irrespective of the conflict over which model for the expansion of medical services should be adopted, government was concerned throughout the interwar years to control costs. In 1922, the government reduced doctors' capitation fees as part of the round of public expenditure cuts and the Minister of Health explicitly threatened to put the doctors back into the hands of the friendly societies' club practice: 'I assume that you do not wish to escape from the Scylla of the Ministry of Health to the Charybdis of the Friendly Societies'.[40] In 1923, GPs resorted to threatening mass resignation from the panel to secure an increase in the level of the capitation fee.

Benefits provided under health insurance were also cut directly. Despite the highly charged debate over the maternal mortality figures and the health and nutrition of childbearing women during the interwar years, married women's national insurance benefits were cut in 1932. Only 10 per cent of married women were in paid employment and therefore insured in their own right, but their sickness and disability rates proved to be extremely high. By 1931–2, married women were experiencing 140 per cent more sickness and 60 per cent more disablement than expected, in comparison with 25 per cent and 65 per cent respectively for unmarried women and a less-than-expected percentage for men. Only part of these differentials can be explained by

---

[39] BMA, *A General Medical Service for the Nation* (London, 1930).
[40] Norman R. Eder, *National Health Insurance and the Medical Profession in Britain, 1913–39* (New York, 1982), p. 125.

administrative changes.[41] Furthermore despite considerable evidence of high morbidity rates among childbearing women and the public outcry about high maternal mortality rates, the government actuary used the statistics as proof of women's 'excessive claims' and successfully argued for a reduction in their benefits. Between them, the government actuary and the exchequer effectively stopped any extension of health insurance during the period.[42] The recommendations of the 1926 Royal Commission on Health Insurance that cover be extended to specialist services was ignored and voluntary hospital finance depended increasingly on the expansion of various non-state insurance schemes, the most important of which was the Hospital Savings Association contribution scheme, and most of all on patient fees. In addition the actuary's influence was reflected in the tightening up of the administration of health insurance. 'Sick visitors' were appointed to check the validity of sickness benefit claims and regional medical officers were given the responsibility of reviewing panel doctors' practice, particularly in respect to prescribing. In 1930, 1,885 doctors were investigated.

Government also ignored the calls of social investigators and women's groups to investigate high levels of morbidity among the unemployed and women. The lead in raising questions concerning the health status of the population during the 1930s was taken first by political lobby groups such as the Children's Minimum Council, the Committee against Malnutrition and the National Unemployed Workers Movement, who called for higher benefit levels to enable families to secure the minimum nutritional requirements set out by the BMA. Second, 'amateur' and 'professional' social investigators set out to explore the incidence of malnutrition, morbidity and mortality in the population. R. M. Titmuss showed that despite the decline in the overall infant mortality rate, a large class differential in mortality persisted[43] and the Women's Health Inquiry Committee's survey of some 1,250 working-class wives concluded that only 31·3 per cent could be considered to be in 'good' health, 22·3 per cent were categorized as 'indifferent', 45·2 per cent as 'bad', and 31·2 per cent as 'very grave'.[44] The high incidence of

[41] Noelle Whiteside, 'Counting the Cost: Sickness and Disability Among Working People in an Era of Industrial Recession, 1920–39', unpublished paper, 1986.

[42] Noelle Whiteside, 'Private Agencies for Public Purposes: Some New Perspectives on Policy Making in Health Insurance Between the Wars', *Journal of Social Policy*, 12 (1984), 165–93; and J. Lewis, *The Politics of Motherhood* (London, 1980), p. 44.

[43] R. M. Titmuss, *Birth, Poverty and Wealth* (London, 1943).

[44] Spring Rice, *Working Class Wives*. The Women's Health Inquiry Committee was chaired by the trade unionist, Gertrude Tuckwell, and included members from leading national women's organizations.

morbidity among childbearing women was confirmed by a few outspoken specialists.[45] Publicly the Ministry of Health stuck by its own Nutrition Advisory Committee Report which set much lower standards of nutrition than had the BMA, and by its conviction that there was no deterioration in the national health. Privately, the Chief Medical Officer was prepared to admit that the ministry could not afford to respond to calls for further investigation. The persistent demands of groups like the Women's Health Inquiry to investigate women's health 'could', he felt, 'have but one ending, namely the demonstration of a great mass of sickness and impairment attributable to childbirth, which would create a demand for organized treatment by the state'.[46] Government confined the extension of provision to the services most closely connected with fears about national fitness and efficiency and in particular to institutional provision for tuberculosis cases and 'mental defectives'.

Women's groups and social investigators were effectively asking that government take a broader view of health care. Women in particular urged government to respond to their demands for access to birth control and for family allowances, both of which they regarded as integral to the promotion of women's health and welfare. However, both government and providers conducted the debate about health-care services within the confines of the existing structures. The Dawson Report had discussed the importance of positive health and physical culture and during the 1930s the Peckham Health Centre promoted the idea that the cultivation of health required a completely different approach from the cure of disease,[47] but these ideas were not actively taken up by either doctors or the ministry. The 1940s did see a brief flowering of 'social medicine' within the medical community, which, although it was not destined to take root, did represent one of the few moments when the nature of medical care was constructively challenged.

The promoters of social medicine were inspired by the work of social investigators and pressure groups during the 1930s. John Ryle, appointed to the first chair in social medicine at Oxford in 1942, paid tribute to the work of the Peckham Health Centre and the Women's Group on Public Welfare, who publicized the poor health of school children evacuated during World War II. Ryle was careful to link social medicine to clinical medicine, seeing it as differing only in terms of the 'social conscience as

---

[45] E.g. James Young, 'The Woman Damaged by Childbearing', *British Medical Journal*, 1 (1929), 891–5 and W. Blair Bell, 'Maternal Disablement', *Lancet*, 1 (1931), 1171–7.

[46] PRO, MH 55/262, Newman to Secretary, 26 October 1932.

[47] J. Lewis and B. Brookes, 'A Reassessment of the Work of the Peckham Health Centre, 1926–51', *Milbank Memorial Quarterly*, 61 (1983), 307–50.

well as scientific interest' with which it pursued its aetiological inquiries.[48] R. M. Titmuss saw it as something more than this: 'Our vision is broadening, men are being pictured against a man-made environment, the multiple factor in disease and disorder is replacing the single causation concept; the study of life is replacing a morbid concentration on death.'[49] The 1944 Goodenough Committee on medical education also perceived social medicine as a means of reorienting the whole medical curriculum: 'To the neglect of the promotion of health, medical practice – and consequently medical education – has been concerned primarily with disease, chiefly as it affects individuals. A radical reorientation of medical education and practice is essential.'[50]

Advocates of social medicine varied in their emphasis: some took up the importance of the relationship between the individual, heredity and environment; some, like Titmuss and J. N. Morris, focused on social factors at the root of diseases such as juvenile rheumatism, and some linked social medicine to the call for a state medical service. The Goodenough Committee believed that 'if medical students are to be fitted to become health advisers and members of a national health service, the ideas of social medicine must permeate the whole of medical education'.[51] However, within the medical schools social medicine made little headway. Increasingly, the concept was narrowed in order to stake a claim to academic respectability. Ryle's own work emphasized the links with clinical medicine and epidemiology at the expense of social science and health policy.

Social medicine was intimately related to the committed discussion of health planning and reconstruction during the war years. However the intense politicking that preceded the establishment of the NHS did not encompass the debate about the nature of medical training and practice. When the Government's White Paper on the proposed NHS was published in 1944, one reviewer in the *Lancet* condemned the proposals on the grounds that they were concerned with medical services rather than with health services. Commenting specifically on the White Paper's proposals regarding the establishment of health centres (which were destined to come to nought), the reviewer wrote:

[48] J. A. Ryle, letter to *British Medical Journal*, 2 (1942), 801.
[49] Titmuss Papers (in the papers of Mrs Kay Titmuss), untitled paper on social medicine, TS 21/12/42.
[50] Ministry of Health and Dept of Health for Scotland, *Report of the Inter-Departmental Committee on Medical Schools* (London, 1944), para. 20.
[51] *Report of the Committee on Medical Schools*, para. 29.

A real health service must surely concern itself first with the way people live, with town and country planning, houses and open spaces, with diet, with playgrounds, gymnasia, baths and halls for active recreation, with workshops, kitchens, gardens and camps, with the education of every child in the care and use of his body, with employment and the restoration to the people of the right and opportunity to do satisfying and creative work. The true 'health centre' can only be a place where the art of healthy living is taught and practised: it is a most ominous and lamentable misuse of words to apply the name to what is and should be called a 'medical centre'.[52]

This commentator was not alone in observing that the NHS appeared to be more a national sickness than a national health service.[53]

Between 1942 and 1948, providers lobbied fiercely to protect their own interests. The 1942 Draft Interim Report of the Medical Planning Commission, inspired by the BMA and comprising seventy-three representatives of professional bodies, included reference not only to the BMA's proposals for extending provision via national insurance, but also to health centres and the possibility of full-time salaried service.[54] The government took this as an indication of more progressive thinking on the part of the BMA, when in fact the inclusion of such ideas owed more to the heterogeneous nature of the body; indeed the Report was noisily buried by the BMA and the Commission never produced a final report. Just as in 1911 the BMA had fought against club practice to further its professional autonomy and control, so from 1942 onward it fought against municipal control and salaried service and was successful in preserving the independent contractor status of the GP virtually intact. The NHS provided universal access to GP services without changing the GP's conditions of work. Public health doctors were plunged into gloom when the Labour government was forced to back away from its commitment to a salaried service under local-authority control. The public health departments' control of municipal hospitals disappeared in 1948 and their clinic work declined drastically as a result of the universal availability of GP services. Public health doctors bewailed 'the remnants that remained', and placed their hopes in the development of health centres, but these failed to materialize.[55] The hospitals, which dominated the health-care system, in terms of training, the resources they absorbed and status (hence the public health doctors' dismay at losing control of

---

[52] 'The White Paper Reviewed, VI', by an urban practitioner, *Lancet*, 1 (1944), 443.

[53] *Annual Report* of the MOH for Salford, 1948.

[54] Medical Planning Commission, 'Draft Interim Report', *British Medical Journal*, 1 (1942), 743–53.

[55] E. J. Johnstone Jervis, 'Has Public Health any Future?', *Public Health*, 59 (1946), 46–9.

the municipal hospitals), were nationalized, thus solving their financial problems. Teaching hospitals retained full control of their affairs under their separate boards of governors, while the hospital management committees of non-teaching hospitals also enjoyed considerable autonomy in matters of day-to-day administration.

During the inter-war years, the centre of the debate was how to extend the provision of personal health-care services to dependants and how to make specialist services more widely available. The key problem was finance. The most radical suggestions from the Labour Party and the Socialist Medical Association involved a salaried state medical service, but none questioned the established hierarchy within the medical profession or the power of the hospital in determining the nature of medical care and treatment. The issue of cost and financing was more acute still in North America where mass unemployment and the absence of any income maintenance provision meant that people could not afford to pay for medical care. In Canada the Commission on Dominion/ Provincial Relations was told that in some areas of the west 'hospitals are so seriously embarrassed that...unless those boards get additional financial assistance within the next few months they individually have no choice except to close the hospital'.[56] Questions of costs and financing were thus at the core of debate over health services in the 1920s and 1930s. In North America priority was given by government to the development of income maintenance provision for the unemployed over the sick, which was logical in terms of the way in which the problem was diagnosed. In the years following the war the Canadian federal government embarked on a programme of hospital building which was envisaged primarily as a public works rather than a health-care programme, and in 1957 introduced an Act whereby it cost-shared hospital insurance with the provinces.[57] Thus the form Canadian health insurance took clearly reflected both the power of the hospital and the North American belief in the importance of direct access to specialist care. In Britain, the hospital became as predominant a force within the NHS. Between 1911 and 1948 Britain had had an essentially tripartite system of health-care services and these divisions were reflected in the bargaining over the shape of the NHS during the mid 1940s. It was the

[56] PAC Ottawa, RG 33/23, vol. 24, Minutes of Evidence to the Rowell Sirois Commission, fol. 6281.

[57] See Carl A. Melicke and Janet L. Storch, *Perspectives on Canadian Health and Social Service Policies: history and emerging trends* (Ann Arbor, MI, 1980), and G. R. Weller and Pranlal Manga, 'The Development of Health Policy in Canada', in M. M. Atkinson and M. A. Chandler (eds.), *The Politics of Canadian Public Policy*, (Toronto, 1983), pp. 223–46.

decision not to unify the services under local-authority control that ensured that the hospital sector would continue to dominate.

The belief that access to a wider spectrum of medical services would result in an improvement in health and the nature of medical care was strengthened in the course of the war-time debates about post-war reconstruction and social reform. William Beveridge for example, assumed that by making access to all health services universal, the NHS would raise health standards and thereby eventually reduce the demands on the service and hence costs.[58] Indeed, one of the reasons why Ffrangcon Roberts'[59] early attack on the NHS proved so influential was that it argued that the demand for health care was infinite.

The NHS froze in place a system of health-care delivery dominated by the medical model which, as Raymond Illsley has observed, contains an implicit set of definitions of the health needs of modern societies; an analysis of the fundamental principles of medical sciences education and organization; and a judgement that these principles are sufficient for the development of health policy and practice.[60] Within such a model there was no formal place accorded the consumer. The impressionistic survey of attitudes towards welfare policies carried out by G. D. H. Cole in 1942 showed health care to be people's first priority and recorded strong negative feelings about the panel system.[61] The NHS proved immediately popular and the popularity has been sustained.[62] Nella Last wrote in the diary she kept for Mass Observation during the war that the NHS would prove a great boon for women in particular[63] and there is no doubt that the women who contributed to the Women's Cooperative Guild's collection of maternity letters and those surveyed by the Women's Health Inquiry would have agreed with her. Yet better access to medical services was accompanied by the imposition of increasingly sophisticated treatments over which women had little control. This was nowhere more true than in the field of obstetrics and gynaecology. During the interwar years domiciliary midwifery practice was reduced sharply and the number of maternity beds increased. In 1920 the ministry estimated that 5 per cent of births needed hospitalization, but by 1944 the

---

[58] PP., Report of the Committee on Social Insurance and Allied Services, Cmd 6404 (London, 1942). [59] Ffrangcon Roberts, *The Cost of Health* (London, 1952).
[60] Raymond Illsey, *Professional or Public Health?*, the Rock Carling Fellowship (Oxford, 1980), p. 86.
[61] Jose Harris, 'G. D. H. Cole's Survey of 1942: did British workers want the welfare state?', in J. M. Winter (ed.), *The Working Class in Modern Britain* (Cambridge, 1983).
[62] Peter Taylor Gooby, *Public Opinion, Ideology and State Welfare* (London, 1985).
[63] R. Broad and Suzie Fleming, *Nella Last's War* (London, 1983).

Royal College of Obstetricians and Gynaecologists had raised this to 70 per cent and undoubtedly this became to some extent a self-fulfilling prophecy irrespective of women's wishes.[64] The failure to build in any mechanisms for patient participation in the NHS has given rise to considerable criticism from consumers in the post-war period, while government has viewed the rise in costs of the medical service with alarm, especially in view of the recent evidence which suggests there is little correlation between the provision of medical care and health status.

Changing assumptions and shifting alliances, 1948–85

In recent years, the issue of spiralling costs and the question mark hanging over the relationship between medical services and health status has resulted in cracks appearing in the belief in the efficacy of scientific medicine and in the role of the state in making it more widely available. Governments in the nineteenth-century struggled to contain costs of poor law medicine and in the twentieth-century of health insurance, coming into conflict with the medical profession in the process. However, in the last decade government has attacked the issue of spiralling costs by attempting to reduce the power of the medical profession. This contrasts with both 1911 and 1946, when the profession's autonomy was reinforced. Furthermore, this pattern is common to both Britain and North America. In doing battle with providers, government has also begun to reduce its own role in medical care in the name of championing the cause of consumer choice.

Charles Webster has estimated that public expenditure on health-care services amounted to 3 per cent of gross national product in 1939 and that the introduction of the NHS resulted in only a small rise to 3·5 per cent, readily explained by the backlog of demand for particular services such as dentures, the increase in nurses' pay and inbuilt inefficiencies such as the overpayment of dentists.[65] This is in line with the view of Titmuss and Abel Smith in 1956 that when the changing age structure of the population and inflation were controlled for, the net diversion of resources to the NHS had been relatively insignificant.[66] Nevertheless,

[64] Lewis, *Politics of Motherhood*, p. 132.
[65] Charles Webster, 'Britain's Experience of Socialized Medicine', Lectures given at Wellcome Unit, Oxford, 1985. See now Charles Webster, *The Health Services Since the War*. vol. I *The Problems of Health Care: The National Health Service before 1957*. (London, 1988). This is the standard work on the NHS.
[66] Brian Abel-Smith and R. M. Titmuss, *The Cost of the NHS*, National Institute of Economic and Social Research Occasional Papers (Cambridge, 1956).

there was a widespread conviction from its inception that the NHS was absorbing ever greater amounts of public money. By the mid 1970s, the service was absorbing 6 per cent of public expenditure and, more significantly, in terms of the future, the hospital sector's share of total costs had risen from a half to two thirds.[67]

Continuing attempts to control costs have focused on the need to control the profession, first by imposing tighter government control over the NHS bureaucracy, and second by advocating a market approach to health-care delivery, designed to lessen the role of government as well as professional dominance. The reorganization of the NHS in 1974 was motivated in large part by the treasury's desire to gain more control over public spending by the Department of Health and Social Security (DHSS).[68] During the 1960s it was widely believed in government that more effective control could be exercised by careful planning, but in the health service planning was frustrated by tripartism. Although in the end less 'managerial' than the 1968 Green Paper promised, the 1974 reorganization aimed to unify the service, increase central control, create a more effective consensus management structure and make possible a better planning system. When this failed to hold down costs in the hospital sector two further reorganizations followed, in 1982 to simplify the bureaucracy by removing one tier in the administrative structure, and in 1984 to identify 'general managers' for each level of the service in the hope that they would be better placed to make firm management decisions than the consensus management teams created in 1974. It was also hoped that the new general managers would be drawn from outside the NHS. Instead of management teams composed of the different health disciplines, decisions would be taken by business personnel. (In fact only about one third of the general manager posts were filled by outsiders.)[69] Parallel attempts to contain health-care costs in North America have led to increased attempts at rationalization by the corporations running US medical services and hence an increase in the power of corporations relative to doctors.[70] In Canada, the federal government brought to a close open-ended cost-sharing agreements with the provincial governments which favoured the development of high technology medicine in 1977, while provincial

---

[67] Kenneth Lee, 'Public Expenditure, Health Services and Health', in *Public Expenditure and Social Policy* (London, 1982), pp. 73–90.

[68] J. Allsop, *Health Policy and the NHS* (London, 1984), and R. C. Brewer, 'Reorganization of the NHS, 1965–74', (TS, 1983, King's Fund Library).

[69] J. Lewis, 'The Changing Fortunes of Community Medicine', *Public Health*, 100 (1986), 3–10.

[70] Starr, *Social Transformation of American Medicine*.

governments have struggled to impose cash limits on hospital boards, more closely negotiate doctors' fee schedules, and develop policies of regionalization as a means of buffering budget cuts.[71]

The effort to curb the autonomy of the medical profession has been inspired by the recognition that doctors are taught in the course of their medical training an absolutist ethic of treatment, which entails the use of professional discretion regarding the latest medical technology. The measure of need for a bone marrow transplant is the individual case and, of course, the result of denial is death. Governments have nevertheless gained confidence in their dealings with the profession as a result of studies which suggest medical services have played very little part in raising the health status of populations. Ivan Illich has gone so far as to argue that modern scientific medicine has positively iatrogenic consequences.[72] More influential still have been Aaron Wildavsky's study in the US and Thomas McKeown's historical study of the decline in mortality in Britain.[73] In McKeown's view, curative medicine comes a poor third, after rising living standards and public health, in accounting for the decline in the death rate. Western governments were able to take up this research in arguing for a shift in resources from the expensive acute sector to preventive medicine, community care and the 'Cinderella' specialities, such as geriatrics and psychiatry. Another major hope of the 1974 NHS reorganization in Britain was that an integrated service would more effectively promote community care. As Titmuss was at pains to point out in the 1950s, good community care does not come cheap.[74] However, cost saving has undoubtedly been uppermost in the minds of the New Right governments of both Britain and the US during the 1980s. Indeed actual expenditure on prevention only accounted for 0·2 per cent of health-care expenditure in 1979–80 and the proportion of expenditure on mental illness actually declined slightly between 1975/6 and 1979/80.[75]

The rhetoric of prevention has nevertheless been harnessed to the cause of cost control. When proponents of social medicine talked about prevention in the 1940s they meant the identification of social and

[71] R. B. Deber and E. Vayda, 'Implementing Policy Change under Universal Health Insurance in Canada. The Ontario Example', in G. Krose (ed.), *Investigative Methods in Public Health*, (Oxford, forthcoming).

[72] Ivan Illich, *Medical Nemesis. The Expropriation of Health* (New York, 1976).

[73] A. Wildavsky, 'Doing Better and Feeling Worse: the Political Pathology of Health Policy', *Daedalus*, 106 (Winter 1977).

[74] R. M. Titmuss, *Commitment to Welfare* (London, 1976), pp. 91–109.

[75] Chris Ham, *Health Policy in Britain* (London, 1982), pp. 40 and 55.

environmental factors inimical to health. However, the concept of prevention in the last decade has concentrated on the individual's responsibility to maintain a healthy life style. Hilary Graham has pointed out the implications of this strategy for mothers who have been identified as 'natural' guardians of their children's and elderly relatives' health by the policy documents of the past decade without close attention being paid to the material constraints under which they may have to operate, which in turn may require considerable sacrifices on the part of women engaged full-time in the work of caring.[76]

Government policy has stressed the importance of containing costs, but it has also sought to invoke the right of consumers to increased choice. However, it has tried to achieve this negatively, by decreasing the power of providers rather than empowering consumers. In 1982 it was suggested that by removing a tier in the bureaucracy the service would become more responsive to local needs. However, the emphasis placed on the importance of local management and decision making was designed to increase the efficiency of the service rather than local accountability. Indeed the consultative document initiating the changes suggested that the only remaining organ of community opinion, the community health councils, might no longer be necessary. And while the consultative document stressed the importance of delegating authority to the local level, the practical outcome of the 1982 and 1984 reorganizations has been, as Rudolf Klein has pointed out, the first systematic attempt in the history of the NHS to call health authorities to account by annual scrutinies of their work and by the use of performance indicators.[77]

Robert Alford has suggested that the effort of government to take control of the health-care system by controlling and redirecting resources is doomed to failure because it would 'require the defeat or consolidation of the social power that has been appropriated by various discrete interest groups and that preserves existing allocations of social values and resources'.[78] Yet in her analysis of contemporary developments in the NHS, Celia Davies sees government pushing hard to achieve above all a reduction in the power of professionals, not just by increased centralization, but also by promoting a more entrepreneurial approach

[76] H. Graham, 'Providers, Negotiators and Mediators: Women as Hidden Carers', in E. Lewin and V. Olesen (eds.), *Women, Health and Healing* (New York, 1985), and J. Finch and D. Groves, *Labour of Love* (London, 1984).

[77] R. Klein, 'The Politics of Ideology and the Reality of Politics: the Case of Britain's NHS in the 1980s', *Milbank Memorial Quarterly*, 62 (1984).

[78] Robert R. Alford, *Health Care Politics* (Chicago, 1975), p. 256.

to health-care provision: 'A consumer-led range of services is a vision beginning to be set against a professional-led care delivery system. In this juxtaposition, the professionals are cast as both careless of resources and as deaf to questions of patient and client choice. Pluralism in welfare is allied with freedom and choice.'[79] This is certainly the message of Green, whose libertarian analysis of the history of medical-care services prior to the state's involvement in health insurance has led him to conclude that a free market in health care did not disadvantage the consumer in the past – friendly societies were able to exercise control over the doctors they employed – and there is no reason why such a system should not work in the future.[80]

However, it is unlikely that promotion of consumer power, inspired as it is by the desire to reduce provider power rather than by a thorough assessment of the position of the consumer, will succeed. It is noticeable for example that the battles of groups such as the Association for Improvements in the Maternity Services to introduce more consumer control have grown more rather than less protracted. The capacity of the women described by Hilary Graham to overcome their isolation as wives and mothers and organize collectively to meet their health needs is no greater now than it was when club doctors refused to treat them in the first decade of the century. It is true that women today have greater expectations of medical services than had their grandmothers,[81] but this is in large measure due to the fact that they have grown up with the idea that the provision of medical care is a right, rather than a reward for deference. In advocating welfare pluralism as a strategy to counter provider power, government also seeks to reduce its own role and therefore minimize any commitment to a broader approach to health problems, such as that advocated by the Black Report which would tackle (in the manner advocated by social investigators and women's groups in the 1930s) problems of nutrition, housing and environmental conditions inimical to health.[82]

While the current debate over the provision of medical care can thus be seen to have many elements in common with those earlier in the century, the differences appear to be of great significance. The debate continues to be constrained by the existing structures of medical care and to revolve around issues of cost and patterns of organization; the attempt

---

[79] C. Davies, 'Things to Come: the NHS in the Next Decade', *Sociology of Health and Illness*, 9 (1987), 302–17.   [80] See note 19 above.

[81] Blaxter and Paterson, *Mothers and Daughters*.

[82] P. Townsend and N. Davidson, *Inequalities in Health* (Harmondsworth, 1982).

to invoke prevention was prompted more by a desire to save money than as a means to reorienting medical care. However, the willingness of the state to attack the medical profession's autonomy and to contemplate a reduction in its own role represents a significant reversal which may result in a significantly different framework for the delivery of health services. These new strategies have been justified by the invocation of consumer sovereignty, albeit that there is still no attempt to involve the consumer in the running of the health services.

The implications of increased life expectancy for family and social life*

ARTHUR E. IMHOF
Translated by Elizabeth Rushden

Introductory remarks

This chapter is characterized by a number of provisos:

1. It should not simply be a catalogue of demands for future research but should present a constructive approach to existing findings.
2. It should demonstrate the relevance of basic biological factors for social history within a changing historical framework.
3. It should contain briefly expressed ideas which would encourage interdisciplinary discussion.

I set myself three further conditions:

4. I wanted to give a presentation that was as clearly outlined and as readily understandable as possible. Short bold strokes seemed more in place than rarified discussions, even if finer differences would have to be overlooked. The proportion of text and diagrams was to be two to one.
5. Since actual life expectancy today, despite an increase, only reaches its maximum biological potential in the case of a minority, it seemed to me to be essential to show where we stand in a continuous process of development and to what changes foreseeable further development might lead. In the same way that historians put present conditions into an historical context, they are also able to see what are apparently constant factors in relation to the future, in relative terms.
6. The main aim of this chapter is, however, to urge the reader to think more deeply. Even if, because of our increased life span, the biological component of our existence no longer constantly impinges to the same extent today as it did in the past, it still remains fundamental. We are all mortal, even if we die somewhat later on. To start thinking about it then is rather late.

* Originally published as 'Die verlängerte Lebenzeit – Auswirkungen aufunser Zusammen-leben', *Saeculum*, 36 (1985). Acknowledgement to publish from the publishers, Karl Alber.

347

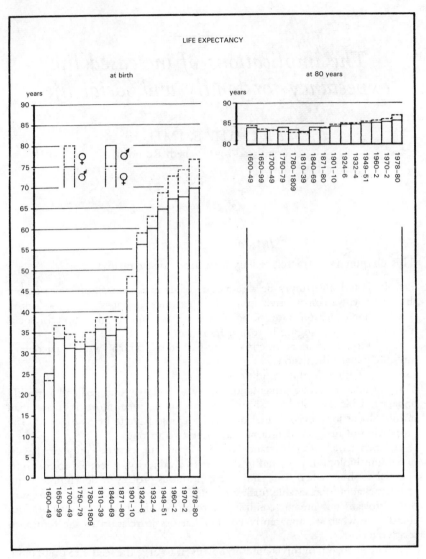

Figure 1 Average life expectancy (i.e. mean age at death) in years from 1600–1900, at birth and, at the age of eighty

Whereas our physiological life expectancy over this period has remained practically the same (see right), our ecological life expectancy has almost trebled (see left). Populations and sources cited: *1600–1869*: Schwalm region in North Hesse: Computer Databank Berlin (based on parish records for circa 30,000 people from the sixteenth to the twentieth century). Because only people who had an entry under baptism as well as burial could be included, and not those who had left or come to the area, we are dealing with minimal values in these calculations – this applies particularly to the life expectancy at birth column. *1871–1934*: Deutsches Reich, *Bevölkerung und Wirtschaft 1872–1972*, hrsg. vom *Statistischen Bundesamt Wiesbaden* (Stuttgart, 1972), p. 110. *1949–80*: Bundesrepublik Deutschland, *Statistisches Jahrbuch 1982 für die Bundesrepublik Deutschland* (Stuttgart, 1982), p. 73.

Two initial clarifications

1. Biological life expectancy has hardly increased over the course of the last few centuries. It is apparent from the right-hand side of Fig. 1 that eighty-year-olds today do not have a life expectancy very much longer than eighty-year-olds three or four centuries ago. Our potential biological life expectancy has remained practically the same, i.e. around eighty-five years. What has increased is the actual life span. (See left-hand column.) In the first half of the seventeenth century it was around twenty-five for all live births regardless of sex or social class; today it is between seventy and eighty.

2. A biologically 'natural death' is a less 'natural death'. Fig. 2 shows the mortality rate of animals which (a) live in the wild, (b) are kept in captivity as domestic animals or in zoos and (c) are protected under good laboratory conditions. The central section of Fig. 2 as well as Fig. 3 show what development central Europeans have undergone between the seventeenth century and today. If our mortality rate three centuries ago was very similar to that of an 'animal population in the wild', then today we are living 'under good laboratory conditions'. Enormous efforts are necessary to maintain this artificially precarious, and dangerously susceptible situation permanently. The demands on and implications for our social life are incontrovertible: peaceful coexistence at a high level of civilization is a *conditio sine qua non*. Guaranteeing this glasshouse atmosphere in the long term is primarily both a collective social as well as an individual personal responsibility. It is only subordinate to this that it can *also be viewed as a matter for public health policy*.

Taking as my basis recent medical gerontological investigations of American researchers, I have outlined in Fig. 2 the final state – as far as it is possible to predict – of this already far advanced development: in the centre, by the so-called 'rectangular curve' 'in the future', and right at the bottom by the relevant distribution of the age of mortality (i.e. in the future, see Fig. 2). It would occur inevitably if 'in the future' most people were able to live out their potential biological life span because of their generally fully utilized biological reserve capacities. After these have lapsed, we would then die a 'natural' death, but hardly a death from old age to be found in Nature. It would be caused by some very minor ailment with no previous long and difficult illness. The symptom-threshold for all those chronic diseases, which today spearhead the statistics for the causes of death such as cancer, diabetes, cirrhosis, arterosclerosis, etc., and which today lead to death in the later years of

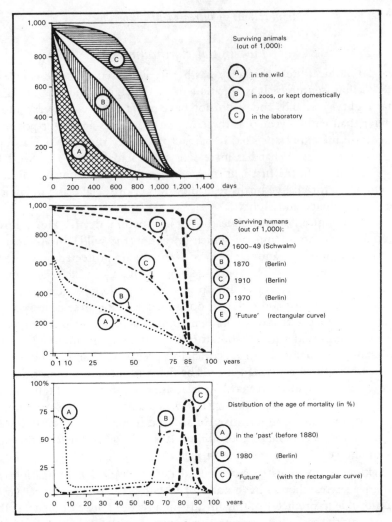

Figure 2 'Natural death': a less 'natural' death

Above: Numbers of surviving animals (out of 1,000), which (A) live in the wild, (B) are kept in zoos or as domestic animals, (C) are kept in protected laboratory conditions. The time axis depicts different families of mouse-like rodents. Source: George A. Sacher, 'Life Table Modification and Life Prolongation', in *Handbook of the Biology of Aging* (New York, 1977), p. 598.

Centre: Number of surviving humans (out of 1,000) from the seventeenth century to the present and projected into 'in the future' when 'the rectangular curve' is reached. Sources: for 1600–49 (Schwalm Region, North Hesse), A. E. Imhof, 'Reconstructing Biological Frameworks of Populations in the Past', in Jerome M. Clubb and K. Scheuch (eds.), *Historical Social Research. The Use of Historical and Process-Produced Data* (Stuttgart, 1980), p. 79. For 1870, 1910, 1970, A. E. Imhof, 'Mortalität in Berlin vom. 18. bis 20. Jahrhundert', in *Berliner Statistik 1977*, p. 141. For the 'future', James F. Fries and Lawrence M. Crapo, *Vitality and Aging. Implications of the Rectangular Curve* (San Francisco, 1981), p. x.

Below: Schematic distribution of the age of mortality in the 'past', today and in the 'future'. Sources: (A) and (B) *Berliner Statistik 1977*, p. 140; (C) Fries and Crapo, *Vitality and Aging*, p. 94.

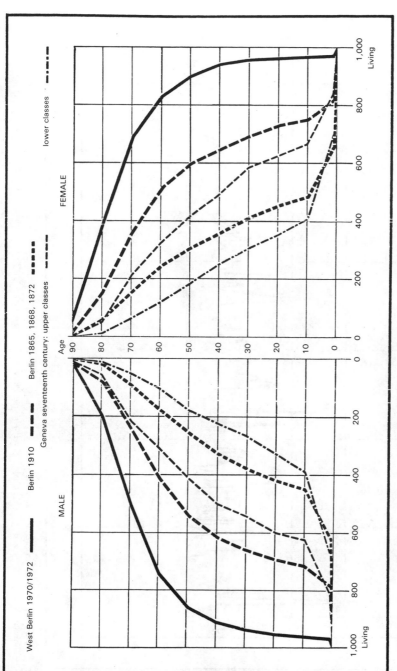

West Berlin 1970/1972 ▬▬▬   Berlin 1910 ▬ ▬ ▬   Berlin 1865, 1868, 1872 ■■■■

Geneva seventeenth century: upper classes ╌ ╌ ╌   lower classes ·╌··╌··

MALE   FEMALE

Age

Living   Living

Figure 3 Surviving men and surviving women (out of 1,000 respectively) from both lower and upper classes in Geneva in the seventeenth century and from Berlin 1865/68/72, 1910 and 1970/72. Both sides of Fig. 3 show that we are now at a very advanced stage of a development that has been taking place over many hundreds of years. The final stage ('rectangular curve') seems to be in sight but has not yet been reached. Source: *Berliner Statistik 1977*, p. 141.

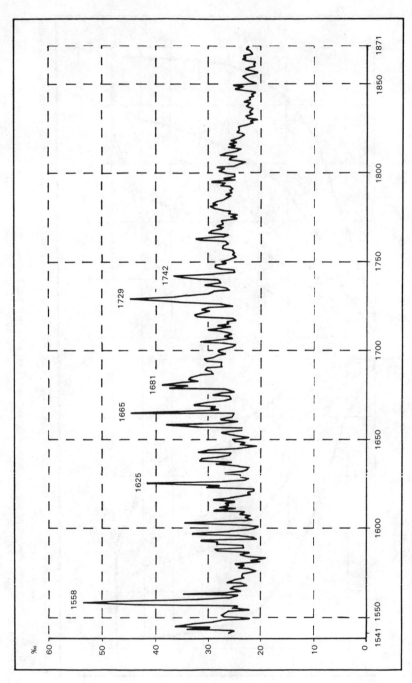

Figure 4a Mortality in England over the years 1541–1871 per 1,000 inhabitants
Source: E. A. Wrigley and R. S. Schofield, *The Population History of England 1541–1871. A Reconstruction* (London, 1981), pp. 531–4.

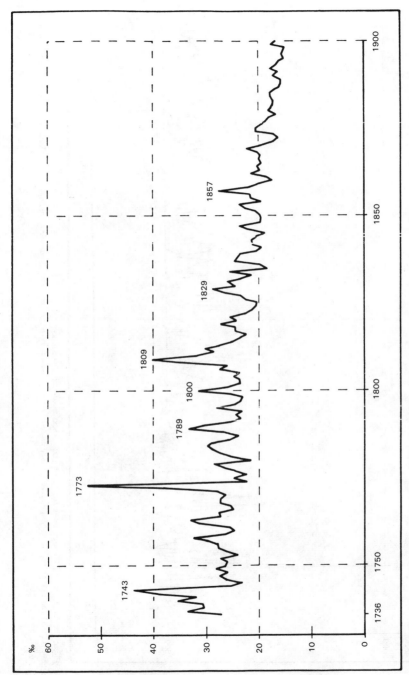

Figure 4b Mortality (not including stillbirths) in Sweden over the years 1736–1900 per 1,000 inhabitants
Source: *Historisk Statistik för Sverige*, vol. 1: *Befolkning*, (Stockholm, 1720–1967; repr. 1969), pp. 866–87.

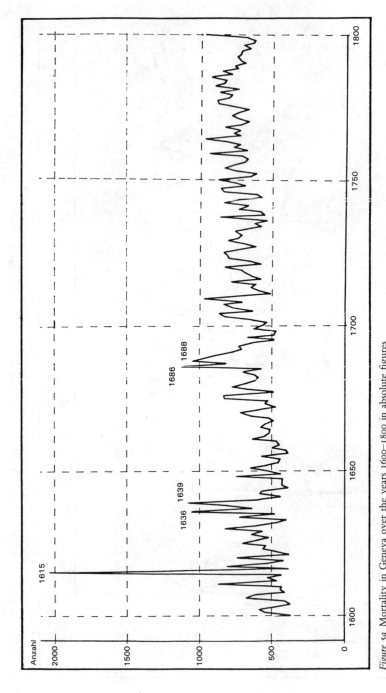

Figure 5a Mortality in Geneva over the years 1600–1800 in absolute figures
Source: Alfred Perrenoud, *La population de Genève du seizième au début du dix-neuvième siècle. Etude démographique*, vol. I: *Structures et mouvements* (Geneva, 1979), pp. 526–30.

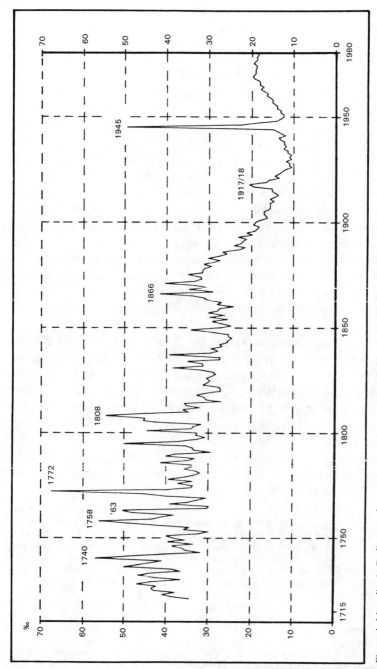

Figure 5b Mortality in Berlin over the years 1721–1980 per 1,000 inhabitants. (1721–1899 includes stillbirths; 1721–1925: Pre-war Berlin; 1926–80: West Berlin)

Sources: *Berliner Statistik 1977*, pp. 138–45 also the title page of the August 1977 edition. For the years 1976–80 expanded on the basis of documentation in the statistical yearbooks for Berlin published by Statistischen Landesamt Berlin (West).

life, would be pushed so far beyond the eighty-five frontier that they could not begin to take effective hold.[1]

What has changed?

The standardization and reduction in the mortality rate

Figures 4 and 5 show the longterm development of the mortality rate in four European populations: in England 1541–1871, in Sweden 1736–1900, in Geneva 1600–1800 and in Berlin 1721–1980. If we try and find a pattern, we can see four distinct phases: in the first phase a generally high rate of mortality with great, sometimes extreme fluctuations from year to year. The peak values with their respective dates can easily be put down to the old death-bearing triad: 'Plague, Hunger and War'. In the second phase, although the mortality rate remained generally high, it did begin increasingly to level off. There were fewer swings of the pendulum and the extreme peaks became smaller and smaller. In the third phase there was a marked change from a generally high to a generally low mortality rate. The fourth and current phase is characterized by a low mortality rate with minor variations from year to year.

If we try and apply this abstract pattern to our fourth example, Berlin, then the first phase would have lasted to about 1810, the second to around 1880, the third to around 1930 and the fourth from then to the present day. Though in Berlin, as it happens, this phasing is broken towards the final stages. Mainly because the effects of the First and Second World Wars do not fit the picture: an indication of the precarious nature of our present and to a far greater extent of our 'future' situation, which cannot be foreseen. 'Plague, Hunger and War' have been held at bay for the time being, but have clearly not been eliminated permanently.

[1] Cf. the two doctors James F. Fries and Lawrence M. Crapo. Their theories of 'natural death from old age' and of the constant biological life span of man (based mainly on the extrapolation of historical data) have not gone unchallenged. As an historian I do not have the competence to take issue with their medical arguments. See, however, for critical comparison, Kenneth G. Manton and Alain Colvez and Jean-Marie Robine, 'Changing Concepts of Morbidity and Mortality in the Elderly Population', *Milbank Memorial Fund Quarterly/Health and Society*, 60: 2 (1982), 183–244. From a sociological standpoint, there is criticism of the liberalist concept of the high degree of individual responsibility and personal control over the chronic processes of decline, 'Lebensverlängerung und Altern ohne Krankheit. Die Untersuchungen von Fries and Crapo', *Zeitschrift für Sozialisationsforschung und Erziehungssoziologie*, 2 (1982) 132–4. It cannot be denied that one must be very careful with such arguments especially in times of noticeable tendencies away from the structuring of the social sphere. We are dealing with basically optimistic-sounding future prospects, not yet with reality. Cf. in this connection, Jürg A. Hauser, 'Ansatz zu einer ganzheitlichen Theorie der Sterblichkeit – eine Skizze', *Zeitschrift für Bevölkerungswissenschaft*, 9 (1983), 159–186.

Implications of increased life expectancy

A fundamental shift in the spectrum of causes of death

The evening out, reduction and stabilization of the mortality rate at a low level are very closely connected with far-reaching shifts in the spectrum of causes of death. Since, as we know, different illnesses present very different features, for example (as many of the infectious diseases which were prevalent in the past) they may last only a short time or (as many of today's chronic ailments) they may last for a long time; some are associated with almost unbearable pain while others are almost symptom-free, some are highly contagious, while others don't affect people who are in close contact. Thus shifts in the panorama of disease obviously have not only grave effects on the ill and dying themselves, but they also have an equal effect on our social life with those afflicted. This applies on an individual or family level to the relationship between the carers and those being cared for, as well as in society as a whole, in the case say of the treatment or segregation of people suffering from infectious and from incurable diseases. Ethical–legal discussions about euthanasia or suicide in old age are at the moment two particularly important topics which are associated with these changes.[2] By way of a real historical example I would like the reader to consider the problems which are inherent in such fundamental changes: in Fig. 6 we can see (above left) the annual distribution of *c.* 40,000 deaths in the parish of Dorotheenstadt in Berlin from 1715 to 1875. Crucial for our considerations is that shortly after 1800, death from smallpox, which was a significant cause of death in infants and young children until that time, was removed from the total spectrum because of the introduction of vaccination against smallpox. (See centre right.) The gap did not remain, however. The other diseases redistributed themselves as had always happened in similar cases. At the time gastro-intestinal (see above right) and respiratory diseases (below right) took their places.[3] The effect on

[2] While the catchword 'euthanasia' is taken up again and again by the mass media and publicized (as in the spring of 1984 with the 'Hackethal case' cf. *Der Spiegel*, 18 (30 April 1984): 'Sterbehalfer Hackethal. Gift für Todkranke'), and there is no shortage of publications on the subject, studies of voluntary euthanasia at an advanced age are more infrequent. But it should make us sit up and think that in 1982 for example, in West Berlin, the group that was at the greatest risk from suicide were the men and women of eighty and over. Even in 1960–4 'incurable disease, depression and mental illness' was deemed in 62·3 per cent of all cases to be the motive for suicide. Cf. Eckart Elsner, 'Selbstmord in Berlin', *Berliner Statistik*, 37 (1983) 230, 234. Elsner also comes to the conclusion that: 'It is not love-sickness which is widely cited as the major problem, but the difficulties of old people, who are often left alone with their fears and see no escape other than suicide', p. 235.

[3] For a bio-medical theory of the so-called pathocenosis (i.e. the totality of all the causes of mortality which form a whole at a particular moment in a particular population) and its dynamics (its historical course – as a concrete example, the rearrangement of the causes, when one of them – as in this case, smallpox – disappears from the total spectrum). Cf. Mirko Drazen Grmek, *Les maladies à l'aube de la civilisation occidentale* (Paris, 1983), pp. 14–17.

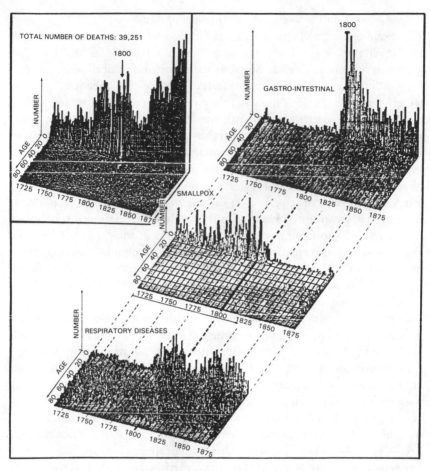

Figure 6 Smallpox as one of the most important causes of death in infants and small children disappeared from the spectrum of causes of death because of the introduction of vaccination shortly after 1800. The empty space was immediately occupied by an increased number of deaths from diseases of the gastro-intestinal tract and the respiratory organs.

Above left: Annual distribution of mortality in the parish of Dorotheenstadt in Berlin according to age of mortality from 1715 to 1875, in absolute figures. Of these, above right: deaths from diseases of the gastro-intestinal tract; centre right: deaths from smallpox; below right: deaths from respiratory diseases.

Source: Computer-Datenbank Berlin (based on death registers of the Berlin parish of Dorotheenstadt; Lutheran Central Archive, West Berlin). On-going research at the Friedrich-Meinecke-Institut der Freien Universität Berlin. All four diagrams are 3-D computer print-outs.

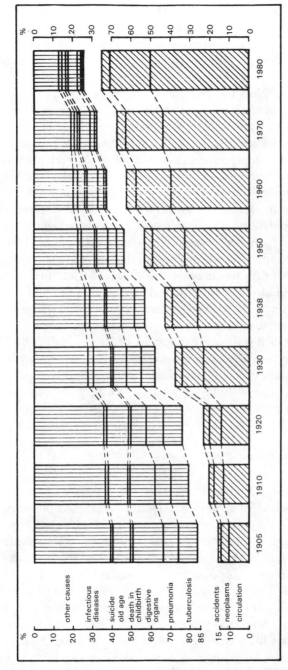

Figure 7 Successive shifts in the distribution frequency of the most important causes of death, or groups of causes, in Germany during the period 1905–80 (the so-called epidemiological transition) shown as a percentage of the total number of deaths in each period Region concerned: 1905–38: German Reich; 1950–80 Federal Republic of Germany. In 1905 deaths from circulatory diseases and neoplasms (cancer) accounted for 14·1 per cent of all deaths; in 1980 the figure was 71 per cent. The rest declined from originally more than four-fifths to a quarter. Infectious diseases were the main diseases to be eliminated.

Sources: *Bevölkerung und Wirtschaft 1872–1972* (Stuttgart, 1972) 120. *Statistisches Jahrbuch 1983 für die Bundesrepublik Deutschland* (Stuttgart, 1983), p. 381.

social life – here particularly the relationship between mothers and children who were mainly affected – meant that on the one hand breastfeeding as an effective protection against gastro-intestinal diseases, and care in the home particularly during the winter months as prevention against respiratory disorders took on a completely new and critical significance. With the two new categories of causes of death, mothers could control to a far greater extent whether their children lived or died, than they had previously been able to do with smallpox.

From Fig. 7 we can see it is not only infants and their mothers who are affected, and not simply historically, but all of us, very directly. In the course of just a few generations, the order of illnesses resulting in death has been completely turned upside down. In 1905 the predominant cause of death for our forebears was still from infectious diseases. Only every sixth person fell prey to cardiac and circulatory disorders or malignant cancerous growths. Today the figure is two out of three. If I relate this change to myself, it simply means that there is a more than 50 per cent probability that I will be in this group. To die of a chronic incurable disease – and to be more than dimly aware of it, and to have to live with it in mind – does not only mean a completely different way of dying for me than was the case in the past with death from an infectious disease which was swift to a greater or lesser degree. This other way of dying will affect my environment. It is questionable whether the old adage 'In the midst of life we are surrounded by death' was not more merciful for many than waiting for a release which is the situation for quite a number of people today.

Effects on our social relationships

In society

In listing biological parameters and their transformation up to the present, I have touched on several occasions on their effect on our social relationships. The following diagrams are set out in such a way that the additional implications cannot fail to strike us. In Fig. 8 I concentrated on the changes in the spectrum of causes of death. The change in the age distribution of the current population is shown very clearly. It is closely connected with the epidemiological transition mentioned above. The suppression of infectious diseases firstly benefited infants and small children and then middle-aged people. More and more babies survived and they became steadily older. This meant that fewer and fewer births were needed in order to achieve a certain number of children or to

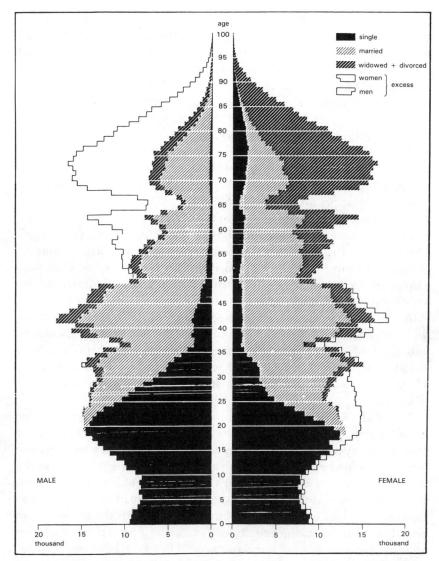

age
100
95
90
85
80
75
70
65
60
55
50
45
40
35
30
25
20
15
10
5
0

■ single
▨ married
▨ widowed + divorced
☐ women ⎫
⬡ men ⎬ excess

MALE

FEMALE

20   15   10   5   0   0   5   10   15   20
thousand   thousand

Figure 8 Population of West Berlin at the end of 1982 according to sex, age and status. Details per 1,000 inhabitants

We can no longer speak of a population pyramid here. In Berlin today there are more old women than young girls. Such an increasingly top-heavy population distribution leads to a large number of problems – individual, family, economic, medical, etc. The reader is referred to three titles, which will give some understanding of the wide-ranging issues which we cannot go into here: Institut National d'Etudes Démographiques (eds.), *Les âges de la vie*, 2 vols. (Paris, 1982 and 1983); Ursula Lehr and W.-F. Schneider, 'Fünf-Generationen-Familie: einige Daten über Ururgrosseltern in der Bundesrepublik Deutschland,' *Zeitschrift für Gerontologie*, 16 (1983), 200–4; Christoph Conrad, 'Geschichte des Alterns: Lebensverhältnisse und sozialpolitische Regulierung' (review article), *Zeitschrift für Sozialisationsforschung und Erziehungssoziologie*, 4 (1984), 143–56 (with numerous references to further reading in European and American publications).

Source: *Berliner Statistik 1983*, p. 260.

361

maintain a certain population level. The once huge base of the population pyramid became visibly smaller, the apex on the other hand became visibly wider. In 1980 there were already as many people aged fifty-five to sixty as there were five- to ten-year-olds in the Federal Republic of Germany, namely 3·6 and 3·5 millions respectively. In 1990 the ratio will be 3·5 to 3 and 1995 4·4 to 3·3 millions in favour of the elderly.[4]

The manifold effects on our present as well as on our future society are topics dealt with so frequently by the media that they do not need to be enumerated in detail here. A few of the recurring headlines will serve as a reminder: 'Pension finance problems', 'Generations agreement' (an agreement that pensions will be paid to people who have retired out of the earnings of people still in employment) 'The burden of the elderly', 'Grey Panthers form their own lobby', 'University of the Third Age', 'More and more families of five generations', 'Inheritance jumps a whole generation'; or with regard to lower birth rates, for examples: 'Bulge shrinks', 'Too few soldiers for the federal army', down to 'Are the Germans becoming extinct?'.

Although these subjects undoubtedly are politically very meaningful and relevant, ranging from social policy, health, the economy, industry and the future to defence, I do not want to go into them here both because they have already been so well aired and for reasons of space. However, I would like to draw attention instead to two less well observed effects.

Firstly I would like to put forward the following idea for consideration. Women today, as we already know from Fig. 1, have a longer life expectancy than men by several years and they are therefore over-represented in the population (see Fig. 8 above right for one of the reasons). There are two aspects to this gender problem. Firstly, it no longer seems justifiable in view of the current population distribution to concern ourselves predominantly or completely with the sexuality and sexual problems of young people only and act as if pensioners or women after the menopause were somehow neutral beings, whom one need not bother about. The factors which have brought about an increase in our life span must also have caused people to be more sexually active and more attractive at a later age. Secondly, bearing in mind the massive imbalance between the sexes especially in the elderly, society should allow these 'surplus' women, often widows, to consider the possibility of entering into sexual relationships other than those previously deemed

[4] *Statistisches Jahrbuch 1983 für die Bundesrepublik Deutschland* (Stuttgart, 1983), p. 69.

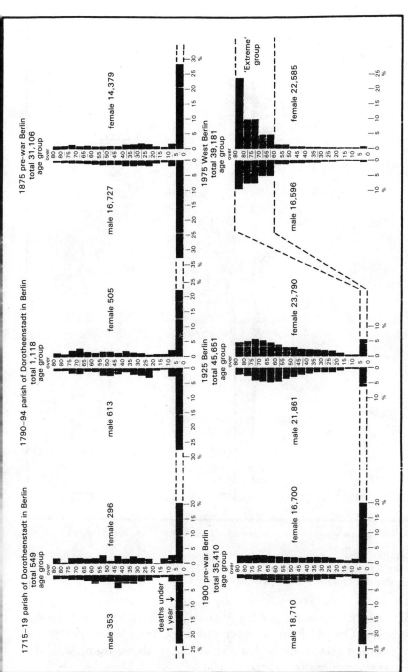

Figure 9 Distribution of mortality according to sex in five-year stages in Berlin during the period 1715–1975, as percentages. 100 per cent is the total number of dead in the period concerned

Dying and death are always concentrated at the extreme end of the age band. While it used to be infants and small children who died in huge numbers, today it is people over sixty. No society can tolerate for any length of time a mortality distribution which endangers the community, as was the case in 1925 (see diagram below centre.) From the point of view of society as a whole, groups at the extreme ends of the age band contribute less. Source: *Berliner Statistik 1977,* p. 140.

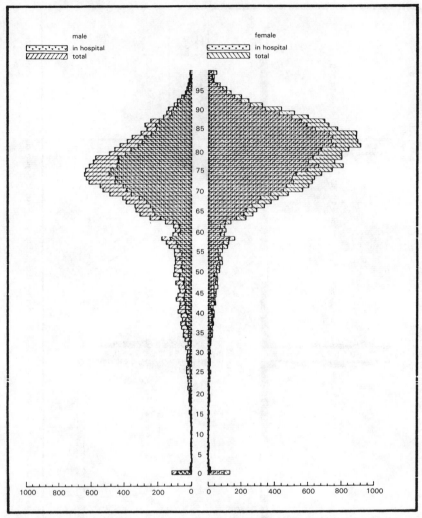

Figure 10 Distribution of mortality according to sex and age in West Berlin, per 1,000 of the population
Total mortality: 36,060, of these 27,413 (= 76%) in hospital; male: 15,189, of these 10,884 (= 71·7%) in hospital. Female: 20,871, of these 16,529 (= 79·2%) in hospital.
Source: Statistische Landesamt Berlin (West).

suitable and, if necessary, society should permit them to form new relationships. On the basis of sheer numbers, the idea of polygamy should not be rejected out of hand. (See Fig. 8 above right, with the distribution according to marital status.)

Implications of increased life expectancy

The second effect of the epidemiological transition, i.e. an increasingly top-heavy population distribution, is not simply ignored out of apathy but is consciously suppressed: it is that dying and death today, as never before in history, are bound up on the one hand with advanced age and on the other with a long chronic incurable infirmity with the need for care, hospitalization and gradual decline. (See Figs. 9 and 10 together with Fig. 7 with the constantly increasing percentage of deaths caused by chronic disease.) These are understandably the less attractive prospects of advanced age for most of us. Since we cannot escape them, we suppress them for as long as we are in our prime. They should play no part if possible in our daily social intercourse. Terminally ill geriatrics are excluded from society. In Berlin death gathers more than three-quarters of its victims in special rooms for the dying behind hospital walls. (Fig. 10 for the year 1978.) Just as death's ripest pickings were once from amongst infants and small children, now they are concentrated on people over sixty. One group on the periphery of the age band has taken the place of the other. To live with groups on the periphery, to cooperate with them and to integrate them has always been a problem for society.

Within the family

Over the last hundred years or more this development has been most dramatic for mothers. Two completely new phases of life have emerged for them. On the one hand they experience today 'post-parental companionship in an empty nest' for some years; on the other hand because of the different life expectancy for men and women they can go through a widowhood which also lasts for several years. (Clearly shown in upper section of Fig. 11.) Neither of these phenomena existed in the past as structural elements.

With regard to partnership, one of the consequences of a long life span becoming standard amongst the parents' generation is that the marriage age in the succeeding generation has increasingly become standardized during the course of the modern period. (See Fig. 12.) Whereas at the beginning of the period under investigation, i.e. at the end of the seventeenth century, it was quite common for people with a great difference in age to marry, today it is more common for people of similar age or, should I say youth, to marry. Today sex appeal in the choice of a partner and sexuality in marriage as the basis for a long, satisfying and fulfilled sex life rightly play a more important role than they did in the era of couples of dissimilar age. In the past, economic or genealogical factors were more critical. Against this background it is

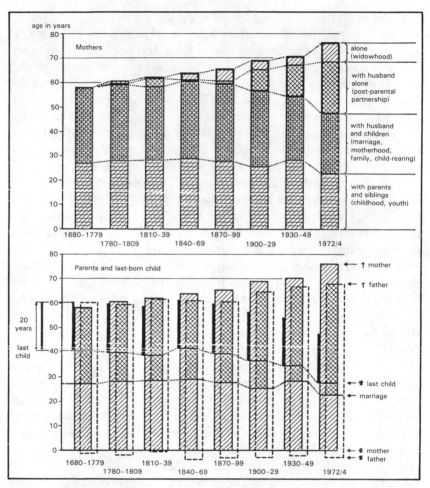

Figure 11 Phases in the lives of parents (below) and of mothers (above) during eight different periods from 1680 to 1974

The emergence and rapid expansion of the new phases, 'post-parental partnership in the empty nest' and 'widowhood' is quite apparent. This is specifically emphasized by the heavy outline in the upper part of the diagrams.

Population and sources: *1680–1949*: life-expectancy: Schwalm region in North Hesse; Computer-Databank Berlin. All the other information: Parish of Gabelbach, 25 kilometers to the west of Augsburg in Swabia. Historical–demographic standard calculations based on Frans Hauf, *Ortssippenbuch Gabelbach* (*Deutsche Ortssippenbüche*, Series B, vol. 8 (Frankfurt am Main, 1975)). *1972/4*: Bundesrepublik Deutschland: *Daten des Gesundheitswesens* (Bonn–Bad Godesburg, 1977), pp. 24–5, 191. Statistischen Bundesamt Wiesbaden, *Die Situation der Kinder in der Bundesrepublik Deutschland* (Stuttgart, 1979), p. 25.

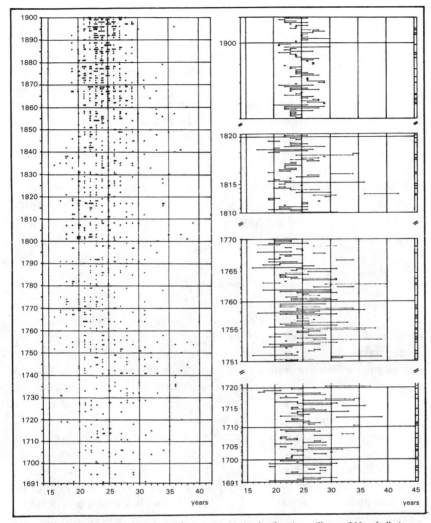

Figure 12 Age, and difference in age, in first marriages in the farming village of Heuchelheim near Giessen in Upper Hesse 1691–1900

Left: Age at first marriage of 1,104 brides (each shown by a dot). Right: Difference in ages of the partners at first-time marriages over four selected periods. Marriages in which the woman was older than the man are shown by dashes and a tiny cross bar at the right-hand edge. The wide distribution of the marriage age to start with and the increased focusing in the course of time are clearly recognizable. Understanding the structure of computer graphics is often just as important as the results of the calculations. In this particular case the 'average' marriage age in the first decade, 1691–1700, was 24·1 for women, 25·8 for men, in the last century, 1891–1900, it was 24·3 for women and 25·4 for men; as though nothing had changed in more than two centuries! For a whole series of observations the gradual standardization of the age of marriage is more important than the fact that the average has remained much the same. For so-called Exploratory Data Analysis, a branch of statistics, cf. John W. Tukey, *Exploratory Data Analysis* (London, 1977), which is still a seminal work.

Source: A. E. Imhof, 'Die namentliche Auswertung der Kirchenbücher. Die Familien von Giessen 1631–1730 und Heuchelheim 1691–1900', in Imhof (ed.), *Historische Demographie als Sozialgeschichte. Giessen und Umgebung vom 17. zum 19. Jahrhundert* (Darmstadt and Marburg, 1975), pp. 315–24, 362–3.

367

understandable that men and women remained closely attached to the male or female community in which they had grown up, even after the marriage. The so-called 'emotional revolution' with regard to married couples seems to me to be a result of the standardization of life expectancy or it is at least one of the prerequisites. In our marital and family life we are much more exclusively attached to one another than was the case in the past. The consequences are all the more serious when it becomes apparent after a certain time that we are unsuited to one another or if we move apart in the later years of marriages which last much longer today with their additional 'empty nest' phase. Psychologists may be better able to judge the consequences of increasing similarity in the age of parents on their life with their children and on their efforts to bring them up.

Summary

The social, political and economic life of a population with an average age of, let us say twenty, is in many respects quite different from one with an average age of forty. One might think of European populations in the sixteenth century on the one hand and on the other in the latter half of the twentieth century or one might compare those in developing countries with those in the industrial nations – not to mention concepts that spring to mind such as 'Youth as a force in the Modern World' or the possible connection between an increasingly aging electorate and a growing tendency towards conservative election results.[5] The population distribution in the Third World is heavily weighted at the bottom, and is thus pyramid-shaped. Because there the population structure is biologically determined, sexuality plays a more decisive role as a means of maintaining the population level than it does in developed countries. Socialization takes place within the context of larger numbers of brothers, sisters and children than it does with us. Contagious diseases are more rampant and death is an everyday occurrence in all age groups, and if a broad social network of neighbours, relations and communities is of

---

[5] This is the title of an essay by Herbert Moller in *Comparative Studies in Society and History*, 10 (1967/8), 237–60. In the elections to the German Parliament in 1980, the lowest poll was amongst the twenty-one to twenty-four-year-olds with 78·9 per cent. It rose steadily with the highest poll amongst the fifty to fifty-nine and sixty to sixty-nine-year-olds with 92·3 and 92·2 per cent respectively. The largest number of voters for the CDU/CSU were men over sixty and the largest number for the SPD were women between eighteen and twenty-four. See *Datenhandbuch zur Geschichte des Deutschen Bundestages 1949 bis 1982*, written and edited by Peter Schindler (Bonn, 1983), pp. 29, 58.

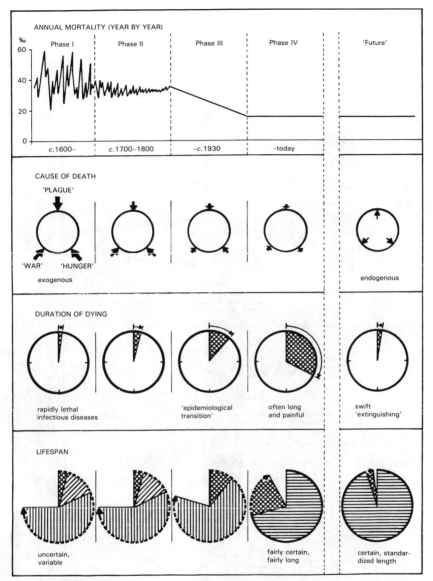

Figure 13 Development of mortality in five phases. Phases I–III: during the last centuries (i.e. from 1600–1930); Phase IV: situation today; Phase V: in 'the future'
The sections of the diagram deal with the following four aspects: (a) mortality: number of deaths from year to year per thousand of the average population; (b) cause of death: change of mortality from exogenous causes due to the old triad 'Plague, Hunger and War' to the physiologically, endogenously determined 'extinguishing' of living functions with no previously long-lasting illness; (c) duration of dying: development from an often rapid death from infectious epidemics, through the often slow and painful death from chronically incurable diseases, to a painless swift 'extinguishing' in 'the future'; (d) life expectancy: development from an uncertain life expectancy with a high concentration of infant and child mortality and a wide range of individual life expectancies to a certain and standardized long life span, which approaches the potential physiological life expectancy.

369

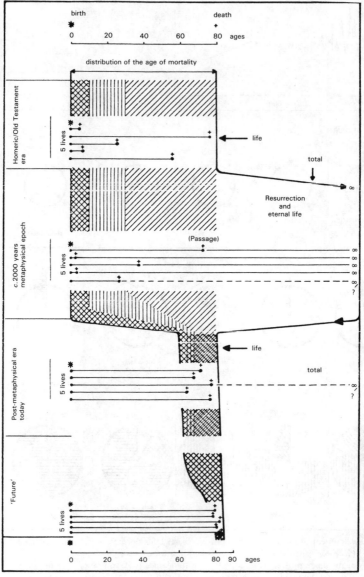

Figure 14 Diagrammatic development of life-extent expectancy of 'Westerners' from Homeric and Old Testament times to the present and 'future'. The idea for this came from Walter Schulz, 'Wandlungen der Einstellung zum Tode', in Johannes Schwartländer (ed.), *Der Mensch und sein Tod* (Göttingen, 1976), pp. 94–107; Schizuteru Ueda, *Der Tod im Zen-Buddhismus*, in *ibid*; pp. 162–172; Alan Jeffrey Spencer, *Death in Ancient Egypt* (Harmondsworth, 1982); Michel Vovelle, *La Mort en l'occident de 1300 à nos jours* (Paris, 1983).

greater importance, grandparents and families with several living generations are less frequently met with – the collective long-term memory has to rely on a smaller number of long-lived individuals. We could go on for a long time enumerating such aspects which are certainly of fundamental significance for the continuance and survival of our society but this would simply mean enumerating a whole host of historical socio-anthropological questions (which, however, was expressly set aside at the outset as being undesirable).[6]

I would like to present my conclusions in a different way. In order to formulate my thesis more easily, I have drawn Figs 13 and 14. In Fig. 13 I show five phases, taking the earlier historical divisions and developing on from them. The first three concern, in very broad outline, the historical development 'during the last centuries'. Phase IV stands for the present, and Phase V (right) for 'the future'. Let us first sum up the development of Phases I–IV. As we remember, mortality was originally very high with characteristically wide swings of the pendulum. Gradually it settled at a high level before it practically halved in the third phase and since then it has remained at a low level without great fluctuations. Regarding the causes of death, during all four phases they were essentially exogenous and could consistently be put down to the effects of the old triad 'Plague' (as an umbrella term for disease in general), 'Hunger' and 'War'. If one then considers the duration of the dying process it was originally relatively short because of the preponderance of rapidly fatal infectious diseases. It became gradually more drawn out during the course of the epidemiological transition and today it is often long and painful with many chronically incurable ailments. Life expectancy was originally extremely variable and despite the concentration of mortality amongst infants and small children, all in all it was very difficult to calculate. It increased with the epidemiological transition, became more certain and is for most people today pretty well

[6] For those interested, the article by André Burguière, which takes in all these questions, 'L'anthropologie historique,' in Jacques Le Goff et. al. *La nouvelle histoire* (Paris, 1978), pp. 37–61, is still highly recommended. The continuing development of this French theory can easily be followed in the wide-ranging 'Anthropologie historique' option, one of the lecture courses of the Paris École des Hautes Études en Sciences Sociales. See also from the American viewpoint, Andrejs Plakans, 'Introduction to Historical Social Anthropology', lecture given at the Freie Universität, Berlin, October 1979. From Germany, see the two collected volumes on this theme: Hans Süssmuth (ed.), *Historische Anthropologie. Der Mensch in der Geschichte* (Göttingen, 1984) and Hans Medick und David Sabean (eds.), *Emotionen und materielle Interessen. Sozialanthropologische und historische Beiträge zur Familienforschung* (Göttingen, 1984). From the physical, anthropological and socio-biological view, see Eckart Voland, 'Human Sex-Ratio Manipulation: Historical Data from a German Parish', *Journal of Human Evolution*, 13 (1984), 99–107. The Göttingen anthropologist comes to grips with the different historical rates of infant mortality between the sexes and in different social classes.

of a standard length. The potential biological life span can be lived out by an increasingly greater number than ever before.

Looking at the 'future' and assuming the gradual attainment of the 'rectangular curve', mortality will remain at the present low level. The causes of death would however be, and this is the critical difference, no longer exogenous but essentially endogenous. More and more people would approach their potential biological limit without serious loss of vitality and they would finally expire without going through a long and difficult illness. Since frailty in advanced age would be drastically diminished, the far-reaching, beneficial effects for the individual as well as for our relationships with our partners, families and society as a whole are obvious. Because of the independence we would gain almost down to our last breath, the numerous dependencies which we fear would disappear. Fears about aging and dying a difficult death would become irrelevant. The cost-intensive care of the elderly would be redundant. Old people's homes and centres for the chronically sick would stand empty in their hundreds, as with the sanatoriums for chest diseases and alpine mountain clinics which flourished a few decades ago.

Should present trends lead to this situation sooner or later, we would have no cause to envy our descendants unreservedly on that account. Even if the millions which are now invested worldwide in medical research were to lead to a decisive breakthrough and the current major causes of death – heart and circulatory disorders and cancer – were replaced by other disorders, if not immediately but steadily, and our descendants died before their symptom-threshold was reached because of their extended organism reserve capacity, this would still only be one aspect of the development. I have referred to the other aspect in Fig. 14 and would like to concentrate more on this, since I am after all an historian and not a futurologist.

On the left-hand side of the diagram, from the example of five lives which are divided into three periods which broadly succeed one another but which at times overlap we can see how the broad distribution of the age of mortality which prevailed for centuries began to focus in recent years on the over-sixty age group. Looking at the 'future' this bunching would continue and having attained the 'rectangular curve' would come to rest at a standardized norm of eighty plus.

The right-hand side of the diagram raises the point that during the period under consideration, a completely different development has taken place. If we look at the most recent past once more, then we have not only, as we often proudly believe, doubled and trebled our average life span, but we have also infinitely reduced our total 'life span' because of the secularization of our ideas about religion and the afterlife, which has taken place alongside. For about 2,000 years, Western thought was shaped by the New Testament and metaphysics. Anchored in it was a belief in the resurrection of the dead and eternal life in the Glory of God. 'Total life' consisted of a longer or shorter and more or less important earthly portion and then the eternal life. Between the two lay, as 'passages', dying and death. Of course it is difficult to say how many of our forefathers shared this belief wholeheartedly. I have tentatively put down four out of five. Today the ratio would be reversed.Certainly most of us are aware of what we have most recently lost. The long-term effects of a 2,000-year-old collective memory cause us a lot of trouble. For many the present stage of development, Phase IV in Fig. 13, is not very satisfying. Our ancestors more than 2,000 years ago, as I have tried to show in Fig. 14 above, were very well aware of their ephemerality. 'The Old Testament does not hide this fact behind all sorts of hypotheses – as for example that only the body dies and not the soul or that death is not final', the Catholic theologian, Hans Urs von Balthasar, said recently, 'it looks the facts straight in the eye'.[7] And the Tübingen philosopher, Walter Schulz says, 'It seems that after the metaphysical era, to which Western Christianity belongs from an historical point of view, has come to an end, we are once again confronted with the possibility and the necessity of recognising the simple fact of transitoriness'.[8] Do the conclusions which we can draw from Fig. 13 and 14, which are the quintessence of the whole chapter, give us cause for optimism?

For me the essential insights into the problem and how they are related are as follows.

The old pattern of the mortality rate which prevailed for centuries, with a wide distribution of individual age of mortality and a very uncertain life span which was hard to predict for the individual, favoured the spread of a value system that went beyond the individual, whether metaphysical, as a belief in an eternal life amongst the heavenly host in the hereafter for 'reasons of justice' (i.e. to compensate) – invented, so it seems to me, for the many who were victim to the everyday occurrence of premature death – or whether related to this life (in the peasant

[7] Hans Urs von Balthasar in his lecture, 'Endlische Zeit innerhalb ewiger Zeit. Zur christlichen Sicht des Menschen,' at the Katholischen Akademie in Bayern. See Extracts in *Zur Debatte* 14: 3 (1984).

[8] Walter Schulz, 'Wandlungen der Einstellung zum Tode', in Johannes Schwartlander (ed.), *Der Mensch und sein Tod* (Göttingen, 1976), pp. 94–107.

societies of the time, whose ethos and behavioural code was determined by the family and agrarian society). Collective rather than individual survival strategies were the logical consequence of these basic biological determinants and shaped a social life which gave mutual support.

As a result of the improved mortality rate and the disappearance of extreme swings of the pendulum, the way for secularization and for the trend towards individualization was smoothed. Little by little the great supplications of the Holy Litany lost their immediacy.

'Save us from "plague", "hunger", and "sudden death", O Lord.' Patron saints of disease lost their justification for existence; their heaven began to be depopulated. After the curve in the mortality rate had smoothed out (what were the causes for this still remain disputed)[9] it was easier to control the remaining degree of mortality and to lower it systematically: an enormous achievement at the time. Along with the fact that it became increasingly easy to calculate individual life spans, the relevance of the traditional broad range of interrelationships diminished. Social behaviour which was mainly collectively orientated loosened its grip and egocentric behaviour gained the upper hand. The impact of secularization led to the abandonment of the life hereafter. This resulted in a complete revaluation of the human body. The perfect functioning of the body became the sole guarantor for the whole of life which was henceforth exclusively here and now. The new and intensified interest in the body received further impetus from the increasing similarity in age of marriage partners, which has probably led to a stronger and longer lasting interest in marital sex life and thus to a strengthening of partnership ties for married couples.

The present pattern of mortality with the majority of deaths concentrated in the over sixties comprises a lengthened and fairly assured life span for most of us for many years to come. At the same time however, because of the epidemiological transition and the standardization of life expectancy, death looms over the final phase of life, i.e. over us in advanced age in many chronically incurable cases as never

[9] For a good short survey of the present state of the debate cf. Alfred Perrenoud, 'Le biologie et l'humain dans le déclin séculaire de la mortalité', TS of lecture given at the collège de France, June 1983. It is particularly disturbing that we don't know why changes in the historical development of mortality over the last centuries worldwide occur simultaneously, i.e. in completely different social, economic and medical conditions, or why certain epidemics, like the plague, have been eliminated. Perrenoud even goes so far as to speak of a 'certain autonomy of mortality'. In any case the simplistic reduction of the debate to the single controversy about medical care versus nutrition only touches the surface. See from Germany on this subject, the so-called McKeown Controversy, the doctor Friedrich-Wilhelm Schwartz, 'Medizinische Versorgung versus Ernährung – Erklärungskonzepte für die historische Zunahme der Lebenswartung' – A critique of *Historical Medical Criticism* by T. McKeown, in: *Medizin, Mensch und Gesellschaft* (September 1984).

before. It reduces both the quality of life and the quality of death. Moreover it is no longer eternity that awaits us but a passing away. We try and suppress both as far as possible. One outcome is a disproportionate interest in the youthful body far away from death and dying, and far removed from any decline, the other is a turning away from old people who are closest to death and to passing away. So many of us live 'back to front' in the true sense of the term, not looking forwards but backwards.

Against this background, reaching the 'rectangular curve' would seem to be doubly worthwhile. For one thing we would no longer need to fear dying, as in the past with the old pattern of mortality, death would be swift but from now on it would occur after a standardized long life at the limits of our potential biological life expectancy.

For another, we could probably come to terms with the loss of belief in eternal life more easily and return once more to the old view of our own ephemerality. If more and more people on earth had everything, including a complete life span in good health, then perhaps eternity would no longer be 'necessary', neither for them nor for those who had previously died prematurely. We would no longer need to have a fixation on youth or be antagonistic to the elderly. They would retain freedom of movement and of choice to the end.

The present pattern of mortality already presents us with a huge chance we have never had before – and this will be even greater when the 'rectangular curve' is reached. Practically every one of us is guaranteed as never before a relatively long life biologically and relatively long-lasting good health. In contrast to our forbears we are able to plan the course of our lives and divide our time. Time has become a fixed, finite and therefore all the more valuable quantity, with which we can and should reckon. It does not seem to me therefore to be very clever to want to remain youthful and live as young people do with an unmapped future.

[10] In view of the strong trend in this direction, it is not to be wondered at that sociologists referring to the present (on the basis of current demographic data, such as the sharp increase in one-person households, the decline in the number of marriages and the increase in relationships outside marriage, which can be dissolved quickly, the reduction in the number of children, etc.) are asking whether we are 'on the road to an autistic society'. ('It is not so much an individual as a social condition that is meant by "autistic" – a condition in which the members of society are becoming loners to an increasing extent and are showing primarily egocentric patterns of thought and behaviour' according to the sociologist Hans-Joachim Hoffmann-Nowotny, professor at the university of Zürich. Cf. (in this connection) the interim report on his long researches, 'Auf dem Wege zu einer Gesellschaft von Einzelgängern?', in *Neue Zürcher Zeitung*, foreign edition no. 155 (7 July 1984), p. 9).

Ancient Israel considered fortunate whoever God had allowed to die 'old and tired of life', Hans Urs von Balthasar[11] tells us once again. Now we are becoming old, but do we tire of life? It is apparently one thing to be able to reach the limit of one's potential biological life expectancy. It is quite another to fill this potential with life, not only so that we have lived to the full physically, but so that it has had meaning and content. The more we become a society of loners because of the individualistic tendencies outlined, the more each one of us is challenged. For what does 'tired of life' mean? What does it mean for this or that individual? For those who remain unmarried, for the divorced, for workers who are already pensioners at fifty-five, for retired university professors? What does it mean in a socialist or a capitalist society?[12] To say that this is just a question for gerontologists is to take the easy way out. But certainly the service they have performed in first opening our eyes to many things should not be denied.[13]

The greatest challenge of increased life expectancy is the challenge to our social life. The extra years we have gained are due to the extensive suppression of the effects of 'Plague, Hunger and War'. The final stage of this development, the 'rectangular curve' is almost within reach. In order to achieve it, indeed merely in order to maintain our present situation long term, 'extensive suppression' is not enough. Above all it is not certain enough. To make it certain it would be necessary to eradicate the causes 'roots and all', an objective in view of the present world situation, which is hard to imagine. We can only live 'under good laboratory conditions' if we ourselves do not destroy those conditions, whether in regard to our environment or to our peaceful coexistence.

[11] Balthasar, 'Endliche Zeit', p. 10.

[12] I would like to mention here my gratitude for a serious and intensive discussion which went on for some hours and which took place after a talk on this subject given at the Central Institute for History of the Academy of Sciences of the GDR in East Berlin on 26 June 1984.

[13] Cf. for example the socio-gerontologist, Leopold Rosenmayer, and also the comprehensive series – which runs to more than fifty volumes – of the German Centre of Questions relating to Old Age, West Berlin (Deutsches Zentrum für Altersfragen): *Beiträge zur Gerontologie und Altenarbeit*.

Index

academic medicine, *see* universities
Abbott, Alexander, 266
Abel-Smith, Brian, 340
Abernethy, John, 237
abscesses, 73, 80
accoucheurs, *see* midwives (male)
Achilles, 16
Achilles the vet, 55
Acilii of Claudiopolis, 42
Ackernecht, Erwin, 203, 253
actors, as healers, 76
Adair, Dr James McKittrick, 105, 106,
   108, 111, 112
Adam, 140, 141
Addams, Jane, 260
addiction, *see* drugs
Addison, Christopher, 328–9
Aegina, civic physician at, 20
ague, 97, 101, 263
AIDS, 313
alchoholism, 304, 309
Alcon (Roman surgeon), 47
Alexander the Great, 27, 28, 29
Alexander of Tralles, 56
Alexandrian medicine, 3, 28, 30, 31–2,
   44, 54
Alford, Robert R., 343
Alfort, France, veterinary school, 175
almoners, hospital, 213
Ambrosius of Puteoli, 56
American colonies, 156; healthiness of,
   127, 132–3; as paradise, 139, 140;
   smallpox inoculation, 190, 192; *see also*
   United States
American Public Health Association, 256
Amiens cathedral school, 66–7
anaesthesia, introduction of, 210, 211

anatomy, Graeco-Roman, 3, 21, 29–30,
   48, 54; *see also* vivisection
Anaxagoras, 23
Anderson, Elizabeth Garrett, 246
Anglo-Saxon medicine, 70
aniline dyes, 310
animals: Graeco-Roman animal
   anatomy, 48, 54; mortality rates in the
   wild and in captivity compared, 349,
   350; notions of health and
   wholesomeness of, in early modern
   England, 142, 144, 145–6
animism, Stahl's theory of, 160, 161,
   162, 164, 165
Annales Médiopsychologiques, 296
Anthimus (Frankish royal doctor), 67
Anthony, Saint, *see* St Anthony's fire
anthrax bacillus, discovery of, 310
antibiotics, 11, 311, 313
Antigonus of Macedon, 30
antimonial remedies, 110
Antioch, 28, 47, 52
antisepsis, 10, 11, 211, 305
Antonius Castor, 52
Antonius Musa, 45
Apollo, 15, 18, 27, 33–4
Apollonius of Citium, 31–2
apothecaries: eighteenth-century, 110,
   184, 223, 225–6; medieval, 80, 81,
   83–4, 85; Scottish, 208; *see also*
   druggists; pharmacy;
   surgeon–apothecaries
Apothecaries Act (1815), 7, 208, 219,
   222, 226, 233–6, 240
apprenticeship, medical, 24 n. 40, 54, 80,
   93, 224, 234
Aquileia, doctors in, 41

377

Index

Beveridge Report, 215
Bicêtre Hospital, Paris, 291
Bichat, Marie-François-Xavier, 308
biliousness, fashionable ailment of, 105
biology, experimental, 308, 310; see also
    bacteriology
Birmingham, 207, 243
birth, see childbirth
blacksmiths, as healers, 230
bleeding, therapeutic technique, 69, 80,
    121, 144, 159, 185; as cure for
    madness, 289, 290; self-bleeding, 97
blind, medieval institutions for, 89
Boer War, public health campaigns
    following, 271, 322, 324, 328
Boerhaave, Herman, 158–9, 162, 163,
    164
Bologna university, medical studies,
    78–9, 80
Bolus of Mende, 32
bone-setting, 69, 80, 93, 94
Bonn, 307; Roman military
    hospital, 51
Bordeaux, 44
Boston, USA, 190, 255
Brieux, Eugène, Les Avariés, 312
Brighton, 271
Bristol, 207, 231
Bristowe, John Syre, 263
Britain: health-care services in twentieth
    century (see also National Health
    Service), 12–13, 317–45; medical
    practitioners and medical reform
    1750–1850, 7–8, 219–47; medical
    research, 310; mortality rates
    1541–1871, 352, 356; public health and
    preventive medicine in nineteenth and
    twentieth centuries, 8–9, 249–75, 325,
    330–3 passim, 337; treatment of
    mentally ill, 9–10, 278–301 passim;
    voluntary reform movement, 176–8,
    179–81; see also England; voluntary
    hospitals
British Hospitals Association, 209
British Institute of Preventive Medicine,
    310
British Lying-In Hospital, 177
British Medical Association, 219, 264,
    332–3, 337
Broderip, William, 226–7, 231

Brontë, Charlotte, treatment of insanity
    in Jane Eyre, 279
Brooke, Henry, 126 n. 17
Brown, John, 165–6
Bruckshaw, Samuel, 117
Bryder, Linda, 324
Buchan, William, 107–8, 110; Domestic
    Medicine (1769), 106, 108, 186, 187,
    188
Buchner, Hans, 314
Bullein, William, Government of Health
    (1558), 132
Bunyan, John, 117
Burdett, Sir Henry, 209
Burton, Robert, 135, 138
Byng, John, Viscount Torrington, 103
Byzantine hospitals, 50 n. 139, 85

Cadogan, William, 177
Caesar, Gaius Julius, 38, 51
Caligula, Roman emperor, 46, 47
Callender, George, 211 n. 50
Calpurnius Asclepiades, Caius, 47
Calvinists, 96, 280
Cambridge University, medical studies,
    219, 230 n. 27, 238
Camden, William, 126
Canada, health-care policies, 330, 338,
    341–2
cancer, 62, 303, 304, 306, 307, 309, 332,
    360
Caracalla, emperor, grant of universal
    Roman citizenship, 43, 45
'carers', 343, 357
Caribbean, hookworm control
    programme, 260
Carlisle, Sir Anthony, 239
Carnegie, Andrew, 260
Carolingian period, 66
Cartesian dualism, 158, 160, 161
Cartwright, Ann, 244
cataracts, 80
cathedral schools, French medieval, 66–7
Catholic Church, 3, 124, 280
Cato the Elder, 35, 36, 50
cattle plague, 174, 175, 263
cell biology, 10, 307, 308
cellular pathology, 251, 307, 308, 309
Celsus, Aulus, 22, 30, 40, 48, 50
census (1911), 272

379

Index

Parkes, Edmund Alexander, 265, 266
Parkinson, John, 139
parks, public, 138, 139
Parmenides, 18, 22
Pasteur, Louis, 9, 266, 309, 310
Pasteur Institute, Paris, 310
Paston, Margaret, 98
patent medicines/nostrums, 110–11, 189
patient–doctor relationship, 1, 10 n. 5, 91–2, 319, 328; in early modern period, 4, 103–4, 109, 157, 185, 188; effect of emergence of scientific medicine on, 6, 10; and National Health Service, 12, 320, 339, 340, 343–4, 345
patriotism/healthiness of native country, 127–9
Patroclus, 16
Paul the Deacon, 71
Pausanias, 33
Peckham Health Centre, 335
pediatrics, 312; see also children
pellagra, 269–70
Pelling, Margaret, 100, 253–4
Pennsylvania Asylum, 300
Pepys, Samuel, 99
Perceval, John Thomas, 116, 118, 287
Percival, Thomas, Medical Ethics (1803), 103
Pergamum, 28, 30, 49, 54
Perkins, William, 124 n. 13
Persia, 18–19, 20, 29, 32, 56
Peterson, M. Jeanne, 320–1
Pettenkofer, Max von, 257, 309, 310
Petty, William, Essays in Political Arithmetic (1687), 176
Phaedrus, 54
pharmacology: ancient Greek, 16, 17, 29, 30; medieval, 60; see also drugs
pharmacy, 83, 224, 226, 228, 241; see also drugs
Pharnaces the rootcutter, 55
Phigalia, plague at, 33
Philadelphia, public health, 255, 266
Philalethae of Men Karou, 42
philanthropy in medicine, 176, 178, 257; and rise of hospitals, 179–80, 199, 200, 201, 204, 213
Philistion, 42
Philo, 31

Philo Judaeus, 31
philosophes, 125, 193
Philosophical Transactions (1714), account of smallpox inoculation, 190
philosophy, association of medicine with, 3, 22–4, 29, 48–9
Phrygia, 40, 42, 55
physicians; in early modern England, 92–3; in eighteenth- and nineteenth-century Britain, 100, 223, 226, 234, 237–40, 241, 243, 246; Enlightenment, 154, 156, 157; medieval, 80, 83, 84, 85; see also medical practitioners; Royal College of Physicians
Physick for Families (1674), 106
Piacenza, 36
pigs, wholesomeness of, 145–6
Pinel, Dr Philippe, 291, 292, 295, 296
Pirquet, Clemens von, 311
Pius, Antoninus, Roman emperor, 47, 52–3
plague, 75, 171, 189, 194, 310; in ancient Greece, 15, 33; in early modern England, 136, 137; in medieval Europe, 8, 61, 62, 83, 86, 87
Planter's Plea (1630), 127
Plato/Platonism, 21, 22, 25–6, 29, 30, 48, 300
Pliny the Elder, 32, 35, 37, 41, 46, 48, 52, 56
Plutarch, 45, 57
Pneumatists, 35
Podalirius, 15, 16
Poitiers cathedral school, 66–7
Poland, care of mentally ill, 280
politics and medicine, 8, 120, 250, 251, 258
pollution, 86, 130, 137–8, 252–3; notions of, in early modern England, 142–3; see also sanitation; street cleaning; water supplies
Polycrates of Samos, 20
Polytheca, 111
poor, the, 5, 132, 251; 'medical police' scheme for, 173–4; medical services for (see also voluntary hospitals; workhouses), 83, 84–5, 100, 101, 208–9, 220; relationship between poverty and disease, 250, 252, 323, 328, 334; as threat to public health,

83, 89; *see also* charitable care of the sick; Poor Law
Poor Law, 94, 264, 327, 330; Amendment Act (1834), 220, 246; Commission, 252, 323; hospitals, 318, 321; medical officers, 242, 321, 325; medical services, 101, 321, 325; *see also* workhouses
Poor Man's Medicine Chest (1791), 106
population: decline, 312; increase, 62, 194–5, 220, 229; structures, 360–5
Porter, Mr (workhouse inmate treated by William Holland), 96, 97
Portugal, care of mentally ill, 280, 283
post-mortems, 6, 203
poultry, wholesomeness of, 146
poverty, *see* poor, the
Pre-Socratic philosophers, 22–3
Precepts, 26–7
preventive medicine, 9, 12, 249, 264–5, 271, 275, 342–3
priest-physicians, eighteenth-century, 187; *see also* clergy
private medicine, 213, 215
Privy Council, Medical Department of, 261, 262, 263
professionalization of medicine, 3, 7, 8, 75; in Britain, 219–47; and rise of hospitals, 199, 203–4; *see also* licensing of medical practitioners
Protestants, 3, 124
Provence, status of doctors in Roman Empire, 44
Providence, Rhode Island, public health programme, 255, 266, 267
Provincial Medical and Surgical Association, 219, 222 n. 6, 224 n. 11
Prudden, T. Mitchell, 266
Prussia, smallpox inoculation of royal household, 193
psychiatry/psychiatric profession, 277, 280, 287–92 *passim*, 295, 296–7, 298–301 *passim*; *see also* asylums; mental illness
Ptolemy VIII, 31
public health: in eighteenth-century Europe, 171, 172–8, 194; impact of bacteriology on, 8–9, 265–71; in Middle Ages, 8, 83, 86–7; in nineteenth-century England, 249, 250,

252–4, 261–6, 270–2, 274–5; in nineteenth-century Europe, 8, 220, 249–54, 261–75 *passim*, 304; schools, 274; in twentieth-century Britain, 325, 330–3 *passim*, 337; in United States, 9, 249, 254–60, 261, 265, 266–70, 272–4, 275; *see also* economic arguments; Public Health Acts
Public Health Acts (Britain), 322, 324; *1848*, 250, 253; *1858*, 262; *1875*, 264
Public Health journal, 272
Public Health Service, United States, 260
pulmonary diseases, report on, 263
purging, 121, 159, 185
Puritan view of doctors, 98
Purkyne, Johannes von, 307
Pythagoreans, 37

quacks/mountebanks, 2, 53; English, 7, 93–4, 102, 110, 222, 223, 227, 232; Enlightenment attitudes, 154, 188–9; *see also* empirics
Quakers, 122, 176, 206, 286
qualifications, medical, 237, 245; *see also* licensing of medical practitioners; medical education
quarantine, 8, 87; *see also* isolation
Queen Charlotte Hospital, London, 177
quinine, 121 n. 3, 305
Quintilian, 49

race, and disease, 313; *see also* eugenics
radiology, 212
Rau, Wilhelm, 172–3
Ray, John, 134
Reece, Richard, 106
Reed, Walter, 259
referral, principle of, 212, 246, 305
reform movement, British, 176–7, 178, 219–47
Regimen of Health, 76
Reichenau monastery, medical manuscripts, 66
Reil, Dr J. C., 291
religion: and deathbed ceremony, 124–5; increased life expectancy and, 13, 373–4, 375; and madness, 116–17, 281–2, 291; and medicine in ancient Greece, 33; religious explanations of

Index

Index